PRINCIPLES OF
HEALTH EDUCATION
and PROMOTION

EIGHTH EDITION

Randall R. Cottrell, DEd, RMCHES®

Retired Professor, Public Health
University of North Carolina Wilmington
Emeritus Professor, Health Promotion and Education
University of Cincinnati

Denise M. Seabert, PhD, MCHES®

Dean, College of Health and Human Services,
California State University, Fresno
Professor Emeritus, Ball State University

Caile E. Spear, PhD, RMCHES®

Professor Emeritus
Boise State University

James F. McKenzie, PhD, MPH, RMCHES®, FAAHE®

Professor Emeritus, Dept. of Physiology & Health Science
Ball State University

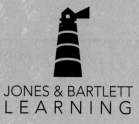

JONES & BARTLETT
LEARNING

World Headquarters
Jones & Bartlett Learning
25 Mall Road, Suite 600
Burlington, MA 01803
978-443-5000
info@jblearning.com
www.jblearning.com

Jones & Bartlett Learning books and products are available through most bookstores and online booksellers. To contact Jones & Bartlett Learning directly, call 800-832-0034, fax 978-443-8000, or visit our website, www.jblearning.com.

Substantial discounts on bulk quantities of Jones & Bartlett Learning publications are available to corporations, professional associations, and other qualified organizations. For details and specific discount information, contact the special sales department at Jones & Bartlett Learning via the above contact information or send an email to specialsales@jblearning.com.

This book was previously published by Pearson Education, Inc.

23134-2

Production Credits
VP, Content Strategy and Implementation: Christine Emerton
Director of Product Management: Cathy Esperti
Product Manager: Whitney Fekete
Content Strategist: Ashley Malone
Content Coordinator: Elena Sorrentino
Project Manager: Kristen Rogers
Project Specialist: Kathryn Leeber
Digital Project Specialist: Rachel DiMaggio
Director of Marketing: Andrea DeFronzo
Content Services Manager: Colleen Lamy
VP, Manufacturing and Inventory Control: Therese Connell
Composition: Exela Technologies
Project Management: Exela Technologies
Cover Design: Theresa Manley
Text Design: Kristin E. Parker
Senior Media Development Editor: Troy Liston
Rights Specialist: Benjamin Roy
Cover Image (Title Page, Chapter Opener):
  © Oxygen/Moment/Getty Images
Printing and Binding: LSC Communications

Library of Congress Cataloging-in-Publication Data
Names: Cottrell, Randall R., author. | Seabert, Denise, author. | Spear, Caile, author. | McKenzie, James F., author.
Title: Principles of health education and promotion / Randall R. Cottrell, DEd, RMCHES, Retired Professor, Public Health,
    University of North Carolina Wilmington, Emeritus Professor, Health Promotion and Education, University of Cincinnati,
    Denise M. Seabert, California State University, Fresno, Professor Emeritus, Ball State University, Caile E. Spear, PhD, RMCHES,
    Professor Emeritus, Boise State University, James F. McKenzie, PhD, MPH, RMCHES, Professor Emeritus, Ball State University.
Other titles: Principles & foundations of health promotion and education
Description: Eighth edition. | Burlington : Jones & Bartlett Learning, [2023] | Revision of: Principles & foundations of health promotion
    and education. 2018. Seventh edition. | Includes bibliographical references and index.
Identifiers: LCCN 2021016305 | ISBN 9781284231250 (paperback)
Subjects: LCSH: Health education. | Health promotion.
Classification: LCC RA440.5 .C685 2023 | DDC 613–dc23
LC record available at https://lccn.loc.gov/2021016305

6048

Printed in the United States of America
25 24 23 22 21   10 9 8 7 6 5 4 3 2 1

We would like to dedicate this book to the people in our lives who mean the most to us: our spouses, Karen, Bonnie, Matt, and Glen; our children, Kyle, Lisa, Kory, Nollis, Anne, Greg, Clark, Nathan, Elias, and Devin; our grandchildren, Kaylee, Anna, Emily, Olivia, Maralee, Marshall, Jonah, Rose, Aevan, Olin, Mitchell, Julia, and Ansley; and our parents, Russell and Edith Cottrell, Gordon and Betty McKenzie, Paul Seabert and Kathy Friedt, and Ellen and Robert Spear.

Brief Contents

Contents

CHAPTER 7 The Settings for Health Education/Promotion. 193

Foreword

Whether you are a student contemplating health education/promotion as a career, have already decided this is the career for you, or are a graduate student entering the field, this text is an invaluable resource you will want to keep. There has never been a more important time in recent history to be a member of the health education/promotion profession. COVID-19 has reminded us all of the importance and value of health education/promotion. The health and well-being of individuals and communities rely on strong health education/promotion organizations and infrastructures.

When thinking about the skills and knowledge needed within the health education/promotion profession, this text provides the foundation. In **Chapter 1**, the value of data in decision making becomes quickly apparent. The development and use of data are key to understanding how health status is measured and can reveal health disparities and inequities. COVID-19 data have drawn attention to the decades of health disparities and social injustice experienced in the United States. Health education/promotion has a vital role in eliminating health disparities and inequities. Understanding the settings in which health education practitioners work (**Chapter 7**), volunteer and professional organization's (**Chapter 8**) and their advocacy work, and societal trends (**Chapter 10**) including policy and political climate are crucial in narrowing these health disparities. History (**Chapter 2**) and understanding how we have managed (or failed to manage) health education/promotion issues can be a guide for future practices and interventions.

Asking the question *why* is a powerful tool for the practitioner. Understanding *why* has contributed to health education/promotion successes of the past. Successes with decreasing traffic fatalities by wearing seat belts in the front and back seats, decreasing dental decay with individual fluoride treatment as well as community water fluoridation, and decreasing use of tobacco and tobacco products all were aided by health education/promotion professionals understanding the *why* of the behavior they were trying to influence. To influence individual, community, and societal behavior changes, **Chapter 4** provides an overview of behavioral theories to better understand the *why* of wearing a face covering/mask during the flu pandemic of 1918 and the recent COVID-19 pandemic. During times of crises (i.e., natural disasters, endemics, pandemics) having a solid ethical guidepost is valuable personally and professionally (**Chapter 5**).

A strength of this textbook lies in **Chapters 6, 7, and 8**. I say this because the authors have expansive and diverse backgrounds as health education/promotion practitioners and are leaders within the profession. Their experience in developing and validating the roles, responsibilities and competencies of health education specialists have become the foundation for professional preparation, development, and credentialing. They have been volunteer leaders in numerous volunteer agencies and held leadership roles in prominent professional health associations/organizations. The authors are exemplar health education/promotion professionals.

There are two key pedagogical features of this text that will provide the reader with insight into the health education/promotion profession. The "Practitioner's Perspective" is written by various practitioners in a variety of settings to give a realistic view of how they work or how they view a specific topic, i.e., credentialing, professional organizations, etc. The other feature is the *Case Study*. Case studies provide a scenario that requires the student to apply their knowledge and provide a solution to the problem. This approach to learning is hands on and allows you, the student, to use what you have learned to effectively solve the problem. What you may find is that solving complex problems requires multifaceted approaches.

This is an exciting time to be studying and entering the profession of health education/ promotion. I encourage you to take advantage of all the opportunities afforded you through this textbook and its resources, as well as through your faculty and university resources. Do not be shy. Talk with your professor about projects you can become a part of. Is there research they are conducting you can be a part of? What about a community health project that needs volunteers? Ask them about professional organizations to join both locally and nationally. Talk with your advisor about ways to be involved on campus through service learning, peer educators, or volunteering at a local health department or nonprofit health agency in the community. If there is not a peer health education group on your campus, take the lead and start one!

Now, more than ever, health education/ promotion needs practitioners and strong leaders, as the challenges we face will require the best minds. It will require those with a solid foundation in health education/ promotion to be leaders in our schools, communities, healthcare and workplace settings, and universities/colleges. This textbook is the first of many building blocks for your health education/promotion foundation.

Enjoy and welcome to health education/ promotion!

Kelli R. Brown, PhD, FASHA, FAAHE
Chancellor, Western Carolina University

Preface

Many students enter the profession of health education/promotion knowing only that they are interested in health and wish to help others improve their health status. Typically, students' interest in health education/promotion is derived from their own desire to live a healthy lifestyle and not from an in-depth understanding of the historical, theoretical, and philosophical foundations of this profession. Other than perhaps a high school health education teacher, many students do not know any health education specialists. In fact, most beginning students are unaware of employment opportunities, the skills needed to practice health education/promotion, and what it would be like to work in a given health education/promotion setting.

This text is written for such students. The contents will be of value to students who are undecided as to whether health education/promotion is the major they want to pursue, as well as for new health education/promotion majors who need information about what health education/promotion is and where health education specialists can be employed. The text is designed for use in an entry-level health education/promotion course in which the major goal is to introduce students to health education/promotion. Students in undergraduate public health programs who are doing a concentration or emphasis in health education will find this book to be essential to their professional preparation. In addition, the book may have value in introducing new health education graduate students, who have undergraduate degrees in fields other than health education/promotion, to the health education/promotion profession.

New to This Edition

This Eighth Edition of *Principles of Health Education and Promotion* (previously published by Pearson as *Principles and Foundations of Health Promotion and Education*) features numerous updates, including significant rewrites to make information flow better in sequence for student use, as well as an updated 7" by 9" trim size and 4-color text. Updates include:

- **Practitioner's Perspective** boxes found throughout the text. They are written by health education/promotion professionals currently working in the field; have been refreshed to offer insights from current practitioners; address such areas as health education certification (CHES), Eta Sigma Gamma, professional associations, internships, and careers in healthcare settings and university wellness centers; among others.

- **Chapter 2** provides updates on current health initiatives, healthcare reform and its impact on health education/promotion; *Healthy People 2030* initiatives; COVID-19; and the Patient Protection and Affordable Care Act, its current status, and its implications for public/community health education.

- **Chapter 4** provides revised information on Planning Models, specifically on the MAPP model.

- **Chapter 6** provides updated coverage on Health Education Specialist Practice Analysis II 2020 (HESPA II), including Appendix B with the new responsibilities, competencies, and subcompetencies of a health education specialist, as well as updated information on program accreditation for freestanding undergraduate public/community health programs.

- **Chapter 7** incorporates "A Day in the Career of…" in each major career setting that now includes information on how COVID-19 may have impacted job responsibilities.
- A NEW! **Appendix A** provides the updated Health Education Code of Ethics.
- A NEW! **Appendix B** provides the HESPA II 2020 responsibilities, competencies and subcompetencies of a health education specialist

Chapter Overview

Chapter 1, "A Background for the Profession," provides an overview of health education/promotion and sets the stage for the remaining chapters.

Chapter 2, "The History of Health and Health Education/Promotion," examines the history of health and health care, as well as the history of health education/promotion. This chapter was written to help students understand the tremendous advances that have been made in keeping people healthy, and it provides perspective on the role of health education/promotion in that effort. One cannot appreciate the present without understanding the past. The chapter will bring students up to date with the most recent happenings in the profession including updated information on the Patient Protection and Affordable Care Act, Healthy People 2030, initiatives in both public and school health education, as well as the COVID-19 pandemic.

Chapters 3, 4, and 5 provide what might best be called the basic foundations. All professions, such as law, medicine, business, and teacher education, must provide students with information related to the philosophy, theory, and ethics inherent in the field.

Chapter 6, "The Health Education Specialist: Roles, Responsibilities, Certifications, and Advanced Study," is designed to acquaint new students with the skills that are needed to practice in the field of health education/promotion. It also explains the certification process to students and encourages them to begin thinking of graduate study early in their undergraduate programs. New information related to changes in the competencies and subcompetencies of a health education specialist based on the Health Education Specialist Practice Analysis II 2020 (HESPA II 2020) study is incorporated into this chapter.

Chapter 7, "The Settings for Health Education/Promotion," introduces students to the job responsibilities inherent in different types of health education/promotion positions and provides a discussion of the pros and cons of working in various health education/promotion settings. Incorporated into each major career setting is, "A Day in the Career of…" section that now includes information on how COVID-19 may have impacted job responsibilities. "Practitioner's Perspective" boxes include perspectives from health education professionals working in the field. This chapter is unique among introductory texts. An important warning is provided to students to be careful about what they post to social networking websites, and information is included on landing one's first job and how to excel in a health education/promotion career. This chapter truly provides students with important insights into the various health education/promotion settings and the overall practice of health education/promotion.

Chapter 8, "Agencies, Associations, and Organizations Associated with Health Education/Promotion," introduces students to the many professional agencies, associations, and organizations that support health education/promotion. This is an extremely important chapter because all health education specialists need to know of these resources and allies. All introductory students are encouraged to join one or more of the professional associations described in this chapter. For that reason, contact information for all of the professional associations discussed is included in the chapter.

Chapter 9, "The Literature of Health Education/Promotion," directs students to the information and resources necessary to work in the field. Included in this chapter is basic information related to the Internet and the World Wide Web that should be especially helpful to new students. With the explosion of knowledge related to health, being able to locate needed resources is a critical skill for health education specialists. Finally, health education/promotion students need to consider what future changes in health knowledge, policy, and funding may mean to those working in health education/promotion. They must learn to project into the future and prepare themselves to meet these challenges.

Chapter 10, "Future Trends in Health Education/Promotion," is an attempt to provide a window into the future for today's health education/promotion students.

As one reads the text, it will be apparent that certain standard features exist in all chapters. These are designed to help the student identify important information, guide the student's learning, and extend the student's understanding beyond the basic content information. Each chapter begins by identifying objectives. Before reading a chapter, students should carefully read the objectives because they will guide the student's learning of the information contained in that chapter. After reading a chapter, it may also be helpful to review the objectives again to be certain major points were understood. Being able to respond to each objective and define each highlighted term in a chapter is typically of great value in understanding the material and preparing for examinations.

Throughout the text, take note of the "Practitioner's Perspective" boxes. These are boxes written by health education/promotion professionals who are currently working in the field. Some of the boxes relate to working in a particular setting, while others focus on such areas as ethics, certification, internships, hiring, Eta Sigma Gamma, and graduate study. There are a total of 17 "Practitioner's Perspective" boxes, 11 of them new to this edition.

At the end of each chapter, the student will find a brief summary of the information contained in that chapter. Following the summary are review questions. Students are encouraged to answer these questions because they provide an additional method for targeting learning and reviewing the chapter's contents. A case study follows the review questions. Case studies allow readers to project themselves into realistic health education situations and problem solve how to handle such situations. Next, readers will find critical thinking questions designed to extend readers' learning beyond what is presented in the chapter. They require readers to apply what they have learned, contemplate major events, and project their learning into the future. A list of activities, designed to extend readers' knowledge beyond what can be obtained by reading the chapter, follows the critical thinking questions. In some activities, students are asked to apply or synthesize the chapter's information. In others, students are encouraged to get actively involved with experiences that will help integrate learning from the text with a practical, real-world setting. By completing these activities, students should have a better understanding of health education/promotion. The activities are followed by Weblinks, which have been updated and expanded for this edition. Weblinks are sites that students can access to read more about a topic, extend their learning, or obtain interesting and important resource materials. Each chapter ends with a list of references the authors used to develop the chapter. All references are cited in the chapter, and students can use the references to obtain more detailed information on a topic from an original source when they desire to do so.

Resources

The following instructor supplements are available with the eighth edition:

- An **Instructor's Manual** that includes a synopsis, an outline, teaching ideas, website activities, and video resources for each chapter.
- A **Test Bank** that includes multiple-choice, true/false, and essay questions for each chapter.
- **Slides in PowerPoint format** that feature chapter outlines and key points from the text.

We readily acknowledge that the information contained in this text represents our bias regarding what material should be taught in an introductory course. There may be important introductory information we have not included, or we may have included information that may not be considered introductory by all users. We welcome and encourage comments and feedback, both positive and negative, from all users of this text. Only with such feedback can we make improvements and include the most appropriate information in future editions.

Randall R. Cottrell
Denise M. Seabert
Caile E. Spear
James F. McKenzie

Acknowledgments

First, we would like to thank all of the health education faculty who have adopted each new edition of our text and all of the students who have used the text. The response we have received has been truly gratifying. Without you, we would not be writing the eighth edition of our text.

We would also like to thank Jones & Bartlett Learning for producing *Principles of Health Education and Promotion, Eighth Edition*. We would especially like to thank Cathy Esperti, Director of Product Management; Whitney Fekete, Product Manager; and Ashley Malone, Content Strategist; for their editorial guidance and their hard work on this project, as well as Kathryn Leeber, Project Specialist; Benjamin Roy, Rights Specialist; and Troy Liston, Senior Media Development Editor.

CHAPTER 1

A Background for the Profession

CHAPTER OBJECTIVES

After reading this chapter and answering the questions at the end, you should be able to:

- Define the terms *health*, *health education*, *health promotion*, *disease prevention*, *public health*, *community health*, *global health promotion*, *population health*, and *wellness*.
- Describe the current status of health education/promotion.
- Define *epidemiology*.
- Explain the means by which health or health status can be measured.
- List and explain the goals and objectives of health education/promotion.
- Identify the practice of health education/promotion.
- Explain the following concepts and principles:
  - Health field concept
  - Levels of prevention
  - Risk factors
  - Health risk reduction
  - Chain of infection
  - Communicable disease model
  - Multicausation disease model
  - Selected principles of health education/promotion—*participation*, *empowerment*, *advocacy*, *social media*, and *cultural competence*

Health education/promotion has come a long way since its beginnings. Health education/promotion as we know it today only dates back about 85 years, but the progress in development has accelerated most rapidly in the past 40 years (Glanz & Rimer, 2008). As the profession has grown and changed, so have the roles and responsibilities of health education specialists. The purpose of this book is to provide those new to this profession with a sense of the past—how the profession was born and on what principles it was developed; a complete understanding of the present—what it is that health education specialists are expected to do, how they should do it, and what guides their work; and a look at the future—where the profession is headed, and how health education specialists can keep pace with changes to be responsive to those whom they serve.

This chapter provides a background in the terminology, concepts, and principles of the profession. It defines many of the key words and terms used in the profession, briefly discusses why health education/promotion is referred to as an emerging profession, looks at the current state of the profession, shows how health and health status have been measured, outlines the goals and objectives of the profession, identifies the practice of health education/promotion, and discusses some of the basic, underlying concepts and principles of the profession.

Key Words, Terms, and Definitions

Each chapter introduces new terminology that is either important to the specific content presented in the chapter or used frequently in the profession. This chapter discusses the more common terms that will be used throughout this text. Like the profession, these words and definitions have evolved over the years. The most recent effort occurred in 2020 (Report of the 2020 Joint Committee on Health Education and Promotion Terminology [Joint Committee], [Joint Committee, 2021]). The 2020 Joint Committee was spearheaded by the Coalition of National Health Education Organizations (see Chapter 8 for information on professional organizations). The Joint Committee is charged with reviewing and updating the terminology of the profession. The members of the 2020 Joint Committee were composed of representatives from the member organizations in the Coalition of National Health Education Organizations (see Chapter 8), the National Commission for Health Education Credentialing, Inc. (see Chapter 6), and the Foundation for the Advancement of Health Education (Joint Committee, 2020). Before this meeting,

there had been eight major terminology reports developed for the profession over the past 90 years with the first dating back to 1927 (Johns, 1973; Joint Committee, 2001, 2012; Joint Committee on Health Education Terminology, 1991a, 1991b; Moss, 1950; Rugen, 1972; Williams, 1934; Yoho, 1962).

Before presenting some of the key terms used in the profession, an in-depth discussion of the word *health* may be helpful. Health is a difficult concept to put into words, but it is one that most people intuitively understand. The World Health Organization (WHO) has defined health as "the state of complete mental, physical and social well-being not merely the absence of disease or infirmity" (WHO, 1947, p. 1). This classic definition is important because it identifies the vital components of health and further implies that health is a holistic concept involving an interaction and interdependence among these various components. A number of years after the writing of the WHO definition, Hanlon (1974) defined health as "a functional state which makes possible the achievement of other goals and activities. Comfort, well-being, and the distinction between physical and mental health differ in social classes, cultures, and religious groups" (p. 73). And more recently, the WHO (1986) has stated that "To reach a state of complete physical, mental, and social well-being, an individual or group must be able to identify and to realize aspirations, to satisfy needs, and to change or cope with the environment. Health is, therefore, seen as a resource for everyday life, not the object of living. Health is a positive concept emphasizing social and personal resources, as well as physical capacities" (p. 5). In other words, good health should not be the goal of life but rather a vehicle to reaching one's goals in life. We feel that these major concepts of health are captured in the definition that states that **health** "is a *constellation of factors – economic, social, political, ecological, and physical – that add up to healthy, high-quality lives for individuals and communities*"

(University of Kansas, 2020, para. 8). As such, health can exist in varying degrees—ranging from good to poor and everywhere in between—and depends on each person's individual circumstances. "For example, a person can be healthy while dying, or a person who is quadriplegic can be healthy in the sense that his or her mental and social well-being is high and physical health is as good as it can be" (Hancock & Minkler, 2005, p. 144).

In addition to the word *health*, it is also important to have an understanding of the following key terms and definitions:

community health—"the health status of a defined group of people and the actions and conditions to promote, protect and preserve their health" (Joint Committee, 2021)

health education—"any combination of planned learning experiences using evidence based practices and/or sound theories that provide the opportunity to acquire knowledge, attitudes, and skills needed [to] adopt and maintain healthy behaviors" (Joint Committee, 2021)

health promotion—"any planned combination of educational, political, environmental, regulatory, or organizational mechanisms that support actions and conditions of living conducive to the health of individuals, groups, and communities" (Joint Committee, 2021) (See **Figure 1.1** for the relationship between health education and health promotion.)

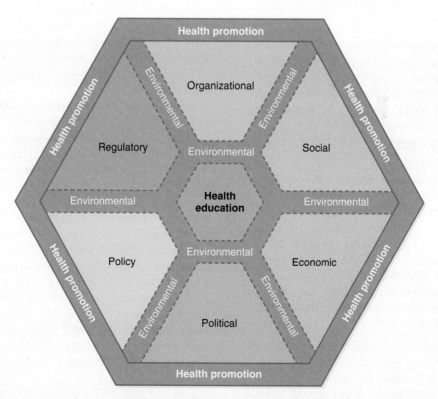

Figure 1.1 The relationship between health education and health promotion.

disease prevention—"the process of reducing risks and alleviating disease to promote, preserve, and restore health and minimize suffering and distress" (Joint Committee, 2001, p. 99).

dimension of health and wellness—"the many aspects of a person's life, including the emotional, physical, occupational, intellectual, financial, social, environmental, and spiritual areas. These dimensions are considered interconnected as one area builds upon another" (Joint Committee, 2021).

public health—"the science and art of preventing disease, prolonging life, and promoting health through the organized efforts and informed choices of society, organizations, communities, and individuals" (Joint Committee, 2021).

global health promotion—"placing priority on improving health and achieving equity for all people worldwide. Work is directed to help all people reach the 'highest attainable standard of health' goal set by the World Health Organization" (Joint Committee, 2021).

population health—"a cohesive, integrated, and comprehensive approach to health care that considers the distribution of health outcomes within a population, the health determinants that influence distribution of care, and the policies and interventions that affect and are affected by the determinants" (Nash et al., 2016, p. 448)

wellness—"whereby an individual actively seeks a collection of preventive practices and processes in which all dimensions of that person's health are addressed to achieve optimal well-being and minimize conditions of illness" (Joint Committee, 2021).

Before we leave the discussion about key words and terms of the profession, it should be noted that there is not complete agreement on terminology. We could easily have found another definition for each of the terms presented here written by either a respected scholar in health education/promotion or a legitimate professional or governmental health agency.

The Health Education/ Promotion Profession

Historically, there have been a number of occasions that can be considered "critical" to the development of health education/promotion. (See Chapter 2 for an in-depth presentation of the history.) But there has been no time in which the status of the profession has been more visible to the average person or as widely accepted by other health professionals as it is today. Much of this notoriety can be attributed to the health promotion era of public health history that began in about 1974 in the United States.

The United States' first public health revolution spanned the late 19th century through the mid-20th century and was aimed at controlling the harm (morbidity and mortality) that came from infectious diseases. By the mid-1950s, many of the infectious diseases in the United States were pretty much under control. This was evidenced by the improved infant mortality rates, the reduction in the number of children who were contracting childhood diseases, the reduction in the overall death rates in the country, and the increase in life expectancy (see **Table 1.1**). With the control of many communicable diseases, the focus moved to the major chronic diseases such as heart disease, cancer, and strokes— diseases that were, in large part, the result of the way people lived.

By the mid-1970s, it became clear that the greatest potential for reducing morbidity,

Table 1.1 **Life Expectancy at Birth, at 65 Years of Age, and at 75 Years of Age, According to Sex: United States, Selected Years 1900–2017**

Year	At Birth			At 65 Years			At 75 Years		
	Both Sexes	Male	Female	Both Sexes	Male	Female	Both Sexes	Male	Female
1900	47.3	46.3	48.3	11.9	11.5	12.2	*	*	*
1950	68.2	65.6	71.1	13.9	12.8	15.0	*	*	*
1980	73.7	70.7	77.4	16.4	14.1	18.3	10.4	8.8	11.5
2010	78.7	76.2	81.0	19.1	17.7	20.3	12.1	11.0	12.9
2017	78.6	76.1	81.1	19.4	18.1	20.6	12.3	11.3	13.0

*= Data not available.
Data from National Center for Health Statistics. (n.d.). *Health, United States, 2018 – Data finder.* Retrieved December 6, 2020, from https://www.cdc.gov/nchs/hus/index.htm

saving lives, and reducing healthcare costs in the United States was to be achieved through health promotion and disease prevention. At the core of this approach was health education/promotion. In 1980, the U.S. Department of Health, Education, and Welfare (USDHEW) presented a blueprint of the health promotion and disease prevention strategy in its first set of health objectives in the document called *Promoting Health/Preventing Disease: Objectives for a Nation* (USDHEW, 1980). This document proposed a total of 226 objectives divided into three main areas—preventive services, health protection, and health promotion. This was the first time a comprehensive national agenda for prevention had been developed, with specific goals and objectives for anticipated gains (McGinnis, 1985). In 1985, it was apparent that only about one half of the objectives established in 1980 would be reached by 1990, another one-fourth would not be reached, and progress on the others could not be judged because of the lack of data (Mason & McGinnis, 1990). Even though not all objectives were reached, the planning process involved in the 1980 report demonstrated the value of setting goals and listing specific objectives as a means of measuring progress in the nation's health and healthcare

services. These goals and objectives published by the U.S. Department of Health and Human Services (USDHHS), now in their fifth generation as *Healthy People 2030*, have defined the nation's health agenda and guided its health policy since their inception. (See Chapter 2 for more on *Healthy People 2030*.)

Now more than 20 years into the 21st century, the health of the people in the United States is better than any time in the past. "By every measure, we are healthier, live longer, and enjoy lives that are less likely to be marked by injuries, ill health, or premature death" (Institute of Medicine [IOM], 2002, p. 2). Yet, we could do better. Four modifiable health risk behaviors—lack of physical activity, poor nutrition, tobacco use, and excessive alcohol use—cause much of the illness, suffering, and early death related to chronic diseases and conditions (Centers for Disease Control and Prevention [CDC], n.d.-a, para. 2). Thus, "behavior patterns represent the single most prominent domain of influence over health prospects in the United States" (McGinnis et al., 2002, p. 82).

As the health agenda has become more clearly defined, so has the health education/promotion profession. In 1998, the U.S. Department of Commerce and Labor formally recognized "health educator" as a distinct occupation, thus demonstrating that the health education/promotion profession is moving in the right direction. More recently, a study titled "Marketing the Health Education Profession: Knowledge, Attitudes, and Hiring Practices of Employers" conducted by Hezel Associates (2007) was conducted. Through this study, the term *health education specialist* has gained favor over the use of the term *health educator*. A **health education specialist** has been defined as "an individual who has met, at a minimum, baccalaureate-level required health education academic preparation qualifications, who serves in a variety of settings, and is able to use appropriate educational strategies and methods to facilitate the development of policies, procedures, interventions, and systems conducive to the health of individuals, groups, and communities" (Joint Committee, 2021). Thus, the term *health education specialist* will be used throughout the remainder of this book.

Clearly, there is a need for health education/promotion interventions provided by health education specialists in the United States both today and in the future.

Measuring Health or Health Status

Although the definition of health is easy to state, trying to quantify the amount of health an individual or a population possesses is not easy. Most measures of health are expressed using health statistics based on the traditional medical model of describing ill health (injury, disease, and death) instead of well health. Thus, the higher the presence of injury, disease, and death indicators, the lower the level of health; the lower the presence of injury, disease, and death indicators, the higher the level of health. Out of necessity, we have defined the level of health with just the opposite—ill health (Seabert, McKenzie & Pinger, 2022).

The information gathered when measuring health is referred to as **epidemiological data**. These data are gathered at the local, state, and national levels to assist with the prevention of disease outbreaks or control those in progress and to plan and assess health education/promotion programs. Epidemiology is one of those disciplines that helps provide the foundation for the health education/promotion profession. **Epidemiology** is defined as "the study of the distribution and determinants of health-related states or events (including disease), and the application of this study to the control of diseases and other health problems" (Centers for Disease Control and Prevention Centers, 2011b). In the following sections, several of the more common epidemiological means by which health, or lack thereof, are described and quantified. (see Practitioner's Perspective).

Rates

A **rate** is "a measure of the frequency with which an event occurs in a defined population over a specified period of time" (CDC, 2011b) Rates are important because they provide an opportunity for comparison of events, diseases, or conditions that occur at different times or places. Some of the more commonly used rates are death rates, birth rates, and morbidity rates. **Death rates** (the number of deaths per 100,000 resident population), sometimes referred to as *mortality* or *fatality rates*, are probably the most frequently used means of quantifying the seriousness of injury or disease. (See **Table 1.2** for death rates and **Table 1.3** for an example of a formula used to tabulate rates.) "The transition from wellness to ill health is often gradual and poorly defined. Because death, in contrast, is a clearly defined event, it has continued to be the most reliable single indicator of health status of a population. Mortality statistics, however, describe only a part of the health status of a population, and often only the endpoint of an illness process" (USDHHS,

Practitioner's Perspective

Epidemiology: Jamie Harding

CURRENT POSITION: Health Promotion Program Manager

EMPLOYER: Central District Health Department, Boise, Idaho

DEGREE/INSTITUTION/YEAR: Master of Health Science, Boise State University, August 2006; Bachelor of Science, Athletic Training and Bachelor of Science, Health Promotion, Boise State University, May 2001.

MAJOR: Health Science—Health Policy emphasis (graduate); Athletic Training (undergraduate); Health Promotion (undergraduate)

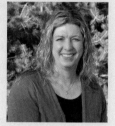
Courtesy of Jamie Harding.

Describe your past and current professional positions and how you came to hold the job you now hold (How did you obtain the position?): During my senior year of undergraduate work, I interned at Saint Alphonsus Regional Medical Center in the Marketing Department. Upon my graduation, the internship position led to a full-time employment opportunity within the same department. I worked in this capacity for approximately one year when I obtained a promotional opportunity to work for the Idaho Department of Health and Welfare (IDHW). I worked in several capacities for the IDHW for 10 years. Specifically, my positions were in the Division of Medicaid in the Regional Medicaid Services office as a Health Resources Coordinator in Medicaid's managed care program, Healthy Connections; in the Diabetes Prevention and Control Program; in the Physical Activity and Nutrition Program as a Health Program Specialist and finally as a Physical Activity and Nutrition Program Manager. These experiences honed my skills in grant writing to agencies such as the CDC and the U.S. Administration of Aging, negotiating and managing contracts, supervising employees, facilitating statewide networks for prevention activities, and creating and overseeing program budgets. Having these skills helped me obtain the Health Promotion Program Manager position at Central District Health Department in April of 2012, where I helped guide the local health department's shift away from working on individual behavior change activities to that of broad-based population impact to increase access to physical activity and healthy eating opportunities.

Describe the duties of your current position: Within the Office of Health Promotion, my staff and I primarily focus on increasing access to physical activity and healthy eating along with reducing tobacco initiation and use. I also oversee the implementation of a senior fall prevention program and an agency worksite wellness program. Additionally, I conduct semiannual and annual performance reviews along with providing regular coaching and mentoring to staff. I lead staff in strategic and policy agenda planning utilizing a policy, systems and environmental change approach to influence broad-based population impact, and negotiate and manage contracts with multiple agencies such as IDHW and nonprofit organizations. These are my major position duties. I'm also involved with staff in providing technical assistance and training to community partners, participating on state and local coalitions, alliances, and advisory boards with a physical activity, nutrition, tobacco prevention, and healthy aging emphasis.

Describe what you like most about this position: After having worked for 10 years at a state agency, I've enjoyed gaining local-level experience. I appreciate the opportunity to work in each community to spend time developing and fostering relationships while gaining an understanding of the specific needs of that community. I have noticed I spend more time fostering partnerships through face-to-face meetings and phone calls than through email communication.

Describe what you like least about this position: Stable and ongoing funding for primary prevention has been problematic for public health. In the past, most funding opportunities came to us in a categorical manner or with a disease-specific focus. Recently, we are starting to see a shift to funding

(continues)

Epidemiology: Jamie Harding

primary prevention work that is focused on mitigating chronic disease risk factors through broad-based population work. Public health funding continues to be inadequate and inconsistently funded so this is an ongoing challenge. Because we are often underfunded, we are limited on available human resources, which results in a challenge to have adequate staff to meet the workload demands.

In addition, we often have problems with programmatic siloes in public health resulting in duplication of effort. Programs tend to work independently of each other, often using the same community-based partners. Unfortunately, in a small state like Idaho, many community-based partners are serving on multiple coalitions and alliances. It is not uncommon for me to attend two different coalition meetings within a short period of time and usually the same core group of people is in attendance. We talk about integration and streamlining efforts among programs and community partners, but it is difficult to put this into practice.

How do you use health data/epidemiology in your current position? We use health data to inform us on the current and changed state of our communities. These data help us determine the priority needs in each community for addressing access to physical activity, healthy eating, and tobacco use prevention. Within our four-county jurisdiction, we are working with several communities to implement the CDC-developed Community Health Assessment and Group Evaluation (CHANGE) Tool. The CHANGE Tool community health assessment affords us an opportunity to assess community strengths, identify areas for improvement, and assist the community with prioritizing community needs related to population-based strategies. Currently, we rely on state-collected data such as the CDC's Behavioral Risk Factor Surveillance System (BRFSS) and Youth Risk Behavior Surveillance System (YRBSS) to assess health behaviors, but we recognize there are health data gaps in Idaho. There are efforts underway to address these data gaps and develop a clearinghouse to store chronic disease risk factor data. We use best practice or evidence-based practices in our community-based work to create lasting, sustainable change. Our goal is to create an environment in which the healthy choice is the default choice for all individuals.

What recommendations/advice do you have for current health education students desiring to become community health educators? I work with interns on a regular basis and am often interviewed by students seeking guidance for entering the public health field. I recommend developing skills to become a strong written and oral communicator. Much of our work is done through written documents and via oral presentations. I'm often asked to present to the Central District Health Department Board of Health or other groups within the community so being organized and comfortable with public speaking is key. Additionally, I write grant applications, reports, contracts, and communicate via email so strong written skills are a necessity. I recommend that students be nimble and flexible in their careers. Students need to know that an entry-level position may not be their dream job but it serves as an opportunity to develop skills and relationships with other individuals working in the field. It is a way to gain experience so when promotional opportunities are available, they can apply for them. It's also critical that students connect with working professionals through local, state, and national societies and associations. Oftentimes, networking opens the door for employment opportunities.

1991, p. 15). Rates can be expressed in three forms: (1) crude, (2) adjusted, and (3) specific. A **crude rate** is the rate expressed for a total population. An **adjusted rate** is also expressed for a total population but is statistically adjusted for a certain characteristic, such as age. A **specific rate** is a rate for a particular population subgroup such as for a particular disease (i.e., disease-specific) or for a particular age of people (i.e., age-specific).

Table 1.2 Crude Death Rates for Selected Causes of Death: United States, 2017

Cause	Deaths per 100,000 Population
All causes	8,863.8
Diseases of the heart	198.8
Malignant neoplasms (cancer)	183.9
Unintentional injuries	52.2
Chronic lower respiratory diseases	49.2
Cerebrovascular diseases (stroke)	44.9
Alzheimer disease	37.3
Diabetes mellitus	25.7
Influenza/pneumonia	17.1
Suicide	15.5

Data from Kochanek, K. D., Murphy, S. L., Xu, J., & Arias, E. (2019). Deaths: Final data for 2017. *National Vital Statistics Reports, 68*(9), 1–77. https://www.cdc.gov/nchs/data/nvsr/nvsr68/nvsr68_09-508.pdf

Table 1.3 Selected Mortality Rates and Their Formulas

Rate	Definition	Example (U.S. 2017)
$Crude\ death\ rate =$	$\dfrac{\text{Number of deaths (all cause)}}{\text{Estimated midyear population}} \times 100{,}000$	863.8 per 100,000
$Age-specific\ death\ rate =$	$\dfrac{\text{Number of deaths, } 45-54}{\text{Estimated midyear population, } 45-54} \times 100{,}000$	401.5 per 100,000
$Cause-specific\ mortality =$	$\dfrac{\text{Number of deaths, (suicide)}}{\text{Estimated midyear population}} \times 100{,}000$	14.5 per 100,000

Data from Heron, M. (2019). Deaths: Leading causes for 2017. *National Vital Statistics Reports, 68*(6), 1–77. https://www.cdc.gov/nchs/data/nvsr/nvsr68/nvsr68_06-508.pdf

Examples include calculating the death rate for heart disease in the United States or the age-specific death rate for 45- to 54-year-old people.

There are three other epidemiological terms that are used to describe the magnitude of a rate of some event, disease, or condition in a unit of population. They are (1) **endemic**—occurs regularly in a population as a matter of course, such as heart disease in the United States; (2) **epidemic**—an unexpectedly large number of cases of an illness, specific health-related behavior, or other health-related event in a population, like the Opioid overdose epidemic in the United States; and (3) **pandemic**—an outbreak over a wide geographic area, such as a continent. The novel coronavirus-2019, or COVID-19, is an example of a current pandemic. As you continue your preparation to become a health education specialist, you will be introduced to more and more epidemiological principles and terms.

Life Expectancy

Life expectancy is another means by which health or health status has been measured. However, it is also based on mortality. Even with this limitation, though, life expectancy has been described as "the most comprehensive indicator of patterns of health and disease, as well as living standards and social development" (CDC, 1994, pp. 2–8). **Life expectancy** is the average number of years of life remaining for persons who have attained a given age. Life expectancy is often presented by sex, race, and Hispanic origin, or other characteristics using age-specific death rates for the population with that characteristic. (NCHS, 2015). The most frequently used times to state life expectancy are at birth, at

age 65, and age 75 (see Table 1.1) It must be remembered that life expectancy is an average for an entire cohort (usually a single birth year) and is not necessarily a useful predictor for any one individual. In terms of evaluating the effect of chronic disease on a population, life expectancies calculated *after* birth have been found to be more useful measures than life expectancy *at* birth because life expectancy at birth reflects infant mortality rates.

Years of Potential Life Lost

A third means by which health or health status has been measured is **years of potential life lost (YPLL)**. YPLL "is a measure of premature mortality" (NCHS, 2015, p. 446) (see **Table 1.4**) and is calculated by subtracting a person's age at death from 75 years. For example, for a person who dies at age 30, the YPLL are 45. Until 1996, the U.S. government used age 65 in calculating YPLL, but

Table 1.4 Age-Adjusted Years of Potential Life Lost (Per 100,000 Population) Before Age 75 for Selected Leading Causes of Death: United States, 1990 and 2018

Cause	1990	2018
Malignant neoplasms	2,003.8	1,151.3
Unintentional injuries (accidents)	1,162.1	1,317.1
Diseases of the heart	1,617.7	916.2
Suicide	393.1	466.6
Homicide	417.4	259.4
Chronic liver disease and cirrhosis	196.9	191.1
Diabetes mellitus	155.9	180.6
Chronic lower respiratory diseases	187.4	156.4
Cerebrovascular diseases (stroke)	259.6	153.6
Influenza and pneumonia	141.5	85.7
HIV	383.8	38.9

Data from U.S. Department of Health and Human Services & Centers for Disease Control and Prevention. (n.d.). *WISQARS: Leading causes of death visualization tool.* Retrieved December 6, 2020, from https://www.cdc.gov/injury/wisqars/index.html

because life expectancy in the United States has continued to increase and is greater than 75 years, that age is now used (NCHS, 2015).

Disability-Adjusted Life Years

The three measures of health and health status noted previously are commonly used in the United States and other developed countries. However, because mortality does not express the burden of living with disability (for example, the resulting paralysis from an automobile crash or the depression that often follows a stroke), the WHO and the World Bank developed a measure called **disability-adjusted life years (DALYs)**. One DALY can be thought of as one lost year of "healthy" life as a result of being in states of poor health or disability (Murray & Lopez, 1996; WHO, 2008).

To calculate total DALYs for a given condition in a population, years of life lost (YLL) and years lived with disability (YLD) of known severity and duration for that condition must each be estimated, then the total summed. For example, to calculate DALYs incurred through road accidents in India in 1990, add the total years of life lost in fatal road accidents and the total years of life lived with disabilities by survivors of such accidents (Murray & Lopez, 1996, p. 7).

Health-Related Quality of Life

Even though DALYs go beyond measuring health in terms of just mortality, they really do not get at the quality of life (QOL). Although QOL refers to a person or group's general well-being, **health-related quality of life (HRQOL)** is "an individual's or a group's perceived physical and mental health over time" (CDC, n.d.-e, para. 1). Healthcare providers have often used HRQOL to measure the effects of chronic disease in their patients to better understand how a disease interferes with a person's daily life. Similarly, public health professionals have used HRQOL to measure the effects of numerous disorders, short- and long-term disabilities, and diseases in different populations. Tracking HRQOL in different populations can identify subgroups with poor physical or mental health and can help guide policies or other interventions to improve their health (CDC, n.d.-e).

Increasingly, health professionals have been using the concept of HRQOL to quantify and track the health status of people. Measures of HRQOL are now included on a number of different health surveys, including the BRFSS and the National Health and Nutrition Examination Survey (NHANES) (see next section for discussion of these surveys). Both the BRFSS and the NHANES use the standard four-item "Healthy" Days core questions (CDC HRQOL-4) created by the Centers for Disease Control and Prevention (CDC) and presented in **Box 1.1**.

Box 1.1 "Healthy" Days Core Questions (CDC HRQOL-4)

---

1. Would you say that in general your health is:
   a. Excellent
   b. Very good
   c. Good
   d. Fair
   e. Poor
2. Now, thinking about your physical health, which includes physical illness and injury, for how many days during the past 30 days was your physical health not good?
3. Now thinking about your mental health, which includes stress, depression, and problems with emotions, for how many days during the past 30 days was your mental health not good?
4. During the past 30 days, for how many days did poor physical or mental health keep you from doing your usual activities, such as self-care, work, or recreation?

Reproduced from Centers for Disease Control and Prevention. (n.d.-e). *Health-related quality of life.* Retrieved October 31, 2018, from http://www.cdc.gov/hrqol/methods.htm

Health Surveys

Data collected through surveys conducted by governmental agencies are other means by which health or health status has been measured in the United States. Six examples are presented here. The first two, the National Health Interview Survey (NHIS) and the National Health and Nutrition Examination Survey (NHANES), are conducted by the National Center for Health Statistics (NCHS). The NHIS, which has been used for more than 60 years, is a household survey in which respondents are asked a number of questions about their health and health behavior. One of the questions, for example, asks the respondents to describe their health status using one of five categories: excellent, very good, good, fair, or poor.

The NHANES data are collected using a mobile examination center. Through personal interviews, physical examinations, and clinical and laboratory testing, data are collected on a representative group of Americans. These examinations result in the most authoritative source of standardized clinical, physical, and physiological data on the U.S. population. Included in the data are the prevalence of specific conditions and diseases and data on blood pressure, blood cholesterol, body mass index, nutritional status and deficiencies, and exposure to environmental toxins (CDC, n.d.-h).

The third example of data collected from surveys actually come from a family of surveys called the National Health Care Surveys. These surveys are designed to "answer key questions of interest to health care policy makers, public health professionals, and researchers" (CDC, n.d.-i, para. 1). The National Health Care Surveys are used to study resource use, including staffing, quality of care, disparities in healthcare services, and diffusion of certain healthcare technologies (CDC, n.d.-i). The fourth example of data collected through a survey is the data collected through the Behavioral Risk Factor Surveillance System (BRFSS). The BRFSS is the nation's premier system of adult health-related data regarding health-related risk behaviors, chronic health conditions, and use of preventive services. Using telephone survey techniques, these data are collected by individual states, territories, and the District of Columbia through cooperative agreements with the CDC (CDC, n.d.-b).

Because of the success of the BRFSS, a similar surveillance system was begun for youth. The Youth Risk Behavior Surveillance System (YRBSS) was developed in 1990 to monitor priority health-risk behaviors that contribute markedly to the leading causes of death, disability, and social problems among youth and adults in the United States. The six categories of priority health-risk behaviors include (1) tobacco use; (2) unhealthy dietary behaviors; (3) inadequate physical activity; (4) alcohol and other drug use; (5) sexual behaviors related to unintended pregnancy and sexually transmitted diseases, including HIV infection; and (6) behaviors that contribute to unintentional injuries and violence (CDC, n.d.-m).

The final survey presented, the National College Health Assessment (NCHA), is one that collects health data about college students. The NCHA is the only one presented here that is not conducted by a government agency. The NCHA is connected to the professional organization American College Health Association (ACHA) (see Chapter 8 for more on this association). The ACHA developed the NCHA, which can be conducted as either a paper-pencil or online survey, to assist schools in collecting data about students' habits, behaviors, and perceptions about topics such as alcohol, tobacco, and other drug use; mental health; weight, nutrition, and exercise; personal safety and violence; and sexual health. The ACHA charges schools for conducting the NCHA, but the schools have the flexibility to select the surveying method, sample size, priority population, and time it is offered (ACHA, 2020).

Using Health Data in Health Education/ Promotion

In this section, we would like to give you an example of how health education specialists may use data. As you will soon learn, a major task of health education specialists is to assist those in the priority population (individuals, groups, and communities) in obtaining, maintaining, and improving their health. Often, this means planning some type of health education/promotion program that can be used by those in the priority population. These programs should be based on the needs of the priority population, and the needs are often described using data.

For example, let's say a health education specialist is working for a local (county) health department at a time when the state health department has just made funds available through a competitive grant process to deal with the high rates of cancer in the state. Because of some past concerns about cancer in the county, their supervisor has suggested they seek funding. Although they have heard some residents express concern about possible higher rates of cancer, they are really not sure about the type of cancer or whether there is a specific group of people affected. Therefore, they need to be able to describe the potential problem and identify a priority population. One approach would be to determine if there are any health disparities associated with cancer in their county. It has long been "recognized that some individuals are healthier than others and that some live longer than others do, and that often these differences are closely associated with social characteristics such as race, ethnicity, gender, location, and socioeconomic status" (King, 2009, p. 339). These gaps between groups have been referred to as *health disparities* (also called health inequalities in some countries). More formally, **health disparity** has been defined as a "higher burden of illness, injury, disability,

and/or mortality that is experienced by one group relative to another due to current or historic disadvantage, oppression, or racism, which is manifested through inequitable social, economic, and environmental systems" (Joint Committee, 2021).

One place to start looking for cancer health disparities would be the cancer mortality rates (i.e., crude and age-adjusted) for the state as a whole compared with the county where the health education specialist works. These data may be available from the NCHS or another center within the CDC, from the state department of health, or from a university research center. Comparisons could also be made based on the mortality rates for various types of cancer. If the health education specialist knew what types of cancers were of greatest concern in the county, they could then examine the data for the county on the basis of certain demographic characteristics that have been associated with certain cancers. So the health education specialist may be using sex-, age-, or race/ethnicity-specific rates to compare various subgroups while looking for disparities. Once the health education specialist identifies a subgroup problem with a type of cancer, they may turn to data from the BRFSS to look for risk behaviors that are known to contribute to or cause the type of cancer identified. Again, the health education specialist may find the needed data in a state or local agency or university as well. Using different sources of data should help the health education specialist find the focus of her program for the priority population and put them in a position to compete for the grant money from the state department of health. Examples of what the health education specialist may have found through this process are higher rates of prostate cancer in African American men between the ages of 45 and 64 years or a higher prevalence of certain types of leukemia in children younger than 15 years of age.

In summary, to get to the point of being able to identify a priority population (i.e., a certain subgroup of people) and program focus (i.e., risk factors associated with a certain type of cancer), several different types of data were used. Initially, the health education specialist used cancer mortality data, then prevalence rates for various types of cancer and different subgroups, and finally risk factor data for various types of cancer.

The Goal and Purpose of the Profession

The ultimate goal of all service professions, including health education/promotion, is to improve the quality of life, even though the quality of life is difficult to quantify (Raphael, Brown, Renwick, & Rootman, 1997). However, many professionals feel that there is a direct relationship between quality of life and health status. Quality of life is usually improved when health status is improved, or, as Ashley Montagu (1968, p. 206) has stated, "The highest goal in life is to die young, at as old an age as possible." To that end, "the goal of health education is to promote, maintain, and improve individual and community health. The teaching-learning process is the hallmark and social agenda that differentiates the practice of health education from that of other helping professions in achieving this goal" (National Commission for Health Education Credentialing, Inc. [NCHEC], 1996, pp. 2–3).

Because quality of life and health status are complex variables, they are not usually changed in a short period of time. To reach these goals, people usually work their way through a number of small steps over a period of time that equip them with all that is necessary to impact both their health status and, in turn, their quality of life. Thus, it is the work of health education specialists to create interventions (programs) that can assist people in working toward better health. This work is reflected in the purpose of health education that "is to positively influence the health behavior of individuals and communities as well as the living and working conditions that influence their health" (New York State as presented at Coalition for National Health Education Organizations [CNHEO], 2007, p. 1).

The Practice of Health Education/Promotion

While the practice of health education specialists is outlined in the responsibilities and competencies presented in Chapter 6, as noted in our discussion of the use of data previously, the primary role of health education specialists is to develop appropriate health education/promotion programs for the people they serve. The practice of health education/promotion is based on the assumption "that beneficial health behavior will result from a combination of planned, consistent, integrated learning opportunities. This assumption rests on the scientific evaluations of health education programs in schools, at worksites, in medical settings, and through mass media" (Green & Ottoson, 1999, pp. 93–94). The results of these *scientific evaluations*, referred to by Green and Ottoson, are one source of data that contribute to a body of data known as evidence. **Evidence** is data that can be used to make decisions about planning. When health education specialists practice in such a way that they systematically find, appraise, and use evidence as the basis for decision making when planning health education/promotion programs, it is referred to as **evidence-informed practices** (Joint Committee, 2021).

Although the practice of health education specialists is easily stated, it is by no means easy to carry out. Much time, effort, practice, and on-the-job training are required to be successful. Even the most experienced health education specialists find program development challenging because of the constant changes in settings, resources, and priority populations (McKenzie, Neiger, & Thackeray, 2016).

The specific steps taken to develop a health education/promotion program vary depending on the planning model used (see Chapter 4); most models include the following steps (McKenzie et al., 2016) (see Figure 4.17):

1. Assessing the needs of the priority population
2. Setting goals and objectives
3. Developing an intervention that considers the peculiarities of the setting
4. Implementing the intervention
5. Evaluating the results

Therefore, it becomes the practice of health education specialists to be able to carry out all that is associated with these tasks.

Over the years, to be educated to serve as a health education specialist, individuals have been trained in three different types of academic programs—community health education, public health education, and school health education. In recent years, mostly because of the profession's movement toward accreditation of all undergraduate programs in health education, there has been a movement to just two preparation tracks as opposed to three in the past. Community health education programs are increasingly switching over to public health education to meet accreditation requirements (see Chapter 6 for more on accreditation).

Basic Underlying Concepts of the Profession

Previously mentioned in this chapter and discussed in greater detail in Chapter 2, the profession of health education/promotion is one that has been built on the principles and concepts of a number of disciplines and professions. Pieces of community development and organizing, education, epidemiology, medicine, psychology, and sociology can be found within health education/promotion. In the sections that follow, we present some of the basic underlying concepts of the profession. Please note that we have not exhausted the discussion of each of these topics but, rather, present sufficient information to allow a basic understanding of each.

The Health Field Concept and the Determinants of Health

Soon after the Canadian government implemented its national health plan that ensured health care for all Canadians, it began to look more closely at the health field as a way of improving Canadians' health. The **health field** is a term the government described as being far more encompassing than the "health-care system." This term was much broader and included all matters that affected health (Lalonde, 1974). Because the health field was such a broad concept, it was decided that there was a need to develop a framework that would subdivide the concept into principal elements so that the elements could be studied. Such a framework was developed and called the **health field concept** (Laframboise, 1973).

The health field concept divided the health field into four elements: (1) human biology, (2) environment, (3) lifestyle, and (4) healthcare organization. These four elements were the result of an assessment of underlying factors of sickness and death and key indicators of overall health in Canada (Lalonde, 1974). **Human biology** is defined as the organic make-up of an individual and all those aspects of health, both physical and mental, which are developed within the human body as a consequence of the basic biology (Lalonde, 1974, p. 31). This not only includes the genetic inheritance of an individual but also the processes of maturation and aging and the complex interaction of the various systems of the human body (Lalonde, 1974). The element of **environment** "includes all those matters related to health which are external to the human body and over which the individual has little or no control" (Lalonde, 1974, p. 32). Some examples of things often included in the element of environment are geography, climate, community size, industrial development, economy, and social norms.

The element of **lifestyle** comprises the combination of decisions which individuals have control, more or less, that impact their health (Lalonde, 1974). In more recent times, lifestyle has been more commonly referred to as **health behavior** (those behaviors that impact a person's health). The fourth element in the health field concept is healthcare organization. **Healthcare organization** "consists of the quantity, quality, arrangement, nature and relationships of people and resources in the provision of health care" (Lalonde, 1974, p. 32). This fourth element is often referred to as the healthcare system.

The utility of the health field concept has proved to be helpful over the years, both in Canada and in the United States. Its greatest importance may have been to bring attention to the concept of health promotion and disease prevention. Before this point in history, the primary focus of health care had been on the cure of disease, not the prevention of disease. In fact, it was stated that the health field concept put human biology, environment, and lifestyle on equal footing with healthcare organization (Lalonde, 1974). Since its development, studies using this concept in both Canada and the United States have provided a greater understanding of what contributes to morbidity and mortality and what health professionals can do to help improve the health of those whom they serve.

Using a similar framework as that of the elements of the health field concept, it is now believed that the health of populations is shaped by five intersecting domains (i.e., the **determinants of health**): (1) genetics (e.g., sex, age, and individual characteristics), (2) individual behavior (e.g., diet, physical activity, and alcohol use), (3) social circumstances (e.g., education, socioeconomic status,

housing, and crime), (4) environmental and physical influences (e.g., safe water, where a person lives, and crowding conditions), and (5) health services (e.g., access to quality health care, cost, and lack of insurance coverage) (IOM, 2001; McGinnis, 2001; McGovern, Miller, & Hughes-Cromwick, 2014; USDHHS, 2020) (also see the discussion of the Multi-causation Disease Model later in the chapter). These domains are dynamic and vary in impact depending on where one is in the life cycle (IOM, 2001).

In addition to understanding the determinants of health as they contribute to a person's current state of health, the **social determinants of health** also play a critical role in the health of people and communities. Social determinants of health are the "conditions in which people are born, live, learn, work, and play, all of which typically would impact their health outcomes. These conditions and outcomes are shaped by the distribution of money, power, and resources at global, national, and local levels" (Joint Committee, 2021). Like the determinants of health, the social determinants of health (see **Figure 1.2**) encompass five areas: (1) economic stability (e.g., poverty, employment, housing stability such as homelessness or foreclosure, and food security); (2) education access and quality (e.g., high school graduation rates, enrollment in higher education, language, and literacy); (3) social and community context (e.g., perceptions of discrimination and equity, civic participation, and incarceration); (4) healthcare access and quality (e.g., access to health care, access to primary care, and health literacy; and (5) neighborhood and built environment (e.g., quality of housing, environmental conditions, access to healthy foods, and crime and violence) (USDHHS, 2020). Addressing these social determinants of health can impact the health of large numbers of people in ways that can be sustained over time.

We know that genetics play a big part in late-onset diseases such as diabetes, cancer,

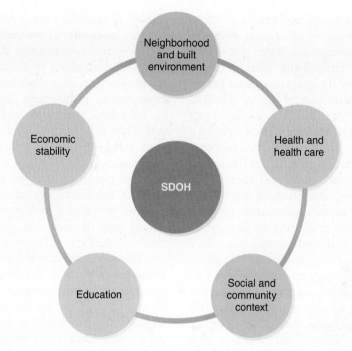

Figure 1.2 Social determinants of health.

and cardiovascular disease, whereas employment and income (social circumstances) have a significant influence on health and health care throughout life. Further, environmental aspects also impact health. For example, families with access to sidewalks and safe neighborhoods (neighborhood and built environment) are more likely to engage in health-enhancing behaviors.

On a population basis, using the best available estimates, the impacts of various domains on early deaths in the United States distribute roughly as follows: genetic predispositions, about 30%; social circumstances, 15%; environmental exposures, 5%; behavioral patterns, 40%; and shortfalls in medical care, approximately 10%. But more important than these proportions is the nature of the influences in play where the domains intersect. Ultimately, the health fate of each of us is determined by factors acting not mostly in isolation but by our experience where domains

interconnect. Whether a gene is expressed can be determined by environmental exposures or behavioral patterns. The nature and consequences of behavioral choices are affected by our social circumstances. Our genetic predispositions affect the health care we need, and our social circumstances affect the health care we receive (McGinnis et al., 2002, p. 83).

The Levels and Limitations of Prevention

The word *prevention* has already been used several times in this chapter. We now want to formally define the term, present the different levels of prevention, and briefly discuss the limitations of prevention. **Prevention**, as it relates to health, has been defined as the planning for and the measures taken to forestall the onset of a disease or other health problem before the occurrence of undesirable health events. This definition presents three distinct levels of prevention: primary, secondary, and tertiary prevention. **Primary prevention** comprises those preventive measures that forestall the onset of illness or injury during the prepathogenesis period (before the disease process begins) (Seabert, McKenzie, & Pinger, 2022). Examples of primary prevention measures include wearing a safety belt, using rubber gloves or a face covering when there is potential for the spread of disease, immunizing against specific diseases, exercising, and brushing one's teeth. Any health education/promotion program aimed specifically at averting the onset of illness or injury is also an example of primary prevention.

Illness and injury cannot always be prevented. In fact, many diseases, such as cancer and heart disease, can establish themselves in humans and cause considerable damage before they are detected and treated. In such cases, the sooner a condition is detected and medical personnel intervene, the greater the chances of limiting disability and preventing death. Such identification and intervention are known as secondary prevention. More specifically, **secondary prevention** includes the preventive measures that lead to an early diagnosis and prompt treatment of a disease or an injury to limit disability and prevent more serious pathogenesis. Good examples of secondary prevention include personal and clinical screenings and examinations such as blood pressure, blood cholesterol, and mammograms. The goal of such screenings and examinations is not to prevent the onset of the disease but rather to detect its presence during early pathogenesis, thus permitting early treatment and limiting disability (Seabert, McKenzie & Pinger, 2022).

The final level of prevention is **tertiary prevention**. It is at this level that health education specialists work to retrain, reeducate, and rehabilitate the individual who has already incurred disability, impairment, or dependency. Examples of some tertiary measures include educating a patient after lung cancer surgery or working with an individual who has diabetes to ensure that the daily insulin injections are taken. **Figure 1.3** provides

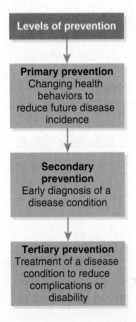

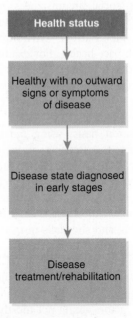

Figure 1.3 Levels of prevention.

a visual representation of the levels of prevention in relation to health status.

Although health education specialists can intervene at any of the three levels of prevention and can have a great deal of success, it should be obvious from the previous discussion of the health field concept and the determinants of health that prevention is not the "magic bullet" for an endless life. Prevention does have its limits. McGinnis (1985) has noted four major categories of limitations: (1) biological, (2) technological, (3) ethical, and (4) economic. Biological limitations center on life span. How long should individuals expect to live healthy lives or, for that matter, how long should they expect to live at all? Even with the best inputs and a bit of luck, one should not expect to live longer than 80 to 110 years. Body parts will eventually wear out from use.

Technological advances also have their limitations. Today, healthcare workers have a vast array of technical equipment available to help them care for their patients, but technology still has not been able to eradicate AIDS or malaria or to explain the cause of Alzheimer's disease.

Prevention is also limited by ethical concerns (see Chapter 5). Even though helmets would increase the chances of survival in automobile crashes, is it ethical to have a law that says all drivers and passengers in automobiles must wear them? Or is it ethical to penalize people via fines, taxes, or surcharges for acting in unhealthy ways, such as driving an automobile without a safety belt on, buying and using tobacco products, or for not having a smoke detector and fire extinguisher in the home?

Finally, prevention has economic limitations. Prevention is limited by the amount of money that is put into it. Although the exact figures are difficult to determine, it is commonly understood that fewer than 5% of all dollars spent on health in the United States each year are spent on essential public health services, government public health activity, and population-based public health

activity (Turnock, 2012). Stated another way, approximately 95% of the 2 trillion plus dollars spent on health in the United States each year is spent on curing ill health, not on health promotion and disease prevention (Sultz & Young, 2011).

Risk Factors

The health field concept, the determinants of health, and the social determinants of health have provided those interested in health issues with a framework from which the health field can be studied. The levels of prevention and their limitations have provided this same group of people with a time frame from which to plan to help forestall the onset of, limit the spread of, and rehabilitate after pathogenesis or another health problem. What none of these concepts fully discloses is the focus at which health promotion and disease prevention programming should be aimed, **risk factors**. A risk factor is any attribute, characteristic or exposure of an individual that increase the likelihood of developing a disease or injury. Risk factors increase the probability of morbidity and premature mortality but do not guarantee that people with a risk factor will suffer the consequences.

Risk factors can be divided into two categories: (1) **modifiable risk factors** (changeable or controllable) and (2) **nonmodifiable risk factors** (nonchangeable or noncontrollable). The former include such factors as sedentary lifestyle, smoking, and poor dietary habits—things that individuals can change or control whereas the latter group includes factors such as age, sex, and inherited genes—things that individuals cannot change or do not have control over. Note that these two categories of risk factors are often interrelated. In fact, the combined potential for harm from a number of risk factors is greater than the sum of their individual potentials. For example, asbestos workers have an increased risk for cancer because of their exposure to this carcinogen. Further, if they smoke, they have a 30 times greater chance of developing lung cancer than their nonsmoking coworkers and 90 times greater chance of getting lung cancer than people who neither work with asbestos nor smoke. The risk increases further if they have an inherited respiratory disease.

Knowledge about the impact of risk behaviors has continued to grow. In looking back over the 20th century, we have seen disease prevention change "from focusing on reducing environmental exposures over which the individual had little control, such as providing potable water, to emphasizing behaviors such as avoiding use of tobacco, fatty foods, and a sedentary lifestyle" (Breslow, 1999, p. 1030). As noted previously, approximately 40% of the early deaths in the United States each year are caused by these behavior patterns that could be modified by preventive interventions (McGinnis et al., 2002). Therefore, much of the focus of the work of health education specialists has been to help individuals identify and control their modifiable risk factors.

Health Risk Reduction

To focus on specific risk factors, health education specialists must have a basic understanding of both communicable (infectious) and noncommunicable (noninfectious) diseases. **Communicable diseases** also referred to as infectious diseases, are illnesses caused by infectious agents or its toxins that are transmissible from one individual to another (Seabert, McKenzie & Pinger, 2022), and **noncommunicable diseases** or illnesses are those that cannot be transmitted from an infected person to a susceptible, healthy one (Seabert, McKenzie & Pinger, 2022). Our intent in this section and the ones that follow is not to present information on all possible diseases and their related risk factors that a health education specialist may have

to develop programs for but rather to provide a general understanding of the spread and cause of disease. (See **Table 1.5** for leading causes of death and their risk factors.)

Before moving on, we would like to make a special note about the data presented in **Figure 1.4**. The term *leading causes of death* is used in this figure. That term refers to "the primary pathophysiological conditions identified at the time of death, as opposed to the root causes" (McGinnis & Foege, 1993, p. 2207). McGinnis and Foege (1993) conducted a study to see if they could identify the root causes of death. What they found was that the leading *actual causes of death* were modifiable behaviors—behaviors that people could change. The behavior that was the leading actual cause of death was tobacco use, accounting for some 400,000, or 19%, of the mortality in 1990. A similar study to that of McGinnis and Foege was conducted by Mokdad, Marks, Stroup, and Gerberding in 2004 using 2000 mortality data. They also found tobacco to be the leading actual cause of death, but that poor diet and physical inactivity killed almost as many (see Figure 1.4). It is now estimated that tobacco is the primary cause of more than 480,000 deaths per year, about one in five deaths annually (CDC, n.d.-j). Figure 1.4 provides evidence that nearly half of all causes of death in the United States could be attributed to a number of largely preventable behaviors and that by improving healthy behaviors, we can significantly reduce the consequences of chronic diseases. "These findings, along with escalating healthcare costs and aging population, argue persuasively that the need to establish a more preventive orientation in the U.S. health care and public health systems has become more urgent" (Mokdad et al., 2004, p. 1238).

The Chain of Infection

The **chain of infection** (see **Figure 1.5**) is a model used to explain the spread of a communicable disease from one host to another.

Table 1.5 **Leading Causes of Death and Associated Risk Factors for all Ages: United States, 2019**

Rank	Cause	Risk Factors
1	Diseases of the heart	Tobacco use, high blood pressure, unhealthy cholesterol levels, diet, diabetes, obesity, lack of physical activity, drinking too much alcohol, genetics (CDC, n.d.-f)
2	Malignant neoplasms (cancer)	Tobacco use, alcohol use, diet, obesity, solar radiation, ionizing radiation, exposure to certain chemicals, genetics (CDC, n.d.-c)
3	Unintentional injuries (accidents)	Alcohol misuse, tobacco use (fires), product design, home hazards, handgun availability, lack of safety restraints, excessive speed, automobile design, roadway design
4	Chronic lower respiratory diseases	Tobacco use, diseases
5	Cerebrovascular diseases (stroke)	Tobacco use, high blood pressure, unhealthy cholesterol levels, diabetes, obesity, genetics (CDC, n.d.-f)
6	Alzheimer's disease	Age, family history, genetics, head injury, heart health, general healthy aging (Alzheimer's Association, n.d.)
7	Diabetes mellitus	Obesity (for type II diabetes), diet, lack of physical activity, genetics (CDC, n.d.-d)
8	Nephritis, nephrotic syndrome, and nephrosis	Infectious agents, drug hypersensitivity, genetics, trauma
9	Influenza and pneumonia	Tobacco use, infectious agents, biological factors
10	Suicide	Family history, previous suicide attempts, history of mental disorders, history of alcohol and substance abuse, cultural and religious beliefs, barriers to accessing mental health treatment (CDC, n.d.-l)

Data from Centers for Disease Control and Prevention. (n.d.). *WISQARS: Leading causes of death visualization tool.* Retrieved April 7, 2021, from https://www.cdc.gov/injury/wisqars/index.html

The basic premise represented in the chain of infection is that individuals can break the chain (reduce the risk) at any point; thus, the spread of disease can be stopped. For example, the spread of some waterborne diseases is stopped when the first link of the chain is broken with the chlorination of the water supply, thus killing the pathogens that cause a disease. The risk is reduced because the pathogen is destroyed before it is consumed. The chain can also be broken by placing a barrier between the means of transmission and the portal of entry, as when healthcare providers protect themselves with surgical masks and rubber gloves. In this case, the risk is reduced because individuals are not exposing themselves to the pathogen. With such information, health education specialists can help create programs that are aimed at "breaking" the chain and reducing the risks.

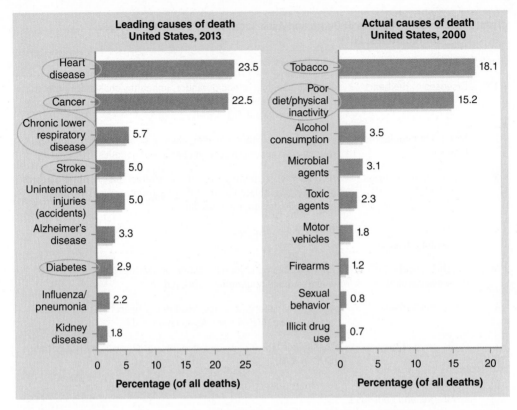

Figure 1.4 Leading versus actual causes of death in the United States.

Data from Mokdad, A. H., Marks, J. S., Stroup, D. F., & Gerberding, J. L. (2005). Correction: Actual causes of death in the United States, 2000. *Journal of the American Medical Association, 293*(3), 293–294. https://doi.org/10.1001/jama.293.3.293; National Center for Health Statistics. (2019). Health, United States: 2018. Retrieved December 6, 2020, from https://www.cdc.gov/nchs/data/hus/hus18.pdf

Communicable Disease Model

A second model used to describe the spread of a communicable disease is the **communicable disease model**. **Figure 1.6** presents the elements of this model—agent, host, and environment. These three elements summarize the minimal requirements for the presence and spread of a communicable disease in a population. The agent is the element (or, using the chain of infection labels, the pathogen) that must be present for a disease to spread—for example, bacteria or a virus. The host is any susceptible organism that can be invaded by the agent. Examples include plants, animals, and humans. The environment includes all other factors that either prohibit or promote disease transmission.

Thus, communicable disease transmission occurs when a susceptible host and a pathogenic agent exist in an environment conducive to disease transmission.

Multicausation Disease Model

Obviously, the chain of infection and communicable disease models are most helpful in trying to prevent disease caused by a pathogen. However, they are not applicable to noncommunicable diseases, which include many of the chronic diseases such as heart disease and cancer. Most of these diseases manifest themselves in people over a period of time and are not caused by a single factor but by combined factors. The concept of "caused by many factors" is referred to as

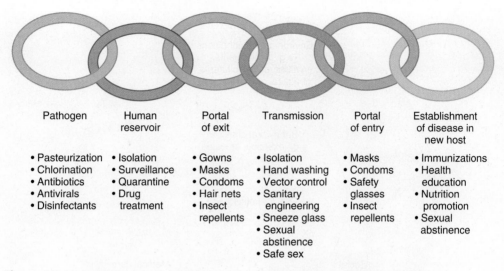

Pathogen	Human reservoir	Portal of exit	Transmission	Portal of entry	Establishment of disease in new host
• Pasteurization • Chlorination • Antibiotics • Antivirals • Disinfectants	• Isolation • Surveillance • Quarantine • Drug treatment	• Gowns • Masks • Condoms • Hair nets • Insect repellents	• Isolation • Hand washing • Vector control • Sanitary engineering • Sneeze glass • Sexual abstinence • Safe sex	• Masks • Condoms • Safety glasses • Insect repellents	• Immunizations • Health education • Nutrition promotion • Sexual abstinence

Figure 1.5 Chain of infection model and strategies for disease prevention and control.

Reproduced from Seabert, D. M., McKenzie, J. F., & Pinger, R. R. (2022). *McKenzie's an introduction to community & public health* (10th ed.). Jones & Bartlett Learning.

the **multicausation disease model** (see **Figure 1.7**). For example, it is known that heart disease is more likely to manifest itself in individuals who are older, who smoke, who do not exercise, who are overweight, who have high blood pressure, who have high cholesterol, and who have immediate family members who have had heart disease. Note that within this list of factors, there are both modifiable and nonmodifiable risk factors.

As when using the chain of infection model, the work of health education specialists is to create programs to help people reduce the risk of disease and injury by helping those in the priority population identify and control as many of the multicausative factors as possible. This model should look familiar to you because it is made up of the five determinants of health discussed previously in this chapter.

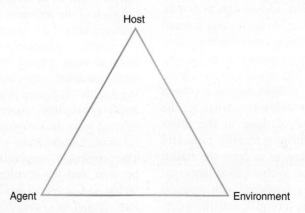

Figure 1.6 Communicable disease model.

Reproduced from Seabert, D. M., McKenzie, J. F., & Pinger, R. R. (2022). *McKenzie's an introduction to community & public health* (10th ed.). Jones & Bartlett Learning.

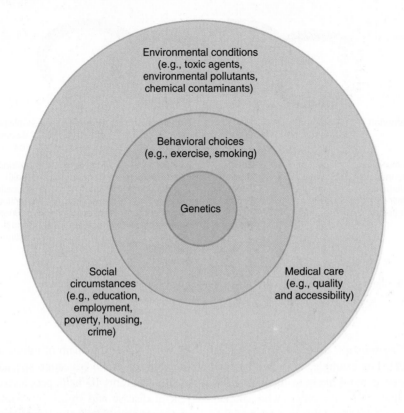

Figure 1.7 Multicausation disease model.

Other Selected Principles

Several other principles of health education/ promotion have been identified as important (Cleary & Neiger, 1998). Health education specialists must address the principles of participation, empowerment, and cultural competency while being culturally responsive if health education/promotion is to be successful. We would like to add two other principles to this list, socio-ecological approach and advocacy. **Participation** refers to the active involvement of those in the priority population in helping identify, plan, and implement programs to address the health problems they face. Without such participation, ethical issues associated with program development come into play, and the priority population probably will not support and feel **ownership** of (responsibility for) the

program. For example, if the health education specialists for a large corporation are creating a health promotion program for all employees, they should not begin to plan without the participation of (or at least representation by) each of the segments (clerical, labor, and management) of the employee population.

Health education/promotion activities have recently placed more emphasis on socio-ecological approaches to improving health. The underlying concept of the **socio-ecological approach** (sometimes referred to as the *ecological perspective*) is that behavior has multiple levels of influences. This approach "emphasizes the interaction between, and the interdependence of factors within and across all levels of a health problem" (Rimer & Glanz, 2005, p. 10). That is to say, seldom does behavior change based on influence from a single level. People live in environments (i.e., physical, social, political, cultural, and economic) that shape behaviors and access to the resources they need to maintain good health (Pellmar, Brandt, & Baird, 2002). Scholars who study and write about the levels of influence have used various labels to describe them. However, commonly used labels include individual and individual's characteristics (e.g., knowledge, attitudes, values, and skills), social relationships, organizational influences, community characteristics, and public policy (McLeroy, Bibeau, Steckler, & Glanz, 1988). Physical environment and culture have recently been added to levels of influence (Simons-Morton, McLeroy, & Wendel, 2012). In practice, behavior change often involves influences on multiple levels. For example, to get a person to begin an exercise program, it may take a conversation with their physician (i.e., social influence), a company policy (i.e., organizational-level influence), and also the county commissioners voting to put walking paths in the community (i.e., community-level influence). Thus, a central conclusion of the socio-ecological approach "is that it usually takes the combination of both individual-level and environmental/policy-level interventions to achieve substantial changes in health behavior" (Sallis, Owen, & Fisher, 2008, p. 467). Therefore, health education specialists must do more than just educate to help to change behavior. As a group, these skills are often called **population-based approaches**. They include policy development, policy advocacy, organizational change, community development, empowerment of individuals, and economic supports.

Consider this example to better understand how a population-based approach works. A state-level voluntary health organization was spending most of its time and resources helping individuals quit using nicotine or preventing others from starting to use nicotine. Recently, the organization has developed a statewide advocacy network to respond to nicotine-related legislation. They are using a population-based approach to influence legislation and policy that will ultimately impact individual nicotine behaviors. They still maintain the more individual approaches to dealing with the nicotine issue but have added the population-based approach.

Advocacy is another principle in which health education specialists have become more involved. **Advocacy** is defined as "any attempt to influence procedures, policy, public opinion, and/or attitudes that directly affect people's lives" (Joint Committee, 2021). Professional associations encourage health education specialists to get involved in advocacy for the profession and for health-related issues (Auld & Dixon-Terry, 2010). As an example, the Society for Public Health Education (see Chapter 8 for more on this organization) sponsors an annual advocacy summit. This annual event allows public health and advocacy professionals and students to gather to learn about and engage in effective advocacy for a common agenda.

If health education/promotion is going to create lasting change, those in the priority population must be empowered as a result of the health education/promotion programming. **Empowerment** is a "social action process for people to gain mastery over their lives and the lives of their communities" (Minkler, Wallerstein, & Wilson, 2008, p. 294). Empowerment can take place at the individual, the organization or group, and the community level. Often, empowerment at one level can influence empowerment at the other levels. An example of empowerment occurred in Indiana—a community with a significantly high rate of obesity and cancer, which have been linked to a lack of physical activity. The Indiana Complete Streets Coalition formed to ensure that communities throughout Indiana have neighborhoods, public spaces, and transportation systems that can support physical activity and healthy living. As a result, individuals and families have been empowered to improve their health because they now live in neighborhoods where it is possible to walk and bike safely

(CDC, n.d.-g). Social media is one growing strategy being used by health education specialists to advocate and empower individuals and communities. **Social media** is any type of "media that uses the Internet and other technologies to allow for social interaction (McKenzie et al., 2012, p. 448). Social media tools can include such things as online video sharing (e.g., YouTube), social networks (e.g., Facebook and Twitter), text messaging, podcasts, virtual worlds, blogs, and podcasts. The use of social media tools is a "powerful channel to reach target audiences with strategic, effective, and user-centric health interventions" (n.d.-k, para. 1). Because the Internet allows for a free flow of information, the CDC has developed guidelines, best practices, and toolkits for health education specialists using and developing social media materials (CDC, n.d.-k, 2011a). Becoming familiar with these various social media tools during your preparation as a health education specialist will prove valuable as doctors' offices, hospitals, state and local health departments, and voluntary agencies are using these tools to communicate with patients, volunteers, employees, and the general public.

There are many factors that impact the effectiveness of health education/promotion programming. Because of the health disparities that exist between and among the various subpopulations in the United States (Selig, Tropiano, & Greene-Moton, 2006) and because of the increasing diversification of the U.S. population (Pérez & Luquis, 2008), much more attention has been placed on understanding the impact of culture (i.e., values, beliefs, attitudes, traditions, and customs) on health and providing culturally appropriate programs (Davis & Rankin, 2006). Cultural factors arise from guidelines (both explicit and implicit) that individuals "inherit" from being a part of a particular society, racial or ethnic group, religious community, or other group. For health education specialists to be effective in a variety of communities, they need to strive to be culturally competent and provide culturally responsive health education (Davis & Rankin, 2006; Luquis, Pérez, & Young, 2006; Selig et al., 2006). **Cultural competence** is "a developmental process defined as a set of values, principles, behaviors, attitudes, and policies that enable health professionals to work effectively across racial, ethnic and linguistically diverse populations" (Joint Committee, 2012, p. 16). Both health education specialists and the community health agencies providing health education/promotion programs need to be **culturally responsive** by providing a "positive, strengths-based approach to health education that is rooted in respect and appreciation for the role of culture in learning and development" (Joint Committee, 2021).

Summary

This introductory chapter presented many of the basic principles of the profession of health education/promotion including definitions of many of the key words and terms used in the profession, including *health, health education, health promotion, disease prevention, community health, global health promotion, population health,* and *wellness*; a look at the current status of health education/promotion; an explanation of how health or health status have been measured, including mortality rates, life expectancy, YPLL, DALYs, HRQOL, and health surveys; an outline of the goal and purpose of the profession; the practice of health education/promotion including planning, implementing, and evaluating programs; some of the basic underlying concepts and principles of the profession including the health field concept, determinants of health, social determinants of health, levels of prevention, risk factors, and health risk reduction via understanding disease; and the principles of participation, ecological approach, advocacy, empowerment, social media, and cultural competence.

Review Questions

1. Define *health, health education, health promotion, disease prevention, public health, community health, global health promotion, population health,* and *wellness.*
2. What is the status of health education/promotion?
3. Explain each of the following means of measuring health or health status.
   - Mortality rates. What is the difference among crude, adjusted, and specific rates?
   - Life expectancy
   - Years of potential life lost (YPLL)
   - Disability-adjusted life years (DALYs)
   - Health-related quality of life (HRQOL)
   - Health surveys
4. Of all the different measures of health presented in this chapter, which one do you think is the best indicator of health? Why?
5. Why are health-related data and epidemiology such an important discipline for health education/promotion?
6. In a given community with a midyear population estimate of 50,000, there were 21 deaths as a result of strokes in the year. What is the rate of stroke deaths per 100,000 population?
7. What is the goal of health education/promotion? What is its purpose?
8. What constitutes the basic practice of health education/promotion?
9. What is the difference between the leading causes of death and the actual causes of death?
10. Briefly explain the following concepts and principles of health education/promotion.
    - Health field concept; determinants of health
    - Levels of prevention
    - Risk factors
    - Health risk reduction
    - Chain of infection
    - Communicable disease model
    - Multicausation disease model
    - Selected principles of health education/promotion—participation, socio-ecological approach, advocacy, empowerment, social media, cultural competence, and culturally responsive.

Case Study

As a health education specialist with the Delaware County Health Department, Jordan (pronouns: he/him/his) has been asked by a local religious leader to give a presentation on preventing HIV and STDs to the Christian youth group (9th to 12th graders) of the community. The request has taken Jordan by surprise because for the past couple of years he has attempted to make similar presentations in the local schools but has been turned away because the superintendent said "the community was too conservative for such matters." Knowing that at least some of the people in the community think HIV and STD prevention education is too controversial but also knowing the information is important for youth to have, Jordan wants to make sure he prepares and delivers a program that is well received. This is finally the chance he has been waiting for to make his entry into the youth population of the community. Jordan has decided to create a presentation on HIV and STD prevention that incorporates information on both risk factors and the chain of infection. To make sure that his presentation is on target, he has asked several other employees of the health department to sit down with him and brainstorm some ideas for his presentation. He begins his session with his colleagues by asking them all to write down information they think he should include in his presentation. Assume that you are one of these other employees of the health department in this meeting. What would you include on your list for Jordan? What would you advise Jordan not to include? Why? He then asks his colleagues for ideas on how to present the information (e.g., lecture, video, or role playing). What do you think would be the best method to use? Why did you select this method? How long do you think Jordan's presentation should be? Why?

Critical Thinking Questions

1. In this chapter, the term *public health* was defined. To what extent do you think that the government, at any level, has the right to legislate good health? For example, do you think a governmental body has the responsibility (or right) to require all motorcycle drivers to wear helmets because statistics show that wearing helmets can save lives? Defend your answer.
2. If you were asked by the CDC to come up with a new measure to describe the health status of an individual, what would you include in such a measure and why?
3. If you had the opportunity to develop three new health education/promotion programs, one at each level of the three levels of prevention (primary, secondary, and tertiary) for the community in which you live, what would they be? Who would be the priority population? Why did you pick the three that you did?

Activities

1. If you have not already done so, access the government document *Healthy People: The Surgeon General's Report on Health Promotion and Disease Prevention*. It provides a good background on the health promotion era in the United States.
2. Write your own definitions for *health, health education*, and *health promotion* using the concepts presented in the chapter.
3. Write one paragraph for each of the following:
   - Why do you think the health field concept was so important in getting people to think about health promotion?
   - At what level of prevention do you think it would be most difficult to change health behavior? Why?
4. In a PowerPoint presentation, use the chain of infection to outline three different means for preventing the spread of COVID-19.
5. In a photo story, use the multicausation disease model to explain how a person develops heart disease.

Weblinks

1. **http://www.cdc.gov/nchs/**

   National Center for Health Statistics (NCHS)

   This site is a rich source of data about health in the United States and the instruments used to collect the data.

2. **http://www.cdc.gov/brfss/**

   Behavioral Risk Factor Surveillance System (BRFSS)

   The BRFSS, the world's largest telephone survey, tracks health risks in the United States. Information from the survey is used to improve the health of U.S. citizens. At this site, you will find general information about the BRFSS, data generated by the BRFSS, copies of the data collection instruments, and more.

3. **http://www.cdc.gov/healthyyouth/**

   Youth Risk Behavioral Surveillance System (YRBSS)

   At this site, you will find general information about the YRBSS, data generated by the YRBSS, copies of the data collection instruments, and more.

4. **https://www.thinkculturalhealth.hhs.gov/**

   Think Cultural Health

   This is a page at the U.S. Department of Health and Human Services, Office of Minority Health website that presents information on cultural competence for health professionals. The site has a tagline of "advancing health equity at every point of contact." Included at the site are educational programs, resources, and other materials.

5. **http://www.bls.gov/ooh/**

   Occupational Outlook Handbook

   This is a page at the U.S. Department of Labor, Bureau of Labor Statistics website that provides the occupational outlook for a wide range of professions. Search for "health educators" to see short explanations of the nature of the work; training, other qualifications, and advancement; employment; job outlook and projections; earnings; wages; and sources of additional information about health education specialists.

6. **http://www.countyhealthrankings.org/**

   County Health Rankings

   This website presents the *County Health Rankings*. This site is a collaboration between the Robert Wood Johnson Foundation and the University of Wisconsin Population Health Institute.

References

Alzheimer's Association. (n.d.). *Causes and risk factors for Alzheimer's disease*. Retrieved December 6, 2020, from https://www.alz.org/alzheimers -dementia/what-is-alzheimers/causes-and-risk -factors

American College Health Association. (2020). *ACHA-NCHA*. Retrieved November 29, 2020, from https://www.acha.org/NCHA/NCHA_Home

Auld, M. E., & Dixon-Terry, E. (2010). The role of health education associations in advocacy. In J. M. Black, S. Furney, H. M. Graf, & A. E. Nolte (Eds.), *Philosophical foundations of health education* (pp. 311–318). Jossey-Bass.

Breslow, L. (1999). From disease prevention to health promotion. *Journal of the American Medical Association, 281*(11), 1030–1033.

Centers for Disease Control and Prevention (CDC). (n.d.-a). *About chronic diseases*. Retrieved April 28, 2021, from https://www.cdc.gov/chronicdisease/about /index.htm

Centers for Disease Control and Prevention (CDC). (n.d.-b). *Behavioral Risk Factor Surveillance System.* Retrieved August 31, 2020, from https://www.cdc.gov/brfss/index.html

Centers for Disease Control and Prevention (CDC). (n.d.-c). *Cancer: How to prevent cancer or find it early.* Retrieved July 29, 2020, from https://www.cdc.gov/cancer/dcpc/prevention/index.htm

Centers for Disease Control and Prevention (CDC). (n.d.-d). *Diabetes: Diabetes risk factors.* Retrieved April 23, 2021, from https://www.cdc.gov/diabetes/basics/risk-factors.html

Centers for Disease Control and Prevention. (CDC). (n.d.-e). *Health-related quality of life (HRQOL).* Retrieved October 31, 2018, from https://www.cdc.gov/hrqol/index.htm

Centers for Disease Control and Prevention (CDC). (n.d.-f). *Heart disease: Know your risk for heart disease.* Retrieved December 9, 2019, from https://www.cdc.gov/heartdisease/risk_factors.htm

Centers for Disease Control and Prevention (CDC). (n.d.-g). *National Comprehensive Cancer Control Program: Success stories.* Retrieved June 26, 2020, from http://www.cdc.gov/cancer/ncccp/state.htm

Centers for Disease Control and Prevention (CDC). (n.d.-h). *National Health and Nutrition Examination Survey.* Retrieved May 27, 2021, from http://www.cdc.gov/nchs/nhanes.htm

Centers for Disease Control and Prevention (CDC). (n.d.-i). *National Health Care Surveys.* Retrieved October 16, 2018, from https://www.cdc.gov/nchs/dhcs/index.htm

Centers for Disease Control and Prevention (CDC). (n.d.-j). *Smoking and tobacco use: Fast facts.* Retrieved May 14, 2021, from https://www.cdc.gov/tobacco/data_statistics/fact_sheets/fast_facts/index.htm#diseases

Centers for Disease Control and Prevention (CDC). (n.d.-k). *Social media at CDC: CDC social media tools, guidelines & best practices.* Retrieved December 27, 2019, from http://www.cdc.gov/socialmedia/tools/guidelines/index.html

Centers for Disease Control and Prevention (CDC). (n.d.-l). *Suicide prevention: Risk and protective factors.* Retrieved May 13, 2021, from https://www.cdc.gov/violenceprevention/suicide/riskprotectivefactors.html

Centers for Disease Control and Prevention (CDC). (n.d.-m). *Youth Risk Behavior Surveillance System (YRBSS).* Retrieved October 27, 2020, from https://www.cdc.gov/healthyyouth/data/yrbs/index.htm

Centers for Disease Control and Prevention (CDC). (1994). *Chronic disease in minority populations.* Atlanta, GA.

Centers for Disease Control and Prevention (CDC). (2011a). *The health communicator's social media toolkit.* Retrieved January 16, 2021, from http://www.cdc.gov/socialmedia/tools/guidelines/pdf/socialmediatoolkit_bm.pdf

Centers for Disease Control and Prevention (CDC). (2011b) *Principles of epidemiology in public health practice* (3rd ed.). U.S. Department of Health and Human Services. (Original work published 2006). https://www.cdc.gov/csels/dsepd/ss1978/index.html

Cleary, M. J., & Neiger, B. L. (1998). *The certified health education specialist: A self-study guide for professional competency* (3rd ed.). Allentown, PA: The National Commission for Health Education Credentialing.

Coalition for National Health Education Organizations (CNHEO). (n.d.). *Employer's guide.* Retrieved April 1, 2021, from http://www.cnheo.org/publications.html

Cottrell, R. R., & McKenzie, J. F. (2011). *Health promotion & education research methods: Using the five chapter thesis/dissertation model* (2nd ed.). Sudbury, MA: Jones and Bartlett Publishers.

Davis, P. C., & Rankin, L. L. (2006). Guidelines for making existing health education programs more culturally appropriate. *American Journal of Health Education, 37*(4), 250–252.

Glanz, K., & Rimer, B. K. (2008). Perspectives on using theory: Past, present, and future. In K. Glanz, B. K. Rimer, & K. Viswanath (Eds.), *Health behavior and health education: Theory, research, and practice* (pp. 509–517). San Francisco: Jossey-Bass.

Green, L. W., & Ottoson, J. M. (1999). *Community and population health* (8th ed.). Boston: WCB/McGraw-Hill.

Hancock, T., & Minkler, M. (2005). Community health assessment or healthy community assessment: Whose community? Whose health? Whose assessment? In M. Minkler (Ed.), *Community organizing and community building for health* (2nd ed., pp. 138–157). New Brunswick, NJ: Rutgers University Press.

Hanlon, J. J. (1974). *Public Health.* St. Louis: Mosby.

Heron M. (2016). Deaths: Leading causes for 2013. *National vital statistics reports, 65* (2). Hyattsville, MD: National Center for Health Statistics.

Hezel Associates. (2007). *Marketing the health education profession: Knowledge, attitudes, and hiring practices of employers.* Retrieved March 7, 2016, from http://cnheo.org/files/ExecSummary_Marketing_the_Health_Education_Profession.pdf

Institute of Medicine (IOM). (2001). *Health and behavior: The interplay of biological, behavioral, and societal influences.* Washington, DC: Academy Press.

Institute of Medicine (IOM); Committee on Assuring the Health of the Public in the 21st Century; Board on Health and Disease Prevention; (2003). *The future of the public's health in the 21st century.* Washington, DC: The National Academies Press.

Johns, E. B. (1973). Joint Committee on Health Education Terminology: Report of the Joint Committee on Health Education Terminology. *Health Education, 4*(6), 25.

Joint Committee on Health Education and Health Promotion Terminology. (2001). Report of the 2000 Joint Committee on Health Education and Health Promotion Terminology. *American Journal of Health Education, 32*(2), 89–94. https://doi.org/10.1080/19325037.2001.10609405

Joint Committee on Health Education and Health Promotion Terminology. (2012). *Report of the 2011 Joint Committee on Health Education and Promotion Terminology.* Reston, VA: AAHE.

Joint Committee on Health Education and Promotion Terminology. (2021). 2020 health education and promotion terminology report. Coalition of National Health Education Organizations. http://www.cnheo.org/2020-joint-committee-on-health-education-terminology.html

Joint Committee on Health Education Terminology. (1991a). Report of the 1990 Joint Committee on Health Education Terminology. *Journal of Health Education, 22*(2), 105–106.

Joint Committee on Health Education Terminology. (1991b). Report of the 1990 Joint Committee on Health Education Terminology. *Journal of School Health, 61*(6), 251–254.

King, N. (2009). Health inequalities and health inequities. In E. E. Morrison (Ed.), *Health care ethics: Critical issues for the 21st century* (pp. 339–354). Sudbury, MA: Jones & Bartlett.

Laframboise, H. L. (1973). Health policy: Breaking it down into more manageable segments. *Canadian Medical Association Journal, 108*(3), 388–393.

Lalonde, M. (1974). *A new perspective on the health of Canadians: A working document.* Ottawa, Canada: Ministry of National Health and Welfare.

Luquis, R., Pèrez, M., & Young, K. (2006). Cultural competence development in health education professional preparation programs. *American Journal of Health Education, 37*(4), 233–241.

Mason, J. O., & McGinnis, J. M. (1990). Healthy people 2000: An overview of the national health promotion disease prevention objectives. *Public Health Reports, 105*(5), 441–446.

McGinnis, J. M. (1985). The limits of prevention. *Public Health Reports, 100*(3), 255–260.

McGinnis, J. M. (2001). United States. In C. E. Koop (Ed.), *Critical issues in global health* (pp. 80–90). San Francisco: Jossey-Bass.

McGinnis, J. M., & Foege, W. H. (1993). Actual causes of death in the United States. *Journal of the American Medical Association, 270*(18), 2207–2212.

McGinnis, J. M., Williams-Russo, P., & Knickman, J. R. (2002). The case for more active policy attention to health promotion. *Health Affairs, 21*(2), 78–93.

McGovern, L., Miller, G., & Hughes-Cromwick, P. (2014). Health policy brief: The relative contribution of multiple determinants of health outcomes. *Health Affairs,* 1–9.

McKenzie, J. F., Neiger, B. L., & Thackeray, R (2016). *Planning, implementing, and evaluating, health promotion programs: A primer* (7th ed.). San Francisco: Pearson.

McLeroy, K. R., Bibeau, D., Steckler, A., &. Glanz, K. (1988). An ecological perspective for health promotion programs. *Health Education Quarterly, 15*(4), 351–377.

Minkler, M., Wallerstein, N., & Wilson, N. (2008). Improving health through community organizing and community building. In K. Glanz, B. K. Rimer, & K. Viswanath (Eds.), *Health behavior and health education practice: Theory, research, and practice* (4th ed., pp. 287–312). San Francisco: Jossey-Bass.

Mokdad, A. H., Marks, J. S., Stroup, D. F., & Gerberding, J. L. (2004). Actual causes of death, in the United States, 2000. *Journal of the American Medical Association, 291*(10), 1238–1245.

Montagu, A. (1968). *Man observed.* New York: G. P. Putnam.

Moss, B. (1950). Joint Committee on Health Education Terminology. *Journal of Physical Education, 21,* 41.

Murray, C. J. L., & Lopez, A. D. (Eds.). (1996). *Summary of the global burden of disease: A comprehensive assessment of mortality and disability from diseases, injuries, and risk factors in 1990 and projected to 2020.* Geneva, Switzerland: World Health Organization.

Nash, D. B., Fabius, R. J., Skoufalos, A., Clarke, J. L., & Horowitz, M. R. (2016). *Population health: Creating a culture of wellness* (2nd ed.). Burlington, MA: Jones & Bartlett Learning.

National Center for Health Statistics (NCHS). (2015). *Health, 2014: With special feature on adults aged 55-64.* Hyattsville, MD.

National Center for Health Statistics (NCHS). (2019). *Health, United States, 2018.* Hyattsville, MD.

National Commission for Health Education Credentialing, Inc. (NCHEC). (1996). *A competency-based framework for professional development of certified health education specialists.* Allentown, PA.

Pellmar, T. C., Brandt, Jr., E. N., & Baird, M. A. (2002). Health and behavior: The interplay of biological, behavioral, and social influences: Summary of an Institute of Medicine Report. *American Journal of Health Promotion, 16*(4), 206–219.

Pérez, M. A., & Luquis, R. R. (2008). Changing U.S. demographics: Challenges and opportunities for health educators. In M. A. Perez & R. R. Luquis (Eds.). *Cultural competence in health education and health promotion* (pp. 1–21). San Francisco: Jossey-Bass.

Pinzon-Perez, H., & Perez, M. A. (1999). Advocacy groups for Hispanic/Latino health issues. *The Health Educator Monograph Series, 17*(2), 29–31.

Raphael, D., Brown, I., Renwick, R., & Rootman, I. (1997). Quality of life: What are the implications for health promotion? *American Journal of Health Behavior, 21*(2), 118–128.

Rimer, B. K., & Glanz, K. (2005). *Theory at a glance: A guide for health promotion practice* (2nd ed). NIH Pub. No. 05-3896. Washington, DC: National Cancer Institute.

Rugen, M. (1972). *A fifty year history of the public health section of American Public Health Association; 1922–1972.* Washington, DC: American Public Health Association, Inc.

Sallis, J. F., Owen, N., & Fisher, E. B. (2008). Ecological models of health behavior. In K. Glanz, B. K. Rimer, & K. Viswanath (Eds.), *Health behavior and health education practice: Theory, research, and practice* (4th ed., pp. 465–485). San Francisco: Jossey-Bass.

Seabert, D. M. (2022). *McKenzie's Introduction to Community and Public Health* (10th ed.). Boston: Jones and Bartlett Publishers.

Selig, S., Tropiano, E., & Greene-Moton, E. (2006). Teaching cultural competence to reduce health disparities. *Health Promotion Practice, 7*(3), 247S–255S.

Simons-Morton, B. G., McLeroy, K. R., & Wendel, M. L. (2012). *Behavior theory in health promotion practice and research.* Burlington, MA: Jones & Bartlett Learning.

Sultz, H. A., & Young, K. M. (2011). *Health care USA: Understanding its organization and delivery* (7th ed.). Sudbury, MA: Jones & Bartlett.

Turnock, B. J. (2012). *Public health: What it is and how it works* (5th ed.). Burlington, MA: Jones & Bartlett Learning.

U.S. Department of Health, Education, and Welfare (USDHEW). (1980). *Promoting health/preventing disease: Objectives for the nation.* Washington, DC: U.S. Government Printing Office.

U.S. Department of Health and Human Services (USDHHS). (1991). *Health status of minorities and low-income groups* (3rd ed.). Washington, DC: U.S. Government Printing Office.

U.S. Department of Health and Human Services (USDHHS). (2020). *Healthy People 2020: Determinants of health.* Retrieved November 29, 2020, from https://www.healthypeople.gov/2020/about/foundation-health-measures/Determinants-of-Health

U.S. Department of Health and Human Services (USDHHS). (2014b). *Healthy People 2020: Social Determinants of Health.* Retrieved March 9, 2016, from https://www.healthypeople.gov/2020/topics-objectives/topic/social-determinants-of-health

University of Kansas [Center for Community Health and Development]. (2020). *Community Tool Box, Chapter 2.* https://ctb.ku.edu/en/table-contents/overview/other-models-promoting-community-health-and-development/preceder-proceder/main

Williams, J. F. (1934). Report of the Health Education Section of the American Physical Education Association: Definitions of terms in health education. *Journal of Physical Education, 5*(16–17), 50–51.

World Health Organization (WHO). (1947). *Constitution of the World Health Organization.* Retrieved March 7, 2016, from http://apps.who.int/gb/bd/PDF/bd47/EN/constitution-en.pdf

World Health Organization (WHO). (1986). *Health promotion sante: Ottawa charter.* Retrieved March 7, 2016, from http://www.euro.who.int/en/who-we-are/policy-documents/ottawa-charter-for-health-promotion,-1986

World Health Organization (WHO). (2008). *The global burden of disease: 2004 update.* Retrieved March 7, 2016, from http://www.who.int/healthinfo/global_burden_disease/GBD_report_2004update_full.pdf

Yoho, R. (1962). Joint Committee on Health Education Terminology: Health education terminology. *Journal of Physical Education and Recreation, 33*(Nov), 27–28.

CHAPTER 2

The History of Health and Health Education/ Promotion

CHAPTER OBJECTIVES

After reading this chapter and answering the questions at the end, you should be able to:

- Discuss how health beliefs and practices have changed from the earliest humans to the present day.
- Identify the dual roots of modern health education/promotion.
- Explain why a need for professional health education specialists emerged.
- Trace the history of public health in the United States.
- Relate the history of school health from the mid-1800s to the present.
- Identify important governmental publications from 1975 to the present and describe how these publications have impacted health promotion and education.

Although the history of health education/ promotion as a profession is slightly more than 100 years old, the concept of educating about health has been around since the dawn of humans. This chapter discusses the history of health, health care, and health education/ promotion from the earliest human records to the present. The main focus is on Northern Africa and Europe. These areas had the greatest influence on the development of health knowledge and health care in the United States. Although other parts of the world—for example, the Far East, Africa, Central America, and South America—contributed to the history of health and health care, their accounts are not as directly relevant to the history of health in the United States.

It is important that students recognize the difference between "educating about health," which can be done by anyone who believes they have knowledge about health to share with someone else, and "health education/ promotion," which is done by a professionally trained health education specialist. The need for professional health education specialists emerged as human knowledge of health and health care increased. This chapter emphasizes the health education/promotion profession during the past 150 years as it evolved from the dual roots of school health and public health. You cannot fully appreciate the health education/promotion profession without understanding its origin. History reveals how progress was made over time. It also depicts the obstacles faced by those who promoted health improvements throughout the years. "At the same time, historical study shows us that despite the difficulties, change is possible, given dedication, organization and persistence. Historical case studies may be able to teach us useful lessons about successful strategies used by public health reformers in the past" (Fee & Brown, 1997, p. 1763).

Early Humans

We assume that the earliest humans learned by trial and error to distinguish between things that were healthful and those that were harmful. They were able to observe how animals bathed to cool their bodies and remove external parasites, apply mud to calm insect bites, consume certain herbs to provide medicinal benefits and avoid other herbs that were poisonous (Goerke & Stebbins, 1968, p. 5).

It does not stretch the imagination too far to see how education about health first took place. Someone may have eaten a particular plant or herb and become ill. That person would then warn (educate) others against eating the same substance. Conversely, someone may have ingested a plant or an herb that produced a desired effect. That person would then encourage (educate) others to use this substance. Through observation, trial, and error, other types of health-related knowledge were discovered. Eventually, this knowledge was transformed into rules or taboos for a given society. Rules about preserving food and how to bury the dead may have been implemented. Perhaps taboos against defecation within the tribe's communal area or near sources of drinking water were established (McKenzie & Pinger, 2015). The trial and error method, which undoubtedly produced serious illness and even death among some

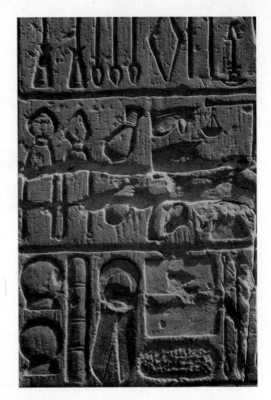

Figure 2.1 Preparation of medicine from honey (the leaf from an Arabic translation of the *Materia Medica of Dioscorides*, dated 1224 Iraq, Baghdad School).

© paintings/Shutterstock.

early humans, gradually became less needed. Knowledge was passed verbally from one generation to the next, preventing at least some of the potential ill effects of everyday life. As society progressed even further, this knowledge was written down and saved (see **Figure 2.1**).

There was still much more unknown than known about protecting health. Disease and death were probably much more common than health and longevity. To early humans, it was puzzling when disease and death occurred for no apparent reason. In an attempt to make these events seem more rational, early man often attributed disease and accidents to magical spirits, which were believed to live in trees, animals, the earth, and the air. When these spirits were angered, they would punish individuals or communities with disease and death (Goerke & Stebbins, 1968). To prevent disease, sacrifices were made to please the spirits or gods, taboos were obeyed, amulets were worn, and "haunted" places were avoided. Charms, spells, and chants were also used as protection from disease (Duncan, 1988). Again, it is likely that some form of rudimentary education about health was taking place to inform people how to keep from provoking the spirits and, thus, prevent disease.

Early Efforts at Public Health

Evidence of broad-scale public health activity has been found in the earliest of civilizations. In India, sites excavated at Mohenjo-Daro and Harappa dating back 4,000 years indicate that bathrooms and drains were common. The streets were broad, paved, and drained by covered sewers (Rosen, 1958). Archeological evidence also shows that the Minoans (3000–1430 B.C.E.) and Myceneans (1430–1150 B.C.E.) built drainage systems, toilets, and water-flushing systems (Pickett & Hanlon, 1990). The oldest written documents related to health care are the **Smith Papyri**, dating from 1600 B.C.E., which describe various surgical techniques. The earliest written record concerning public health is the **Code of Hammurabi** (see **Box 2.1**), named after the king of Babylon. It contained laws pertaining to health practices and physicians, including the first known fee schedule (Rubinson & Alles, 1984).

Early Cultures

The medical lore of the distant past was handed down from generation to generation. In virtually every culture for which there are documented historical accounts, people turned to some type of a physician or medicine man for health information (education

---

Box 2.1 **The Rights and Duties of the Surgeon of 2080 B.C.E.: from the *Code of Hammurabi***

"If a physician operate on a man for a severe wound (or make a severe wound upon a man), with a bronze lancet, and save the man's life; or if he open an abscess (in the eye) of a man, with a bronze lancet, and save the man's eye, he shall receive ten shekels of silver (as his fee)."

"If he be a freeman,* he shall receive five shekels."

"If it be a man's slave, the owner of the slave shall give two shekels of silver to the physician."

"If a physician operate on a man for a severe wound, with a bronze lancet, and cause the man's death; or open an abscess (in the eye) of a man with a bronze lancet, and destroy the man's eye, they shall cut off his hands."

"If a physician operate on a slave of a freeman for a severe wound, with a bronze lancet, and cause his death, he shall restore a slave of equal value."

"If he open an abscess (in his eye), with a bronze lancet, and destroy his eye, he shall pay silver to the extent of one half of his price."

"If a physician set a broken bone for a man or cure his diseased bowels, the patient shall give five shekels of silver to the physician."

"If he be a freeman, he shall give three shekels."

"If it be a man's slave, the owner of the slave shall give two shekels of silver to the physician."

"If a veterinary physician operates on an ox or ass for a severe wound and save its life, the owner of the ox or ass shall give the physician, as his fee, one sixth of a shekel of silver."

"If he operate on an ox or an ass for a severe wound, and cause its death, he shall give to the owner of the ox or ass one fourth its value."

---

*Freeman indicates a rank intermediate between that of "man" (or gentleman) and that of "slave."
Harper, R. F. (1904). *The code of Hammurabi.* University of Chicago Press.

about health), treatments, and cures (Green & Simons-Morton, 1990). In Egypt, as in many other cultures, this role was held by the priests. Eventually, the various incantations, spells, exorcisms, prescriptions, and clinical observations were compiled into written format, some of which survive in our museums and libraries (Libby, 1922).

The Egyptians made substantial progress in the area of public health. They possessed a strong sense of personal cleanliness and were considered to be the healthiest people of their time (see **Figure 2.2**). They used numerous pharmaceutical preparations and constructed earth privies for sewage, as well as public drainage pipes (Pickett & Hanlon, 1990). Nevertheless, they relied primarily on priests for their health information and used remedies such as "dung of the gazelle and the crocodile, the fat of a serpent, mammalian entrails and other excreta, tissues and organs" (Libby, 1922, p. 6).

In approximately 1500 B.C.E., the Hebrews extended Egyptian hygienic thought and formulated (in the biblical book of Leviticus) what is probably the world's first written hygienic code. It dealt with a variety of personal and community responsibilities, including cleanliness of the body, protection against the spread of contagious diseases, isolation of lepers, disinfection of dwellings after illness, sanitation of campsites, disposal of excreta and refuse, protection of water and food supplies, and specific hygiene rules for menstruating women and women who had recently delivered a child.

The history of health and health care in the Greek culture (1000–400 B.C.E.) is intriguing as well as relevant to modern healthcare philosophy. The Greeks were perhaps the first people to put as much emphasis on disease prevention as they did on the treatment of disease conditions. Balance among the physical, mental, and spiritual aspects of the person was emphasized. Among the early Greeks, religion played an important role in health care. However, the role of the physician began to take on a more defined shape, and a more scientific view of medicine emerged.

In the early stages of Greek culture, as represented in the *Iliad* and the *Odyssey*, the priesthood played a role in the healing arts. In the *Iliad*, **Asclepius** was a Thessalian chief

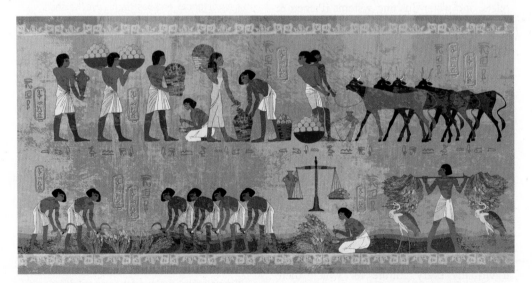

Figure 2.2 The Egyptians were known for their cleanliness and were considered the healthiest people of the time.

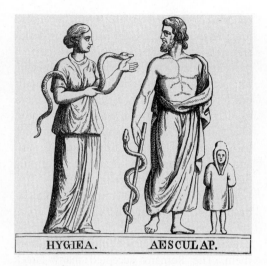

HYGIEA.   AESCULAP.

Figure 2.3 Asclepius and Hygeia.

© ZU_09/DigitalVision Vectors/Getty Images.

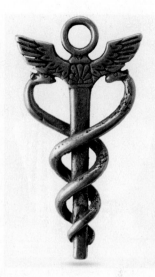

Figure 2.4 Illustration of a caduceus, a symbol that shows two snakes braided around a staff. It is representative of the medical profession and has its earliest association with Asclepius, the Greek healer.

© Oleg Krugliak/Shutterstock.

who had received instruction in the use of drugs. By the beginning of the eighth century B.C.E., tradition had enshrined him as the god of medicine. He had two daughters who also had health-related powers. **Hygeia** was given the power to prevent disease, whereas **Panacea** was given the ability to treat disease. Hygeia was the more prominent figure and was often pictured with her father in sculptures and illustrations of the time (Schouten, 1967) (see **Figure 2.3**). The words *hygiene* and *panacea* can be traced back to these daughters of Asclepius (Libby, 1922).

Eventually, hundreds of elaborate temples were built throughout Greece to worship Asclepius. These temples were typically on beautiful sites overlooking the sea or beside healing fountains. The temple priests practiced their healing arts, which often involved fraud. The temple priests should not be confused with the **Asclepiads**. The Asclepiads were a brotherhood of men present at the temples who initially claimed descent from Asclepius. Although some of the Asclepiads probably helped the priests with their trickery, others broke away from the priests and began to practice medicine based on more rational principles. These ancient temples of Asclepius

left their symbol as a permanent reminder of the past—the staff and serpent of the physician, known as the **caduceus** (Rubinson & Alles, 1984) (see **Figure 2.4**).

The famous Greek physician **Hippocrates** came from the Asclepian tradition. He lived from about 460 B.C.E. until 377 B.C.E. (See **Figure 2.5**.) Hippocrates developed a theory of disease causation consistent with the philosophy of nature held by leading philosophers of his day. Hippocrates taught that health was the result of balance, and disease was the result of an imbalance. To the Greeks, the ideal person was perfectly balanced in mind, body, and spirit. Thus, study and practice related to philosophy, athletics, and theology were all important to maintain balance. To do this, however, took a tremendous commitment of time and energy. Each day required physical activity, study, and philosophical discussion while maintaining proper nutrition and rest. Few people could afford to lead such a life. Those who did were the

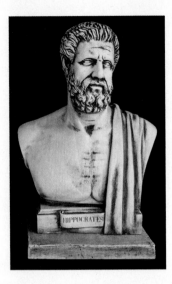

Figure 2.5 Hippocrates, 460–375 B.C.E., "Father of Western Medicine".

© Repina Valeriya/Shutterstock.

aristocratic upper class leading a life of leisure supported by a slave economy (Rosen, 1958). The ideal Greek human being that is so often mentioned was, in fact, a small percentage of the Greek population.

Hippocrates holds an important place in the history of medicine. His theory of health and disease was still being taught in medical schools as a valid theory of disease causation as recently as the first quarter of the 20th century. Hippocrates, however, did more than just theorize about disease. He carefully observed and recorded associations between certain diseases and such factors as geography, climate, diet, and living conditions. Duncan (1988) noted, "One of his [Hippocrates's] most noteworthy contributions is the distinction between 'endemic' diseases, which vary in prevalence from place to place, and 'epidemic' diseases, which vary in prevalence over time" (p. 12). The traditional Hippocratic Oath is still used today and is the basis for medical ethics. Hippocrates and the Asclepiads moved health care away from religion and priests and attempted to establish a more rational basis to explain health and disease. Hippocrates's

concept of balance in life is still promoted today as the best means for maintaining health and well-being.

Hippocrates has been credited with being the first epidemiologist and the father of modern medicine (Duncan, 1988). It is not hard to imagine that he was also a health educator. One can easily see Hippocrates educating his friends and patients about diet, exercise, rest, and the importance of balance in preventing disease and promoting health.

The Romans conquered the Mediterranean world, including the Greeks. In doing so, however, the Romans did not destroy the cultures they conquered but learned from them. The Romans accepted many Greek ideas, including those related to health and medicine. As medical practitioners, the Romans copied much of what they had learned from the Greeks. Where the Romans really excelled was in engineering and administration. They developed water transport systems to move large quantities of fresh safe water to population centers and sewage systems to remove waste. These were major public health advancements (Rosen, 1958). (See **Figure 2.6**.)

The Roman Empire (500 B.C.E.–C.E. 500) built an extensive and efficient aqueduct system. Evidence of some 200 Roman aqueducts remains today, from Spain to Syria and from Northern Europe to North Africa (McKenzie & Pinger, 2015). The total capacity of the 13 aqueducts delivering water to the city of Rome has been estimated at 222 million gallons every 24 hours. At the height of the empire, this would have been enough to provide each citizen of Rome with at least 40 gallons of fresh water per day. Additionally, attention was paid to water purity. At specific points along the aqueduct, generally near the middle and end, settling basins were located, in which sediment might be deposited (Rosen, 1958).

The Romans also developed an extensive system of underground sewers. These served to carry off both surface water and sewage. The main sewer in Rome that emptied into the

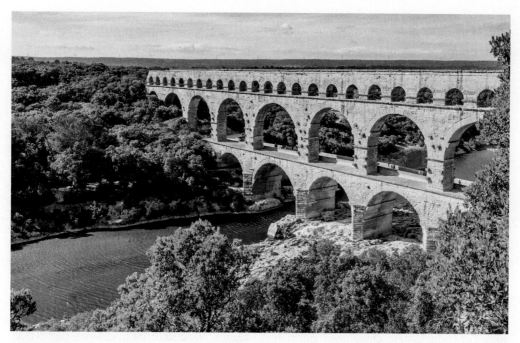

Figure 2.6 Roman aqueducts.
© kavram/Shutterstock.

Tiber River was 10 feet wide and 12 feet high; it was still part of the Roman sewer system during the 20th century.

The Romans made other health advancements. They observed the effect of occupational hazards on health, and they were the first to build hospitals. By the second century C.E., a public medical service was set up whereby physicians were appointed to various towns and institutions. A system of private medical practice also developed during the Roman era (Rosen, 1958).

The Romans furthered the work of the Greeks in the study of human anatomy and the practice of surgery. Some Roman anatomists even dissected living human beings to further their knowledge of anatomy (Libby, 1922). In quoting the Latin writer Cornelius, Libby noted that these anatomists "procured criminals out of prison, by royal permission, and dissecting them alive, contemplated, while they were still breathing, the parts which nature had before concealed, considering their position, color, figure, size, order, hardness, softness, smoothness, and asperity" (Libby, 1922, p. 54). Although some opposed this hideous practice, others supported it, holding "it is by no means cruel as most people represent it, by the tortures of a few guilty, to search after remedies for the whole innocent race of mankind in all ages" (Libby, 1922, p. 54).

Middle Ages

The era from the collapse of the Roman Empire to about 1500 C.E. is known as the Middle Ages or Dark Ages. This was a time of political and social unrest, when many health advancements of previous cultures were lost. Rosen (1958) notes that, "the problem that confronted the medieval world was to weld together the culture of the barbarian invaders with the classical heritage of the defunct [Roman] Empire and with the beliefs and teachings of the Christian religion" (p. 52). This proved to be no easy task.

With the Roman Empire no longer able to protect settlements, each city had to defend itself against its enemies. For safety, people lived within city walls along with their domesticated animals. As the population grew, expansion was difficult and overcrowding was common (Rosen, 1958). Lack of fresh water and sewage removal were major problems for many medieval cities; Roman public health advancements were lost.

To make matters worse, there was little emphasis on cleanliness or hygiene. The new religion, Christianity, found its disciples among the lower classes, where personal hygiene was not practiced, and as a consequence, an entirely different attitude toward the human body developed. Excessive care of the body, that is, man's earthly and mutable part, was unimportant in the Christian dualistic concept, which separated body from soul. For some Eastern churchmen and holy men, living in filth was regarded as evidence of sanctity: cleanliness was thought to betoken pride, and filthiness humility. (Goerke & Stebbins, 1968, p. 9)

Fortunately, as Christianity matured so did its concept of the human body. Eventually, Christians came to believe that the body is the soul's earthly dwelling; thus, permitting better care of it.

Early Christians also reinforced the notion that disease was caused by sin or disobeying God. This propelled priests and religious leaders back into the position of preventing and treating disease. The health-related advancements of the Greco-Roman era were abandoned and shunned. Entire libraries were burned, and knowledge about the human body was seen as sinful.

The Middle Ages were characterized by great epidemics. Perhaps the cruelest of these was leprosy, a disease characterized by severe facial and extremity disfigurement. A highly contagious and virulent disease, all Western countries issued edicts against anyone suspected of having leprosy and regulated every aspect of the sufferer's life. In some

communities, lepers were given the last rites of the church, forced to leave the city, made to wear identifying clothing, and required to carry a rod identifying them as lepers. Other lepers were forced to wear a bell around their necks and to ring it as a warning when other people came near. Such isolation usually brought about a relatively quick death resulting from hunger and exposure (Goerke & Stebbins, 1968). Eventually, leprosy hospitals were founded to treat the inflicted. It has been estimated that by 1200 C.E., there were 1,900 leper houses and leprosaria in Europe (Rosen, 1958).

The bubonic plague, known as the Black Death, may have been the most severe epidemic the world has ever known. The death toll was higher and the disruption of society greater than from any war, famine, or natural disaster in history. "At Constantinople, the plague raged with such violence that 5,000, and even 10,000 persons are said to have died in a single day" (Donan, 1898, p. 94). Estimates of casualties vary from 20 to 35 million, with Europe losing one quarter to one third of its entire population. In Avignon, France, 60,000 people died. As a result, the pope was forced to consecrate the Rhone River so that bodies might be thrown into it, because the churchyards were filled (Goerke & Stebbins, 1968).

Imagine what it must have been like to live through the plague. Literally one out of every three or four people you knew contracted the disease and died. The cause of the disease was unknown, creating widespread fear and superstition. Often, religious leaders and doctors were some of the first victims. They were exposed to the disease early in the epidemic through their contact with infected sufferers. This left many communities with no religious or medical leadership.

People reacted to the plague in different ways. Some became extremely pious, turned away from earthly pleasures, and practiced extreme self-denial in hopes of pleasing God. Others took the opposite approach, lost faith in God, and disregarded legal, moral, and sexual restraints (Goerke & Stebbins, 1968). The Brotherhood of the Flagellants was a group of religious zealots who believed the plague could be avoided by admitting to their sins and then ritualistically beating themselves in atonement. Today, such a group would most likely be labeled a religious cult. Members of this group marched in long, two-column lines from city to city. In each city, they would chant a litany and conduct their ritualistic ceremony. At a signal from the group's master, the Flagellants would strip to the waist and march in a circle until they received another signal from the master. Upon receiving the second signal, they would throw themselves to the ground with their body position indicating the specific sin they had committed. The master would move among the bodies, thrashing those who had committed certain sins or had offended the discipline of the Flagellants in some way. This would be followed by a collective flagellation in which the group members would rhythmically beat their own backs and breasts with a heavy scourge made of three or four leather thongs tipped with metal studs. According to eyewitness accounts, the Flagellants lashed themselves until their bodies became swollen and blue, and blood dripped to the ground. Further complicating the health consequences of such punishment was a rule prohibiting bathing, washing, or changing clothes. When joining the Brotherhood, group members had to pledge to scourge themselves three times daily for 33 days and eight hours, which represented one day for each year of Christ's earthly life (Ziegler, 1969). In other words, to complete the Flagellant pledge, one would have to undergo the ritualistic beating 100 times.

Debate existed during the Middle Ages concerning the cause of the plague. In 1348, Jehan Jacme wrote that the disease was caused by five factors: (1) the wrath of God, (2) the corruption of dead bodies, (3) waters and vapors formed in the interior of the earth, (4) unnatural hot and humid winds, and (5) the conjunction of stars and planets (Winslow, 1944).

Another story concerning the origins of the disease had Italian merchants trapped in a city on the Black Sea that was under siege by a local Mongol prince. The prince was forced to call off the siege because large numbers of his army were dying of a strange disease. Before leaving, the prince ordered his army to catapult the dead, diseased bodies into the city. Within days, the people inside the city began to die. Afraid, the Italian merchants set sail for Italy, but not before infected rats had boarded the ship. Soon many of the sailors became sick. The ship tried to dock in several cities but was denied permission because of the illness. Finally, permission was granted to dock in Sicily where the rats came on shore and the plague began (De'ath, 1995).

Despite the disagreement that existed on the cause of the disease, contemporaries believed that the disease was contagious. In other words, it was passed from person to person in some unknown way. Although this concept of contagion had been around for many years and was discussed in the Bible, it was not until the Middle Ages and the epidemics of leprosy and bubonic plague that it started to become more universally accepted. The contagion concept opened the door to new interest in science and severely weakened the argument of those promoting the sin-disease theory.

The Middle Ages also saw epidemics of other communicable diseases, including smallpox, diphtheria, measles, influenza, tuberculosis, anthrax, and trachoma. The last major epidemic disease of this period was syphilis, which appeared in 1492. As with other epidemics, syphilis killed thousands of people (McKenzie et al., 2018).

Although there were no professional health education specialists during the Middle Ages, education about health continued to exist. Priests, medical doctors, and community leaders attempted to "educate" anyone who would listen to their ideas about health and disease prevention. Given the rudimentary level of health knowledge and the lack of consensus on prevention and causation of disease, a professional health education specialist would probably have contributed little to the general population's health in the Middle Ages.

Renaissance

The Renaissance, which means "rebirth," lasted roughly from 1500 c.e. to 1700 c.e. This time period was characterized by a gradual change in thinking. People began to view the world and humankind in a more naturalistic and holistic fashion. Although progress was slow, science again emerged as a legitimate field of inquiry, and numerous scientific advancements were made. The world did not change overnight from the superstitious and backward beliefs of the Dark Ages to a completely enlightened society in the Renaissance. Disease and plague still ravaged Europe and overall medical care was still rudimentary. Bloodletting was a major form of treatment for everything from the common cold to tuberculosis. Popular remedies included crabs' eyes, foxes' lungs, oil of anise, oil of spiders, and oil of earthworms. A major means of diagnosing a patient's condition consisted of examining the urine for changes in color. The inspection of a patient's urine by a true physician was known as "water casting." For many years, this was the principal diagnostic procedure utilized by the medical profession.

Much surgery and dentistry was performed by barbers because they had the best chairs and sharpest instruments available. Some barbers dispensed health information, as can be seen in the following example from a Danish barber-surgeon: "It is very good for persons to drink themselves intoxicated once a month for the excellent reasons that it frees their strength, furthers sound sleep, eases the passing of water, increases perspiration, and stimulates general well-being" (Durant, 1961, pp. 495–496). Unfortunately, few were probably moderate enough to restrict their binges to once a month.

Rosen (1958) notes that although the Renaissance "is characterized by the rapid growth and spread of science in various fields public health as a practiced activity received very little, if any, direct benefit from these advances" (p. 84). Evidence of the poor public health conditions can be seen in this note describing the average English household floor of the 16th century:

> As to floors, they are usually made with clay, covered with rushes that grow in the fens and which are so seldom removed that the lower part remains sometimes for twenty years and has in it a collection of spittle, vomit, urine of dogs and humans, beer, scraps of fish and other filthiness not to be named (Pickett & Hanlon, 1990, p. 25).

Although living conditions among the English royalty were certainly better than for those of the laboring class, health-related problems were still prevalent. Disposal of human waste was a major problem. Those who lived in old castles located their latrines in large projections on the face of walls. The excrement was discharged from these projections into deep-walled pits, moats, or streams near the walls of the castle. Those less fortunate used chamber pots and simply tossed their contents out the nearest window. Even among royalty, basic hygiene left much to be desired. Few monarchs bathed more frequently than once a week. Much of the material used in royal apparel, such as silk, velvet, and ermine, could not be washed; thus, it simply accumulated dirt and perspiration. Cloaking scents were used to try to renew the clothing, but they were not effective (Hansen, 1980).

On the positive side, the Renaissance was a period of exploration and expanded trade.

The search for knowledge, characteristic of the Greek and Roman eras, was revitalized. Superstitions of the Middle Ages were slowly replaced with a more systematic inquiry into cause and effect. In the middle of the 15th century, learning gained momentum as a result of Johannes Gutenberg's invention of the printing press with moveable type. This allowed the great classical works of Hippocrates and Galen to be reproduced and distributed to larger audiences (Gordon, 1959).

There were also scientific advancements during the Renaissance. The human body was again considered appropriate for study, and realistic anatomical drawings were produced. John Hunter, the father of modern surgery, undertook a more orderly exploration of the workings of the human body. Antonie van Leeuwenhoek discovered the microscope and proved there were life forms too small for the human eye to see. These life forms, however, were not yet associated with disease. John Graunt forwarded the fields of statistics and epidemiology. Through studying the *Bills of Mortality*, published weekly in London, Graunt found that more males than females were born, higher death rates during the first years of life than later in life, and higher death rates among urban dwellers than rural dwellers (Goerke & Stebbins, 1968).

In Italy, many cities had instituted health boards to fight the plague. It did not take long, however, for their responsibilities to be expanded. By the middle of the 16th century, numerous matters had fallen under the control and jurisdiction of these health boards. These included "the marketing of meat, fish, shellfish, game, fruit, grain, sausages, oil, wine and water; the sewage system; the activity of the hospitals; beggars and prostitutes; burials, cemeteries, and pesthouses; the professional activity of physicians, surgeons and apothecaries; the preparation and sale of drugs; the activity of hostelries and the Jewish community" (Cipolla, 1976, p. 32).

Age of Enlightenment

The 1700s were a period of revolution, industrialization, and growth of cities. Both the French and American Revolutions took place during this century. Plague and other epidemics continued to be a problem. Science had not yet discovered that these diseases were produced by microscopic organisms. The general belief was that disease was formed in filth and that epidemics were caused by some type of poison that developed in the putrefaction process. The vapors, or "miasmas," rising from this rotting refuse could travel through the air for great distances and were believed to result in disease when inhaled. This concept, known as the **miasmas theory**, remained popular throughout much of the 19th century. As preventive measures, herbs and incense were often used to perfume the air, supposedly filling the nose and crowding out any miasmas (Duncan, 1988). It was still not known that contaminated water could cause disease infection.

Scientific advancements continued throughout the period. Dr. James Lind, a Royal Navy surgeon, discovered that scurvy could be controlled on long sea voyages by having sailors consume lime juice. To this day, British sailors are known as "limeys." Edward Jenner discovered a vaccine procedure against smallpox. Bernardino Ramazzini wrote on trade and industrial diseases. Theorists of the time conceived of the mind and body not as separate entities, but as dependent on each other. Philosophers of the 18th century, such as Diderot, Locke, Rousseau, and Voltaire, all "promoted the worth of each human life and the importance of individual health for the well-being of society" (Rubinson & Alles, 1984, p. 5).

Although progress was made during this time, health education/promotion in itself still did not emerge as a profession. With the rudimentary state of medical knowledge in the 16th, 17th, and 18th centuries, there would have been little for a health education specialist to do other than promote the misconceptions and half-truths that predominated during the time period. However, health boards, the forerunner of today's health departments, did develop as scientific and medical knowledge increased. The roots of modern health education/promotion were planted, and the first sprouts would soon emerge.

The 1800s

In the first half of the 1800s, little happened to improve the public's health. In England, the streets of London were filthy with animal and human waste. Overcrowding and industrialization added to the problem. These conditions, under which so many people lived and worked, had dire results. Smallpox, cholera, typhoid, tuberculosis, and many other diseases reached high endemic levels (Pickett & Hanlon, 1990).

In 1842, a momentous event occurred in the history of public health when Edwin Chadwick published his *Report on an Inquiry into the Sanitary Conditions of the Labouring Population of Great Britain*. In the report, he documented the deplorable living conditions of Britain's laboring class, made a strong case that these conditions were the cause of much disease and suffering, and called for government intervention. This report eventually led to the formation of a General Board of Health for England in 1848 (Goerke & Stebbins, 1968).

Extraordinary advancements in biology and bacteriology took place by the middle of the 19th century in England and throughout Europe. In 1849, Dr. John Snow, who laboriously studied epidemiological data related to a cholera epidemic in London, hypothesized that the disease was caused by microorganisms in the drinking water from one particular water pump located on Broad Street (see **Figure 2.7**). He removed the pump's handle to keep people from using the water source, and the epidemic abated. Snow's action was remarkable because it predated the discovery that microorganisms cause disease and was in opposition to the prevailing miasmas theory of the time (Johnson, 2006).

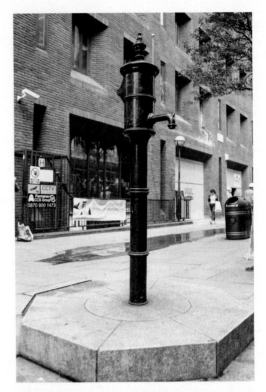

Figure 2.7 By removing the handle of this pump, which is still in place on Broad Street in London, John Snow interrupted a cholera pandemic.

© Nathaniel Noir/Alamy Stock Photo.

In 1862, Louis Pasteur of France proposed his germ theory of disease. After this, advancements in bacteriology greatly accelerated. Over the next 20 years, Pasteur discovered how microorganisms reproduce, introduced the first scientific approach to immunization, and developed a technique to pasteurize milk. Robert Koch, a German scientist, developed the criteria and procedures necessary to establish that a particular microbe, and no other, caused a particular disease. Joseph Lister, an English surgeon, developed the antiseptic method of treating wounds by using carbolic acid, and he introduced the principle of asepsis to surgery. These are just a few of the tremendous advancements in bacteriology made during the second half of the 19th century. As a result, the years from 1875 to 1900 became known as the **bacteriological period of public health** (McKenzie et al., 2018).

Public Health in the United States

1700s

During the 1700s, health conditions in the United States were similar to those in Europe—deplorable. Diseases such as smallpox, cholera, and diphtheria were prevalent. Because of the slave trade, diseases such as yaws, yellow fever, and malaria were common in southern states (Marr, 1982). Large numbers of immigrants were entering the ports, cities were growing, overcrowding was common, and the Industrial Revolution was about to begin.

The primary means of controlling disease were quarantine and regulations on environmental cleanliness. For example, as early as 1647, the Massachusetts Bay Colony enacted regulations to prevent pollution of Boston Harbor. In 1701, Massachusetts passed laws allowing for the isolation of smallpox patients and for ship quarantine, as needed. However, there was no overseeing body or agency to enforce compliance.

In an attempt to address health problems, some cities formed local health boards (Pickett & Hanlon, 1990). Prominent citizens who advised elected officials on health-related matters made up these boards. They had no paid staff, no budget, and no authority to enforce regulations. According to tradition, the first health board was formed in Boston in 1799, with Paul Revere as chairman. This is contested, however, by other cities claiming earlier health boards, including Petersburg, Virginia (1780), Baltimore (1793), Philadelphia (1794), and New York (1796).

Life expectancy is one measure of health status for a given population. It is defined as "the average number of years a person from a specific cohort is projected to live from a given point in time" (McKenzie & Pinger, p. 608). The first life expectancy tables were developed for the United States in 1789 by Dr. Edward Wigglesworth (Ravenel, 1970). **Table 2.1** shows Wigglesworth's table. It provides strong evidence of the prevailing health conditions. In 1789, life expectancy at birth was only 28.15 years. By 2020, the projected life expectancy at birth in the United States was 79.5 years (U.S. National Center for Health Statistics, 2009).

1800s

From 1800 to 1850, health status improved little. Conditions of overcrowding, poverty, and filth worsened as the Industrial Revolution encouraged more and more people to move to the cities. Epidemics of smallpox, yellow fever, cholera, typhoid, and typhus were

Table 2.1 Expectation of Life According to Wigglesworth Life Table—1789

Current Age	Expected Remaining Years of Life	Current Age	Expected Remaining Years of Life
At birth	28.15	At Age 50	21.16
At Age 5	40.87	At age 55	18.35
At age 10	39.23	At age 60	15.43
At age 15	36.16	At age 65	12.43
At age 20	34.21	At age 70	10.06
At age 25	32.32	At age 75	7.83
At age 30	30.24	At age 80	5.85
At age 35	28.22	At age 85	4.73
At age 40	26.04	At age 90	3.37
At age 45	23/92	At age 95	1.62

Reproduced from Ravenel, M. P. (1921). *A half century of public health.* American Public Health Association.

common. Tuberculosis and malaria reached exceptionally high levels. For example, in 1850, the Massachusetts tuberculosis death rate was 300 per 100,000 population, and the infant mortality was about 200 per 1,000 live births. Conditions were so bad that life expectancy actually decreased in some cities during this period of time. In Boston, the average age at death dropped from 27.85 years in 1820–1825 to 21.43 in 1840–1845. In New York during the same period, the average age of death decreased from 26.15 to 19.69 (Shattuck, 1850).

Public health reform in the United States was slow to begin. Interestingly, a major report helped jump-start the public health reform movement in the United States, just as Chadwick's landmark 1842 report stimulated public health reform in Britain. Lemuel Shattuck's 1850 *Report of the Sanitary Commission of Massachusetts* contained remarkable insights about the public health issues of Massachusetts, including how to approach and solve these problems. Shattuck was a bookseller and publisher from Boston. He retired early at age 46 and dedicated the remainder of his life to his interest in community affairs (American Public Health Association [APHA], 1959). His report is remarkable because no national or state public health programs existed at the time, and local health agencies that did exist were functioning at a minimal level. Shattuck visualized how to improve the public's health through the initiation of state and local level health departments. "Shattuck made 50 recommendations in his report to improve public health practice." Of those 50 recommendations, 36 are still accepted principles of public health practice today (Goerke & Stebbins, 1968). Among his many recommendations were the keeping of vital statistics, environmental sanitation, control of food and drugs, teaching prevention and sanitary science in medical schools, smoke control in cities, control of alcoholism, the supervision of mental disease, exposure of nostrums, preaching health from pulpits, routine

physical exams, and the establishment of nurse training schools (APHA, 1959; Pickett & Hanlon, 1990).

The publication of Shattuck's report did not mean an end to the public health problems in the United States. In fact, the report went largely unnoticed for 19 years until 1869, when the Commonwealth of Massachusetts established a state board of health made up of physicians and laymen exactly as Shattuck had envisioned. One year later, Virginia and California formed their own state boards of health (Ravenel, 1970). By 1900, 38 states had established state boards of health. Today, every U.S. state has a state board or department of health.

Despite the formation of state boards of health, these state-level agencies could not meet health needs on a more local level. With limited resources, there was simply too much to accomplish. As a result, the first full-time county health departments were formed in Guilford County, North Carolina, and Yakima County, Washington, in 1911. Some sources have cited Jefferson County, Kentucky, as the first county health department, set up in 1908 (Pickett & Hanlon, 1990).

As states initiated boards of health, board members had to interact, communicate, and develop their skills. These needs led to the founding of the American Public Health Association (APHA). (See Chapter 8 for more APHA information.) Following a series of national conventions on quarantine held from 1857 through 1860, "Stephen Smith invited a group of 'refined gentlemen' to discuss informally the possibility of a national sanitary association" (Bernstein, 1972, p. 2). Smith's suggestion of an association for health officials and interested citizens was well received. A decision was made to establish a committee to work on a permanent organization. One year later, in 1873, the first annual meeting was held in Cincinnati, Ohio, and 70 new members were elected. Smith remained active in the association throughout his life. At the age of 99, he walked

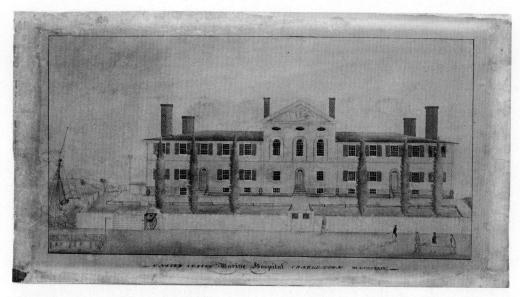

Figure 2.8 Old Marine Hospital in Charleston, South Carolina, 1934.
Courtesy of the U.S. Naval Academy Museum, Annapolis, Maryland.

to the podium unassisted to speak at the 50th anniversary celebration of the APHA.

The federal government started a public health service that dates back to 1798, when Congress passed the Marine Hospital Service Act. Previously, sailors in the merchant marine had nowhere to turn for health care. Because they paid no local or state taxes, ill or injured sailors generally were not welcomed in port cities. The Marine Hospital Service Act required the owners of every ship to pay the tax collector 20 cents per month for every seaman they employed. This money was used to build hospitals and provide medical services in all major seaport cities (see **Figure 2.8**). This act created the first prepaid hospital and medical insurance system. Eventually the plan came under the administrative control of a national public health agency (Pickett & Hanlon, 1990).

Successive legislation throughout the 19th century gradually expanded the scope of the Marine Hospital Service. In 1902, Congress retitled it the Public Health and Marine Hospital Service and gave it a definite organizational structure under the direction of the surgeon general. In 1912, "Marine Hospital" was dropped from the name, and the service became known as it is today, the U.S. Public Health Service. "The mission of the U.S. Public Health Service Commissioned Corps is to protect, promote, and advance the health and safety of our Nation" (U.S. Public Health Service, 2020). The Commissioned Corps comprises over 6,100 health professionals who proudly wear the uniform of the U.S. Public Health Service (see **Figure 2.9**). These professionals serve in 800 locations within the United States and abroad.

In 1879, Congress created the National Board of Health. The board was composed of seven members appointed by the president, including representatives of the army, navy, Marine Hospital Service, and Justice Department. Its functions were to obtain information on all matters related to public health and provide grants-in-aid to state boards of health. The National Board also provided money to university scientists for health-related research. Unfortunately, the board

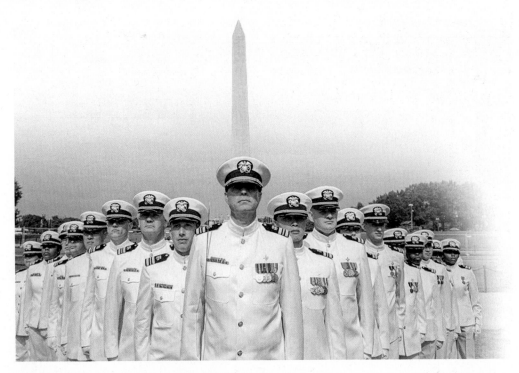

Figure 2.9 Uniform of the U.S. Public Health Service.

Courtesy of U.S. Department of Health and Human Services.

was short-lived. In administering quarantine functions, the board incurred opposition from state agencies and private shipping concerns. Others in positions of power were not in favor of the research grant program and felt such expenditures were extravagant. Thus, in 1882, the board's appropriations were transferred to the Marine Hospital Service, which carried on with the quarantine functions but discontinued the grant program (U.S. Department of Health, Education, and Welfare [USDHEW], 1976).

1900 to Present

The period from 1900 to 1920 is known as the **reform phase of public health** (McKenzie, Pinger & Seabert 2018). During this time, urban areas expanded, and many people lived and worked in deplorable conditions. To address these concerns, federal regulations were passed concerning the food

industry, states passed workers' compensation laws, the U.S. Bureau of Mines and the U.S. Department of Labor were created, and the first clinic for occupational diseases was established. By the end of the 1920s, the movement for healthier workplace conditions was well established, and the average life expectancy had risen to 59.7 years.

Also during this period, the first national voluntary health agencies were formed. They were run primarily by volunteers along with a few paid staff. Each of these agencies was designed to address a specific health problem. For example, the National Association for the Study and Prevention of Tuberculosis was established in 1902, and the American Cancer Society was founded in 1913. Today, volunteer agencies continue to be important players in the prevention of disease and the promotion of health (McKenzie, Pinger & Seabert 2018). They often hire health education specialists.

The 1920s were a relatively quiet period in public health. Progress continued, but at a slower pace. However, the Public Health Education Section of the APHA was founded in 1922 (Bernstein, 1972). This is the APHA section to which most health education specialists belong. Its mission is, "To be a strong advocate for health education and health promotion for individuals, groups and communities, and systems and support efforts to achieve health equity in all activities of the Association" (APHA, 2020).

The need for health education/promotion existed in the early 20th century as many questionable and fraudulent health practices were being promoted. Moore's book about public health in the United States (1923) included two chapters on questionable and unreliable health activities. One of the most interesting examples involved a cure-all product known as Tanlac. The May 11, 1917, edition of the *Holyoke Daily Transcript* contained Fred Wicks' testimonial in a Tanlac advertisement, as well as his obituary (Moore, 1923, pp. 173–174).

Other examples of questionable health practices also abound. William Harvey Kellogg and his younger brother W. K., founders of the Kellogg cereal company, were best known in the early 1900s for the sanitarium they established and operated in Battle Creek, Michigan. The rich and famous came from all over the world to be treated at the sanitarium. Many of the treatment modalities, however, would be considered questionable and even quackery by today's standards. For example, they used some 200 different types of hydrotherapy along with therapeutic enemas, electric horses, vibrators, and cold air (Butler, Thornton, & Stoltz, 1994). However, the sanitarium did promote exercise and good nutrition as ways to prevent and treat disease. (See **Figure 2.10**.) The concept of prevention was again gaining prominence.

Tension between preventive medicine and curative medicine began to appear in the United States during the early 20th century.

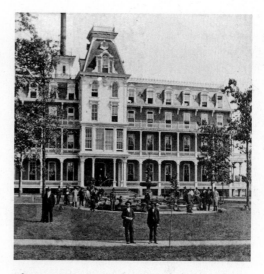

Figure 2.10 Kellogg Sanitarium in Battle Creek, Michigan.

Reproduced from Butler, M., Thornton, F., & Stoltz, D. (1994). *The Battle Creek idea.* Heritage Publications.

Moore (1923) related a story about a town in which public health work had banished malaria. A physician was asked how his profession had been affected by this public health advancement. He replied off-handedly, "If it hadn't been for the influenza, I'd have gone broke. That saved us" (p. 373).

In a more rational manner, Newsholme (1936) noted three reasons why treatment formed a larger part of public health efforts than prevention and why it would continue to do so in the future. First, the knowledge to prevent disease and death was only partial. Medical workers simply did not have the knowledge and skills to prevent many disease states. Second, even when knowledge to prevent disease did exist, many people did not know about it, and those who did know found it difficult to make those changes necessary to prevent disease. Third, there were such a large number of sick people needing prompt medical treatment that it was difficult to focus attention on prevention. Many of the same arguments are used today to account for the emphasis on traditional medical interventions instead of prevention.

From 1930 through World War II, the role of the federal government in social programs expanded. Prior to the Great Depression, medical services were self-funded or funded by relatives and friends, as well as by religious organizations and some voluntary agencies. During the Depression; however, private resources could not meet the demands of those requiring assistance. In 1933, President Franklin D. Roosevelt created numerous agencies and programs as part of his New Deal, which improved the plight of the disadvantaged. Much of the money was used for public health efforts, including the control of malaria, the building of hospitals, and the construction of municipal water and sewage systems.

The Social Security Act of 1935 was a real milestone and the beginning of the federal government's involvement in social issues, including health. The act provided support for state health departments and their programs.

Funding was made available to develop sanitary facilities and to improve maternal and child health.

Two major public health agencies were formed at this time. On May 26, 1930, the Ransdell Act converted the Hygienic Laboratory to the National Institute of Health, with a broad mandate to learn the cause, prevention, and cure of disease (USDHEW, 1976). The National Institutes of Health, as it is called today, is now one of the premiere—if not *the* premiere—medical research facilities in the world. In 1946, the Communicable Disease Center was established in Atlanta, Georgia. Now called the Centers for Disease Control and Prevention (CDC), it is one of the world's leading epidemiological centers. (See **Figure 2.11**.) The CDC is also a major training facility for health communications and educational methods (Pickett & Hanlon, 1990). The

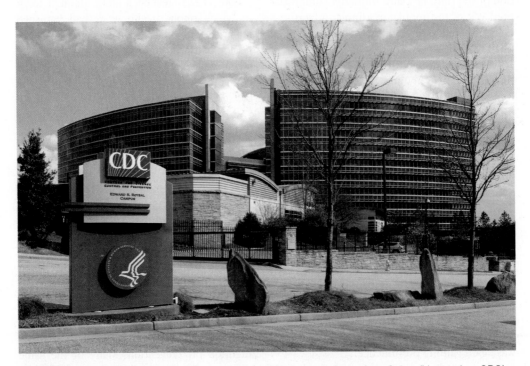

Figure 2.11 CDC's "Arlen Specter Headquarters and Emergency Operations Center" located on CDC's Roybal Campus in Atlanta, Georgia.

© Katherine Welles/Shutterstock.

CDC's mission is "to protect America from health, safety and security threats, both foreign and in the U.S." (CDC, n.d.-c)

Following World War II, concern rose over the number of healthcare facilities and the adequacy of the care they provided. In 1946, Congress passed the National Hospital Survey and Construction Act, also known as the Hill-Burton Act, to improve the distribution and enhance the quality of hospitals. From the passage of the Hill-Burton Act through the 1960s, new hospital construction occurred rapidly. Little thought, however, was given to planning. As a result, hospitals were built too close together and provided overlapping and unnecessary services (McKenzie, Pinger & Seabert 2018).

In 1954, Dr. Mayhew Derryberry, the first chief of health education in the federal government, noted, "The health problems of greatest significance today are the chronic diseases.... The extent of chronic diseases, various disabling conditions, and the economic burden that they impose have been thoroughly documented" (*Voices From the Past,* 2004, p. 368). Before the 1950s, the major emphasis of public health had been on communicable or contagious diseases. However, through improved public health services, medical care, and immunization programs, many contagious diseases no longer threatened as they once had, and the focus shifted ever so slowly to the prevention of chronic diseases. Derryberry predicted how this change of focus would impact health education: "Health education and health educators will be expected to contribute to the reduction of the negative impact of such major health problems as heart disease, cancer, dental disease, mental illness and other neurological disturbances, obesity, accidents and the adjustments necessary to a productive old age" (*Voices From the Past,* 2004, p. 368). Although the seed may have been planted for health education specialists to play a greater role in the prevention of chronic diseases, it was not until the 1970s that the seed finally sprouted.

In 1965, the federal government again passed major legislation designed to improve the health of the U.S. population. Although major improvements were made in health facilities and the quality of health care, there were still many underserved people. Most of these people were either poor or elderly. In response, Congress passed the Medicare and Medicaid bills as amendments to the Social Security Act of 1935. **Medicare** was created to assist in the payment of medical bills for the elderly, whereas **Medicaid** did the same for the poor. These bills provided medical care for millions of people who could not otherwise have obtained such services.

It was evident by the 1970s that disease prevention held the greatest potential for improving Americans' health and reducing healthcare costs. The first national effort to promote the health of citizens through a more preventive approach took place in Canada. In 1974, the Canadian Ministry of Health and Welfare released a publication titled *A New Perspective on the Health of Canadians* (Lalonde, 1974). This document, often called the *Lalonde Report,* presented epidemiological evidence that supported the importance of lifestyle and environmental factors. It called for numerous national health promotion strategies that encouraged Canadians to be more responsible for their own health. (See Chapter 1 for information on the Health Field Concept associated with this publication.) The Lalonde Report influenced many U.S. health professionals to rethink their assumptions that focused on high-technology, treatment-based medicine. So important was this report that Bates and Winder (1984) likened it to a re-emergence of Hygeia and the beginning of the second public health revolution (p. 24).

Healthy People Initiatives and Public Health Standards

In the United States, the government publication *Healthy People* was the first major recognition of the importance of lifestyle in promoting health and well-being (U.S. Public Health Service, 1979). This publication supported a shift from the traditional medical model toward lifestyle and environmental strategies that emphasized prevention.

In 1980, *Promoting Health/Preventing Disease: Objectives for the Nation* was released. This federal document contained 226 U.S. health objectives for the United States, divided into three areas: preventive services, health protection, and health promotion. These objectives provided the framework for public health efforts during the 1980s. They allowed public health professionals to focus on key areas while providing baseline data for measuring progress (U.S. Department of Health and Human Services [USDHHS], 1980). Although not all of these objectives were met, the planning and evaluation process used to develop them became a valuable way to measure progress in U.S. health and healthcare services. This led to the practice of developing U.S. health objectives each decade from the 1990s through the 2020s.

The Healthy People initiative has evolved into an important strategic planning tool for public health professionals at the federal, state, and local levels. Formal reviews measure the progress of these objectives at mid-course (halfway through the 10-year period) and again at the end of 10 years.

Healthy People 2030, the fifth iteration of the Healthy People public health objectives, was released on August 18, 2020, and includes 355 measurable objectives (CDC, n.d.-a). It will guide U.S. public health practice and health education specialists through the decade of the 2020s. Health education specialists need to be familiar with these objectives and use them in their respective practice settings. The Healthypeople.gov website is user friendly and permits the entire report to be searched and accessed. The vision, mission, foundational principles, and overarching goals of Healthy People 2030 can be seen in **Table 2.2**. (CDC, n.d.-b, d).

For *Healthy People 2030* to be effective, programs must be developed and initiated to meet the established objectives. This means that partner states, counties, communities, organizations, and individuals must get involved. It is important to note that when discussing implementation of the Healthy People 2030 Objectives, the CDC suggests a four-step process that includes the major responsibilities of a health education specialist. The four steps are 1) Identifying the needs and priority populations, 2) set targets, 3) utilize evidence-based resources and tools, and 4) Monitor progress (CDC, n.d.-g). You will learn more about the Responsibilities of a Certified Health Education Specialist (CHES) in Chapter 6 of this text.

To inform and guide public health's working toward the Healthy People 2030 objectives, it is imperative that the "10 Essential Public Health Services" be included in all communities (CDC, n.d.-f) (see **Figure 2.12**). The "10 Essential Public Health Services" was revised in 2020 to include equity at the center of the framework. From a health education perspective, it is important to note that one of the 10 Essential Public Health Services is to "communicate effectively to inform and educate people about health, factors that influence it, and how to improve it." With "communication being one of the eight responsibilities of a health education specialist, this confirms the essential role health education specialists play in public health."

Another important initiative designed, in part, to improve the effectiveness of public health departments working on the Healthy People 2030 objectives is the National Public Health Performance Standards (NPHPS) (CDC, n.d.-e). This is a partnership initiative to develop performance standards; collect, monitor, and analyze data; and ultimately improve public health performance. It is important in that it provides a common, systematic strategy for measuring public health

Table 2.2 *Healthy People 2030* Vision, Mission, Foundational Principles, and Overarching Goals

Overarching Goals	
Vision	A society in which all people can achieve their full potential for health and well-being across the lifespan.
Mission	To promote, strengthen, and evaluate the nation's efforts to improve the health and well-being of all people.
Foundational Principles	The following foundational principles guide decisions about Healthy People 2030: <ul><li>The health and well-being of all people and communities is essential to a thriving, equitable society.</li><li>Promoting health and well-being and preventing disease are linked efforts that encompass physical, mental, and social health dimensions.</li><li>Investing to achieve the full potential for health and well-being for all provides valuable benefits to society.</li><li>Achieving health and well-being requires eliminating health disparities, achieving health equity, and attaining health literacy.</li><li>Healthy physical, social, and economic environments strengthen the potential to achieve health and well-being.</li><li>Promoting and achieving health and well-being nationwide is a shared responsibility that is distributed across the national, state, tribal, and community levels, including the public, private, and not-for-profit sectors.</li><li>Working to attain the full potential for health and well-being of the population is a component of decision making and policy formulation across all sectors.</li></ul>
Overarching Goals	Achieving these broad and ambitious goals requires setting, working toward, and achieving a wide variety of much more specific goals. Healthy People 2030's overarching goals are to: <ul><li>Attain healthy, thriving lives and well-being free of preventable disease, disability, injury, and premature death.</li><li>Eliminate health disparities, achieve health equity, and attain health literacy to improve the health and well-being of all.</li><li>Create social, physical, and economic environments that promote attaining the full potential for health and well-being for all.</li><li>Promote healthy development, healthy behaviors, and well-being across all life stages.</li><li>Engage leadership, key constituents, and the public across multiple sectors to take action and design policies that improve the health and well-being of all.</li></ul>

Reproduced from U.S. Department of Health and Human Services. (n.d.). *Healthy people 2030 framework.* https://health.gov/healthypeople/about/healthy-people-2030-framework

performance. Local and state health departments are encouraged to use these performance standard assessments to conduct their own self-assessments. Through this process, weaknesses can be identified and improvements can be made to enhance the overall performance of public health departments (CDC, n.d.-e).

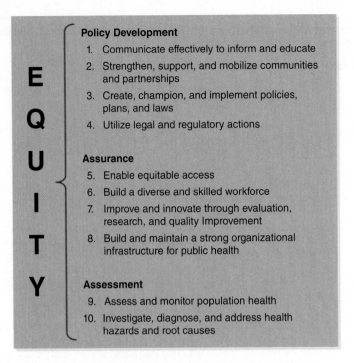

Policy Development

1. Communicate effectively to inform and educate
2. Strengthen, support, and mobilize communities and partnerships
3. Create, champion, and implement policies, plans, and laws
4. Utilize legal and regulatory actions

Assurance

5. Enable equitable access
6. Build a diverse and skilled workforce
7. Improve and innovate through evaluation, research, and quality Improvement
8. Build and maintain a strong organizational infrastructure for public health

Assessment

9. Assess and monitor population health
10. Investigate, diagnose, and address health hazards and root causes

E
Q
U
I
T
Y

Figure 2.12 Ten essential public health services.

Data from Centers for Disease Control and Prevention. (n.d.). *10 Essential Public Health Services*. Retrieved July 1, 2021, from https://www.cdc.gov/publichealthgateway/publichealthservices/essentialhealthservices.html

Health Education/Promotion: A Recognized Profession

One more important historical event for health education/promotion occurred on October 27, 1997, when the Standard Occupational Classification (SOC) Policy Review Committee approved the creation of a new, distinct classification for the occupation of health educator (Auld, 1997/1998). Health educators had pursued this goal for more than 25 years. Health educators were previously included in the category "Instructional Coordinator," a broad, primarily education-related category that failed to consider the many varied and unique responsibilities of health education specialists. Approval of health education as a separate occupational classification means that the Department of Labor's Bureau of Labor Statistics, the Department of Commerce's Bureau of the Census,

and all other federal agencies that collect occupational data now collect data on health education specialists. Many state and local governments also maintain data on health education/promotion. For the first time, it is possible to determine the number of health education specialists employed and the outlook for future health education/promotion positions. This approval is one more sign that health education/promotion is gaining the respect and recognition it deserves.

In summary, tremendous advancements in public health and health education/promotion took place during the 20th century. It could reasonably be argued that the total number of advancements in public health during the 20th century were equal to or greater than the total number of public health advancements in all prior time. In reflecting on these great successes of public health, the

Department of Health and Human Services identified 10 public health achievements they believed had the greatest impact on major causes of morbidity and mortality of the 20th century. **Box 2.2** lists these 10 achievements. Imagine what life would be like today if none of these achievements had been realized. Think of the role health education/promotion has played in these advancements.

Box 2.3 depicts what are considered to be the greatest public health achievements in the United States from 2001–2010. It is interesting that many of the achievements noted in the first decade of the 21st Century mirror or are closely related to the great achievements of the 20th Century. Further advancements in these overlapping areas means that there has been continued advancement and progress. It is especially interesting that development and distribution of vaccinations continues to be a major public health advancement; especially with the emphasis on vaccine development and distribution during the COVID-19 pandemic of 2020.

Box 2.2 **10 Great Public Health Achievements in the United States, 1900–1999**

- Vaccination
- Motor vehicle safety
- Safer workplaces
- Control of infectious diseases
- Decline in deaths from coronary (heart) disease and stroke
- Safer and healthier foods
- Healthier mothers and babies
- Family planning
- Fluoridation of drinking water
- Recognition of tobacco use as a health hazard

Centers for Disease Control and Prevention. (1999). Changes in the public health system. *Morbidity and Mortality Weekly Report, 48*(50), 1141–1147. https://www.cdc.gov/mmwr/preview/mmwrhtml/mm4850a1.htm

---

Box 2.3 **Greatest Public Health Achievements—United States, 2001–2010**

- Vaccine for preventable diseases
- Prevention and control of infectious diseases
- Tobacco control
- Maternal and infant health
- Motor vehicle safety
- Cardiovascular disease prevention
- Occupational safety
- Cancer prevention
- Childhood lead poisoning prevention
- Public health preparedness and response

Centers for Disease Control and Prevention. (2011, May 20). Ten great public health achievements—United States, 2001–2010. *Morbidity and Mortality Weekly Report, 60*(19), 619–623. https://www.cdc.gov/mmwr/preview/mmwrhtml/mm6019a5.htm

School Health in the United States

Life in early America was hard, and there was little time for education. The labor of building homes, clearing forests, tilling fields, hunting, and preparing food filled the days. Most people lived under primitive conditions. Settlements were few and far between. Travel and transportation were costly, slow, and limited to foot, horseback, boat, or wagon.

In the mid-1600s, as communities became more established, the call for education was soon heard. Religion had always been an important part of life in America, and it was the religious leaders who led the drive for education. They believed that Satan benefited when people were illiterate, because they could not read the scriptures. In 1647, Massachusetts passed the "Old Deluder" law to prevent Satan from deluding the people by keeping them from reading the Bible. The law specified that a town with 50 families should establish an elementary school, and a town with 100 households should set up a Latin grammar secondary school (Means, 1962).

The curriculum in these early schools was largely derived from the educational practices in England. Essentially, reading, as the avenue to religious understanding, was the primary subject. Writing, spelling, grammar, and arithmetic supplemented reading. Later, geography and history were added, but the teaching of health was not part of the early education system in the United States.

Because only boys attended these early schools, and working for the family was still a major concern, daily sessions were by necessity of short duration. The length of the school term was usually only a few months. Teachers lacked preparation, with their basic qualifications being only to (1) read, (2) know more of the Bible than the students, (3) work cheap, and (4) keep the students under control. Teachers were totally dependent on the rod for classroom management (Means, 1962). Girls were not sent to school as it was generally felt they could learn everything they needed to know about cleaning, sewing, cooking,

and tending to a home and family from their mothers.

School buildings typically were inadequate (see **Figure 2.13**). They were poorly built, inaccessible, and sometimes temporary structures. Their interiors were inadequately lighted, were furnished with uncomfortable seating, had no sanitary facilities, and were heated with wood-burning stoves. These schools were not even close to meeting modern standards for school construction (Means, 1962).

The schools and their curricula remained much the same until the 1800s. By the mid-1800s, most schools had become tax supported, and attendance was compulsory. Those concerned about public health pointed out the numerous health and safety problems in the schools. These concerns helped bring attention to the conditions of the schools and ultimately paved the way for health instruction in the curriculum (Means, 1962).

Horace Mann, whose writings and speeches promoted the importance of education in general, was perhaps the first

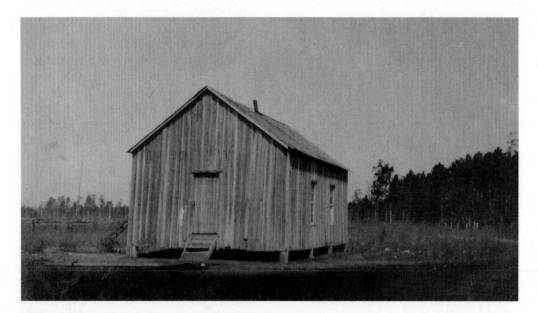

Figure 2.13 An old one-room schoolhouse.

spokesperson for teaching health in schools. He was the elected secretary of the Massachusetts State Board of Education in 1837. Beginning in 1837 with the publication of his *First Annual Report* and continuing through the publication of the *Sixth Annual Report* in 1843, Mann called for mandatory hygiene programs that would help students understand their bodies and the relationship between their behaviors and health (Rubinson & Alles, 1984).

Another momentous event in the development of school health occurred in 1850, when Lemuel Shattuck from Massachusetts wrote his *Report on the Sanitary Commission of Massachusetts* (1850). (This is the same report discussed previously in reference to public health.) Although the report has become a classic in the field of public health, it also provided strong support for school health (Means, 1975). In the report, Shattuck (1850) eloquently supports the teaching of physiology, as the term *health education* had yet to be coined:

> It has recently been recommended that the science of physiology be taught in the public schools; and the recommendation should be universally approved and carried into effect as soon as persons can be found capable of teaching it....Every child should be taught early in life, that to preserve his own life and his own health and the lives and health of others, is one of the most important and constantly abiding duties. By obeying certain laws or performing certain acts, his life and health may be preserved; by disobedience, or performing certain other acts, they will both be destroyed. By knowing and avoiding the causes of disease, disease itself will be avoided, and he may enjoy health and live; by ignorance of these causes and exposure to them, he may contract disease, ruin

his health, and die. Everything connected with wealth, happiness and long life depend upon health; and even the great duties of morals and religion are performed more acceptably in a healthy than a sickly condition. (pp. 178–179)

Aside from local and state attempts to promote the teaching of health-related curricula in the schools, no concerted national effort existed until that of the Women's Christian Temperance Union. Originally founded in 1874, the union expounded on the evils of alcohol, narcotics, and tobacco through every conceivable means and was one of the most effective lobbying organizations ever (Means, 1962). Between 1880 and 1890, every state in the union passed a law requiring instruction concerning the effects of alcohol and narcotics due to stimulus from the Temperance Movement (Turner, Sellery, & Smith, 1957).

Other national movements soon followed. In 1915, the National Tuberculosis Association introduced the "Modern Health Crusade" as a device for promoting the health of school children. It was based on promotion to "knighthood" for those who followed certain health habits. The Child Health Organization of America encouraged the nation to adopt more functional health education/promotion programs. One of its active leaders, Sally Lucas Jean, was ultimately responsible for changing the name from hygiene education to health education (Means, 1962). With this name change, the focus of health education shifted from that of physiology and hygiene, which was factual and unrelated to everyday living, to an emphasis on healthy living and health behavior.

Despite these advancements, health education from 1900 to 1920 was generally characterized by inconsistency and awkward progress. World War I provided the impetus for widespread acceptance of school health education as a discipline in its own right (Turner et al., 1957). Out of 2,510,706 men examined as potential military draftees during World War I, 730,756 (29%) were rejected on physical grounds. A large portion of these physical deficiencies could have been prevented if the schools had been doing their part to train children concerning health and fitness (Andress & Bragg, 1922). In the immediate postwar years, 16 states required hygiene instruction in their public schools; 12 of these states made provisions for the preparation of health teachers in the teacher training schools supported by the state (Rogers, 1936).

Significant research and demonstration projects related to school health education were conducted in the 1920s and 1930s. Examples include the Malden, Massachusetts, project, done in cooperation with the Massachusetts Institute of Technology; the Mansfield, Ohio, project supported by the American Red Cross; the Fargo, North Dakota, project sponsored by the Commonwealth Fund; and the Cattaraugus County, New York, project financed by the Milband Memorial Fund. According to Turner and colleagues (1957), "these programs showed that habits could be changed and health improved through health education" (p. 27).

In the 1930s, the drive for health education from the public slowed. Health education continued to address the major health issues of the time but without the enthusiasm brought on by World War I. Notable research studies supplemented authoritative opinion in helping to point out difficulties and offer solutions related to the teaching of health education. Several important conferences were held on health education and youth health at the national level (Means, 1962). The profession was moving forward.

Professional organizations emerged during the 1900s that still exist today. School health education, long associated with physical education, received official recognition in 1937, when the American Physical Education Association became the American Association for Health and Physical Education, which eventually evolved into the American Association for Health, Physical Education and Recreation and Dance (AAHPERD). In the 1990s, AAHPERD changed from an association to an alliance of national and district associations. The national association that represented health education specialists was the American Association for Health Education (AAHE). For many years, AAHE was a major force in the health education field. At their 2013 National Convention, AAHPERD dropped the association structure and went back to one organization. The name AAHPERD was changed to "SHAPE America" with a mission to, "advance professional practice and promote research related to health and physical education, physical activity, dance and sport." (SHAPE America, 2020). This means that AAHE is no longer in existence. Although SHAPE America still intends to service those school health educators that also teach physical education, most health education specialists, including those focused on school health, have joined another professional association such as the Society for Public Health Education, which represents all health education specialists in all practice settings, or the American School Health Association.

The American School Health Association evolved from the American Association of School Physicians, which was founded in 1927. Over the next 10 years, this association of school physicians expanded its functions, interests, and scope of activity. As a result, it broadened its membership to include school health personnel other than physicians. In 1938, its name was changed to the American School Health Association to reflect these changes. Today, the mission of the American School Health Association is to "transform all schools into places where every student learns and thrives." (American School Health Association, 2020)

The American Public Health Association had long been an organization interested in and supportive of school health. In fact, many of the earliest supporters of health education in the schools had been leaders in public health. Appropriately, the organization established a separate section within its administrative structure to focus on school health interests. In 1942, the School Health Section of the American Public Health Association was formed. (Chapter 8 discusses all of these professional associations in greater detail.)

With the bombing of Pearl Harbor on December 7, 1941, the United States found itself at war. Once again, national focus turned to physical fitness and health. With no major threats of war in the previous 20 years, the physical status of young U.S. men had again degenerated. Of the approximately 2 million men examined for induction into the nation's armed forces, almost 50% were disqualified. Of those disqualified, 90% were found to be physically or mentally unfit (American Youth Commission, 1942). This unfortunate situation helped greatly to stimulate interest in the health of high school students and provided strong motivation for health education/promotion classes.

After World War II, school health education continued to grow as a profession. As Means (1975) observed, "This period from 1940 into the 1970s was one of appraisal, re-evaluation, and consolidation with respect to research accomplished in school health education. During this time leaders in the field attempted to look back, review, and take stock of what was known as a determinant of future action" (p. 107).

The **School Health Education Study** was a major study of significance to school health education. Directed by Dr. Elena M. Sliepcevich (1964), the study included 135 randomly selected school systems involving 1,460 schools and 840,832 students in 38 states. Health behavior inventories were administered to students in grades 6, 9, and 12. The results were appalling. Health misconceptions among students at all levels prevailed.

Questionnaires were distributed to school administrators throughout the country to obtain data on organizational procedures and instructional practices related to school health education. Again, the results indicated major problems in the organization and administration of health programs. Cortese (1993) noted, "...some health topics were omitted while others were repeated grade after grade at the same level of sophistication. No logical rationale placed learning exercises at various grade levels, and a need existed for a challenging and meaningful curriculum" (p. 21).

The second phase of the school Health Education Study established a curriculum writing team to develop a school health education curriculum based on needs identified from the first phase of the study. The team consisted of prominent names in school health education at the time, including Gus T. Dalis, Edward B. Johns, Richard K. Means, Ann E. Nolte, Marion B. Pollock, and Robert D. Russell (Means, 1975). Over the next eight years, the writing team developed a comprehensive curriculum package that schools could implement.

The **School Health Education Evaluation Study** of the Los Angeles area was one more important study. Its purpose was to evaluate the effectiveness of school health work in selected schools and colleges of the area. More specifically, the project aimed at the appraisal of the entire school health program, including administrative organization, school health services, health instruction, and healthful school environment. Furthermore, it examined the students' health knowledge, attitudes, and behavior. The study resulted in 11 conclusions and 17 important recommendations for the field. (Means, 1975).

School health programs have continued to evolve from the mid-1970s to the present. Several important events and trends have impacted school health education and overall school health programs. In 1978, the Office of Comprehensive School Health was established within the U.S. Department of Education. The primary purpose of the office was policy development for health issues that affected children and youth. Although the office held great promise for school health education efforts, unfortunately, it was never fully funded. A director was named, Peter Cortese, but the office was finally deactivated with the budget cuts during President Reagan's administration (Rubinson & Alles, 1984).

The 1980s saw the emergence of two important concepts: coordinated school health programs and comprehensive school health instruction. Based on the initial ideas of Turner and colleagues (1957), and later refined by Allensworth and Kolbe (1987), a **coordinated school health program** consisting of eight interactive components that work together to enhance the health and well-being of the students, faculty, staff, and community was devised. The eight components consisted of health education, physical education, health services, nutrition services, counseling, psychology and social services, healthy school environment, staff health promotion and family, and community involvement.

The original eight component coordinated school health program model has been expanded and revised to now include 10 components, and is known as the Whole School, Whole Community, Whole Child Model (WSCC) (CDC, n.d.-h). To arrive at the 10 WSCC components, the original Healthy School Environment component was split into the social and emotional climate component and the physical environment component. The original family/community involvement component was split into the community involvement component and family engagement component. The WSCC model recognizes the importance of establishing healthy behaviors in youth. To accomplish this, the model promotes the cooperation and collaboration of government agencies, community organizations, schools, community members, and families (See **Figure 2.14**).

Comprehensive school health education is actually the health curriculum component of the WSCC model. **Box 2.4** identifies factors that need to be in place for the development and delivery of a planned, sequential, effective school health education program. Emphasis should be placed on six specific adolescent risk behaviors that are monitored by the Youth Risk Behavior Surveillance System (YRBSS) (CDC, n.d.-i). These six behaviors contribute to the leading causes of death and disability among youth and adults. These behaviors usually are established during childhood, persist into adulthood, are inter-related, and are preventable. These risk behaviors are as follows:

- Behaviors that contribute to unintentional injuries and violence
- Sexual behaviors that contribute to unintended pregnancy and sexually transmitted diseases, including HIV infection
- Alcohol and other drug use
- Tobacco use
- Unhealthy dietary behaviors
- Inadequate physical activity (CDC, n.d.-i)

In 2006, with support from the American Cancer Society, the Joint Committee on National Health Education Standards was formed. Committee members included representation from the American Association for Health Education, The American Public Health Association, The American School Health Association, and the Society of State Leaders of Health and Physical Education. The standards can be seen in **Box 2.5**. The goal of the National Health Education Standards is improved educational achievement for students and improved health in the United States. The standards promote **health literacy**, the capacity of individuals to access, interpret, and understand basic health information and services, and the skills to use the information and services to promote health. The standards provide a foundation for curriculum development, instruction, and assessment of student performance. A rationale and numerous

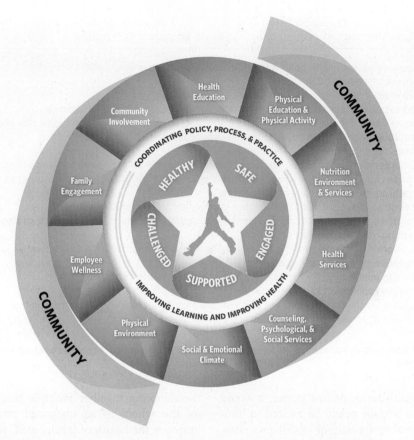

Figure 2.14 CDC diagram of Whole School, Whole Community, Whole Child (WSCC).

Reproduced from Centers for Disease Control and Prevention. (n.d.). *Whole school, whole community, whole child (WSCC).* https://www.cdc.gov/healthyschools/wscc/index.htm

performance indicators, broken down by grade-level groupings, accompany each of the eight standards. The National Health Education Standards also provide an important guide for colleges and universities to enhance pre-professional preparation as well as the continuing education of health education/promotion teachers (CDC, n.d.-d).

The National Board for Professional Teaching Standards, founded in 1987, developed national standards for school health education teachers. These standards go beyond the requirements for state teacher licensure. Since the fall of 2008, individuals with three years of full-time health education/promotion teaching experience and a valid state teacher's license for those three years may voluntarily complete a rigorous evaluation process to become a National Board Certified Health Education Teacher. This National Board Certification places school health education on an equal level with other teaching fields and allows highly qualified and dedicated health education teachers to be recognized for their work. Some states or districts may provide salary bonuses for these highly qualified teachers who obtain National Board Certification (National Board for Professional Teaching Standards, 2020). It is expected that many exceptional and highly dedicated health education/promotion teachers will seek National Board Certification.

Since 1987, the concept of a coordinated school health program has dominated the

Box 2.4 Characteristics of an Effective Health Education Curriculum

1. Focuses on clear health goals and related behavioral outcomes.
2. Is research based and theory-driven.
3. Addresses individual values, attitudes, and beliefs.
4. Addresses individual and group norms that support health-enhancing behaviors.
5. Focuses on reinforcing protective factors and increasing perceptions of personal risk and harmfulness of engaging in specific unhealthy practices and behaviors.
6. Addresses social pressures and influences.
7. Builds personal competence, social competence, and self-efficacy by addressing skills.
8. Provides functional health knowledge that is basic, accurate, and directly contributes to health-promoting decisions and behaviors.
9. Uses strategies designed to personalize information and engage students.
10. Provides age-appropriate and developmentally appropriate information, learning strategies, teaching methods, and materials.
11. Incorporates learning strategies, teaching methods and materials that are culturally inclusive.
12. Provides time for instruction and learning.
13. Provides opportunities to reinforce skills and positive health behaviors.
14. Provides opportunities to make positive connections with influential others.
15. Includes teacher information and plans for professional development and training that enhance effectiveness of instruction and student learning.

Centers for Disease Control and Prevention. (n.d.). *Characteristics of an effective health education curriculum.* https://www.cdc.gov/healthyschools/sher/characteristics/

school health arena. At first glance, it would seem that schools would be excited to initiate comprehensive school health programs. How could they not embrace a concept that would bring together multiple components of the school in an integrated attempt to improve the health of faculty, staff, students, and the community? A healthy child taught

Box 2.5 National Health Education Standards

Health Education Standard 1—Students will understand concepts related to health promotion and disease prevention to enhance health.

Health Education Standard 2—Students will analyze the influence of family, peers, culture, media, technology, and other factors on health behaviors.

Health Education Standard 3—Students will demonstrate the ability to access valid information and products and services to enhance health.

Health Education Standard 4—Students will demonstrate the ability to use interpersonal communication skills to enhance health and avoid or reduce health risks.

Health Education Standard 5—Students will demonstrate the ability to use decision-making skills to enhance health.

Health Education Standard 6—Students will demonstrate the ability to use goal-setting skills to enhance health.

Health Education Standard 7—Students will demonstrate the ability to practice health-enhancing behaviors and avoid or reduce health risks.

Health Education Standard 8—Students will demonstrate the ability to advocate for personal, family, and community health.

Centers for Disease Control and Prevention. (n.d.). *National health education standards.* https://www.cdc.gov/healthyschools/sher/standards/index.htm

by a healthy teacher in a health-conscious community should forward the school's overall mission to provide each child with the best education possible. Unfortunately, the full potential of coordinated school health programs has never been realized in most school districts. Factors may include the low priority placed on health by many school administrators; a lack of leadership to promote, coordinate, and oversee school health programs; and an overemphasis on competency testing. Another dynamic could be the adverse reactions from conservative groups that perceive coordinated school health as a means of incorporating sex education into the curriculum. New optimism has emerged with release of the Whole School, Whole Community, Whole Child movement (CDC, n.d.-h). Time will tell if this expanded and more comprehensive model will gain further traction than the coordinated school health program model of the past.

Another positive support for the future of school health is the bipartisan passage of the 2015 *Every Child Achieves Act*, which recognizes both health education and physical education as "core subjects" in schools (US Department of Education, 2015). Health education specialists had been calling for this recognition for many years (Gambescia, 2006; SOPHE, 2011). Previously both health education and physical education were not considered "core subjects" by federal mandates, which allowed schools to minimize their importance while placing more focus on those subjects such as math, science, and English that were considered core subjects. The passage of this act reflects a growing awareness of the importance of health education to the academic success and overall well-being of students. It will be interesting to watch how passage of this act will actually influence school health education in the future.

Despite the apparent lack of success with coordinated school health programs, schools still hold tremendous promise for health education/promotion efforts. With nearly all young people under 19 years of age attending schools, health education specialists must remain diligent in their effort to bring effective health promotion and education programs to this population. Every health education specialist should be advocating for the Whole School, Whole Community, Whole Child movement with national and state education agencies, federal and state government representatives, and local school boards.

Patient Protection and Affordable Care Act

On March 23, 2010, amid both fanfare and criticism, President Barack Obama signed into law the **Patient Protection and Affordable Care Act** (referred to as the Affordable Care Act or ACA—Also nicknamed Obamacare). Through a combination of cost controls, subsidies, and mandates, it expanded healthcare coverage to 20 million uninsured Americans (Goodnough et al., 2020). Another important feature was the act's focus on prevention and prevention services (Koh & Sebelius, 2010). The bill provided better access to clinical prevention services by removing cost barriers. Furthermore, the bill encouraged, promoted and provided funding for worksite wellness programs, evidence-based community prevention and wellness programs, and school-based health centers. This bill should have created new and expanded opportunities for health education specialists to promote health. More importantly, it was good for the health of Americans. As Koh and Sebelius (2010) stated: "In short, to prevent disease and promote health and wellness, the Act breaks new ground.... Moving prevention toward the mainstream of health may well be one of the most lasting legacies of this landmark legislation" (p. 5).

As of 2020, 20 million Americans had gained health insurance coverage through the ACA (Rapfogel, Gee, & Calsyn, 2020). It was estimated that by 2023, the number of uninsured in the United States would be half the size as in 2012. The ACA, however, was met with much criticism and has faced several legal challenges that reduced its effectiveness. After the 2016 Presidential elections, even more legal challenges were initiated. It is important to note, however, that as of November 2020, the ACA has neither been repealed nor replaced. Perhaps the most significant outcome of the lawsuits is that the ACA's individual mandate tax/penalty was eliminated at the end of 2018. While this had a significant impact on funding for the ACA, it did not eliminate any other features. In December, 2019, a Texas Appellate court ruled that the individual mandate was no longer constitutional since the tax penalty was eliminated. Courts are now considering whether the remainder of the ACA should also be struck down as those opposing the ACA maintain that the mandate is not severable from the remainder of the ACA (Musumeci, 2020). In November, 2020, the Supreme Court heard an appeal of the Texas case with President Trump's Justice Department testifying in favor of the Texas position. In a rare move, the Biden Administration's Justice Department sent a letter to the Supreme Court Justices in February of 2021 stating that they were reversing the position of the former Justice Department and they no longer believed the ACA to be unconstitutional (Liptak, 2021). No decision had been rendered by the Supreme Court as of April of 2021.

COVID-19 Pandemic

COVID-19 was identified in Wuhan, China, in December of 2019. Since then it has spread to become a worldwide pandemic (CDC, 2020). As of April 1, 2021, there were approximately 130 million cases and nearly 3 million deaths worldwide. In the United States, there were approximately 30.5 million cases with over 552 thousand deaths (Johns Hopkins University, 2021). As a result of the pandemic, public health has become more visible. Public health officials are in the news daily. Health education specialists working in public health settings have important roles to play in addressing the COVID-19 pandemic. Public health education professionals are needed to inform the public about the disease and how it may be prevented and controlled (Brisolara & Smigh, 2020). Behavior change programs and campaigns are needed to encourage mask wearing, handwashing, and social distancing. Further public health professionals are needed to serve as contact tracers and to accurately, concisely and thoroughly translate complex epidemiological data to the general public.

Summary

The history of health and health education/promotion is important to the professional development of health education specialists. By understanding the past, you can appreciate the present and become a leader in this emerging profession.

Today's concept of health education/promotion is relatively new, dating back only to the middle to late 1800s. Since ancient times; however, humans have been searching for ways to keep themselves healthy and free of disease. Without knowledge of disease causation or medical treatment, it was only natural to rely on superstition and spiritualism for answers. The concept of prevention was intriguing, but the knowledge and skills to prevent disease were unknown.

Progress in preventing and treating disease is evident in the early civilizations of Egypt, Greece, and Rome. These cultures recognized a need for humans to maintain sound minds and bodies. Systems of rudimentary pharmacology, better waste disposal, and safer drinking water were among some of the most noteworthy improvements.

During the Middle Ages, much of what had been previously learned was lost. Society took a giant step backward. Science and knowledge were shunned, while religion gained new favor as the preferred means of preventing and treating disease. Great epidemics struck the European continent, and millions of people lost their lives.

The Renaissance witnessed a rebirth of interest in knowledge. Science again flourished, and healthcare advancements were made. Understanding of disease, however, was still rudimentary, and the effects of treatments were often worse than the diseases. Sanitary conditions were deplorable and would remain so through the 1800s. The emergence of health education/promotion as a profession was still more than a century away.

The Age of Enlightenment saw tremendous growth in cities as the Industrial Revolution got underway in both England and in the United States. Unfortunately, this population growth compounded sanitation problems related to overcrowding. Epidemics were still prevalent. In addition, employment conditions of the working class were frequently unsafe and unhealthy.

By the mid-1850s, conditions were ripe for the birth of public health in Great Britain and the United States. The contagion theory of disease emerged, and early reformers called for the government to take control of environmental conditions that led to disease. Health departments at city, state, and county levels were established and began to monitor and regulate food safety, water quality, and waste disposal. Professional organizations for health personnel were created, and voluntary agencies were formed. Major pieces of legislation were passed as the government sought to improve working conditions and took greater responsibility for the poor and infirm. During the mid-1900s, emphasis was placed on building new medical facilities

and enhancing the technology required to treat disease.

By the 1970s, the cost of medical treatment had escalated, and concern for prevention was enhanced. This set the stage for the development of national health objectives for the decades of the 1980s, 1990s, and 2000s. *Healthy People 2030* is now in place and identifies the objectives for the current decade. Health education/promotion has made and continues to make great strides as a profession.

In the mid-1800s, as public health was starting to make important strides, school health education was also budding. In addition to reading, writing, and arithmetic, early pioneers saw the need to educate students about health-related matters. In the early 1900s, groups such as the National Tuberculosis Association, the American Cancer Society, and the Women's Christian Temperance Union strongly supported educating school children about health. Both World War I and World War II provided important impetus for health-related instruction and physical training in the schools.

During the 1960s and 1970s, several important studies supported the need for school health education and documented its effectiveness. Coordinated school health programs, created in the 1980s and 1990s, have evolved into the expanded whole school, whole community, whole child concept. School Health Program Guidelines, national health education standards, and identifying the six leading causes of death and disability helped promote health education/promotion.

Although health and school health education have made great strides since the first humans contemplated how to treat and prevent disease, there is still a long way to go. Both in the United States and worldwide, there are many people who do not have access to medical care or the important information and skills of professionally trained health education specialists. Heart disease, cancers, diabetes, obesity, and HIV are prevalent in both developed and developing countries, and traditional infectious diseases, parasitic infections, poor sanitation, unsafe water, and malnutrition continue to affect people in low- and middle-income countries. Further with the COVID-19 Pandemic of 2020, additional stresses and strains have been placed on the medical and public health systems in the United States and abroad. The need for accurate, honest, transparent information in public health has never been greater. Health education specialists are uniquely trained to assist in addressing issues surrounding the prevention and control of COVID-19.

As in the past, health education professionals of today must envision what *can* be and strive to make that vision a reality. Turner et al. (1957) noted the following:

> As society looks ahead, it can conceive the hope that someday almost every human being will be well, intelligent, physically vigorous, mentally alert, emotionally stable, socially reasonable and ethically sound. At least, society must concern itself with progress toward that goal. (p. 18)

Health education specialists must be important players in this process. Health education specialists must continue their important work through community, worksite, and school-based programs.

Review Questions

1. Describe the earliest efforts at health care and informal health education/promotion.
2. Compare and contrast the great societies of ancient Egypt, Greece, and Rome. How are these cultures similar in relation to health? How are they different?
3. What were the major epidemics of the Middle Ages? Why were they so feared? What factors contributed to their spread? What were some strategies people used to prevent these diseases?
4. Discuss the Renaissance and why it is important to the history of health and health care.
5. Who wrote the *Report of the Sanitary Commission of Massachusetts* (1850)? Explain how this report was important to the history of both school health and public health.
6. Identify at least five major groups or events that forwarded school health programs.
7. What Canadian publication and its U.S. counterpart helped focus attention on the importance of disease prevention and health promotion?
8. What are *national health objectives*? Where can they be found? Why are they so important?
9. Describe the initiatives that have shaped school health education programs over the past 10 years.
10. Explain how the Affordable Health Care Act may serve to improve the public's health and advance the health education/promotion profession in the United States.
11. Discuss how the COVID-19 pandemic has impacted health, health care, and health education practice.

Case Study

Rory (she/her/hers) is a health education specialist employed by the local health department. In this role, she meets with the news media on a regular basis as a means to educate the public about important health issues. The local TV station wants to interview her about COVID-19, how it has impacted the health department, and what the average person can do to keep from contracting the disease. Rory wants to develop an outline of important points she would like to make. Your task, as Rory's student intern, is to develop the first draft of these important talking points.

Critical Thinking Questions

1. If a health educator is simply considered someone who educates others about health, who would be considered humanity's first health educators? Defend your answer.
2. If a health education specialist trained in the year 2013 could time-travel back to the Middle Ages, what impact could that person have on the health problems of that era? What positive factors would work in the health education specialist's favor? What negative factors would work against the health education specialist?
3. When the first schools were being established in Massachusetts, do you believe health education/promotion would have been accepted as an academic subject? Why or why not? Do you believe health education/promotion is accepted as an academic subject at the present time? Why or why not?
4. Go online and find a copy of the new *Healthy People 2030* objectives. Read the introduction and overview. Find the objectives for one of the topic areas and review them. Next, select one objective in that topic area that you feel strongly about, and explain why you feel it will or will not be met by the year 2030. What role might a health education specialist have in meeting the objective you selected?

Activities

1. Develop a timeline using 100-year increments from the early Egyptians to the current year. Mark all of the important health-related events as they occurred along the timeline. Next, continue your timeline 100 years into the future. Predict and mark important health-related events. Explain why you believe these predictions will come true.
2. Imagine what it would have been like to live through an outbreak of the Black Death in the Middle Ages. Write a five-day personal diary, with daily entries depicting what you might have seen or heard and how you might have felt. How would the experience of living through the Black Plague be similar and different from living through the COVID-19 pandemic?
3. Interview several individuals who are at least 80 years old concerning the health care they received as young children. Ask them to describe any health education/promotion they can remember. When was it? Where did it occur? Who provided the education? Was it effective?
4. Contact your high school health teacher. Ask if they are aware of the National Standards for Health Education and to what extent the curriculum in the school district has been based on these standards. Ask the health teacher if they are aware of the Whole School, Whole Community, Whole Child movement. If so, what has been done to implement this model at the local level? Who coordinates the effort? What programs or initiatives are a result of the effort? If nothing has been done, ask why? Try to determine the barriers to initiating the Whole School, Whole Community, Whole Child program in the district.

Weblinks

1. **http://www.cdc.gov/museum/timeline /index.html**

   Centers for Disease Control and Prevention

   This CDC website provides a "timeline" to learn about important events in the history of the CDC from its founding in 1946 to the present. Take note of the many important contributions to public health by this illustrious organization. Give special attention to the 2020s and note the CDC's role in addressing the COVID-19 pandemic.

2. **https://history.nih.gov/exhibits /history/index.html**

   National Institutes of Health, Office of History

   This National Institutes of Health (NIH) website provides a brief history of this organization, highlighting some of its more important accomplishments.

3. **https://www.nytimes.com/2020/03/23 /health/obamacare-aca-coverage-cost -history.html**

   This New York Times article provides an excellent overview of the Affordable Care Act and what has happened since it was signed into law. It addresses both the positives and negatives of the act and discusses some of the legal challenges it has faced.

4. **https://health.gov/healthypeople**

   Healthy People 2030

   This is the home page for the *Healthy People 2030* goals and objectives. From this page, you should be able to access the actual *Healthy People 2030* objectives, as well as information on how the objectives were developed and organized.

5. **http://www.cdc.gov/healthyschools /wscc/index.htm**

   Education Development Center, Inc.

   This website provides a detailed description of the Whole School, Whole Community, Whole Child initiative including a description of various components and how they can be integrated into the school program. Additional information on health & academics, data & statistics, tools, and resources are available at this site. There is even a Virtual Healthy School tour that you can take. This information is important for health education specialists who want to work in schools and make a difference in the lives of their students.

6. **https://www.youtube.com/watch ?v=AweoZYsiCu4**

   A full-length movie about Father Damien and the Kalaupapa, Molokai, Leper Colony, the last leper colony still functioning in the United States.

7. **https://vimeo.com/32226544**

   Watch this video on the history of public health in the United States.

References

Allensworth, D. D., & Kolbe, L. J. (1987). The comprehensive school health program: Exploring an expanded concept. *Journal of School Health, 57*(10), 409–412.

American Public Health Association. (1959). Lemuel Shattuck (1793–1859): Prophet of American Public Health. *American Journal of Public Health Nations Health, 49*(5), 676–677.

American Public Health Association. (2020). *Public Health Education and Health Promotion*. Retrieved November 11, 2020, from https://www.apha.org/apha-communities/member-sections/public-health-education-and-health-promotion

American School Health Association. (2020). *About the American School Health Association*. Retrieved November 12, 2020, from http://www.ashaweb.org/about/

American Youth Commission. (1942). *"Health and fitness," youth and the future*. Washington, DC: American Council on Education.

Andress, M. J., & Bragg, M. C. (1922). *Suggestions for a program for health teaching in the elementary schools*. U.S. Department of the Interior, Bureau of Education, Health Education No. 10, Washington, DC: U.S. Government Printing Office.

Auld, E. (Winter 1997/1998). Executive edge. *SOPHE News & Views, 24*(4), 4.

Bates, I. J., & Winder, A. E. (1984). *Introduction to health education*. San Francisco: Mayfield.

Bernstein, N. R. (1972). *APHA: The first one hundred years*. Washington, DC: American Public Health Association.

Brisolara, K. F., & Smith, D. G. (2020). Preparing students for a more public health–aware market in response to COVID-19. *Preventing Chronic Disease, 17*, 200251. doi: http://dx.doi.org/10.5888/pcd17.200251

Butler, M., Thornton, F., & Stoltz, D. (1994). *The Battle Creek idea*. Battle Creek, MI: Heritage Publications.

Centers for Disease Control and Prevention (CDC). (2020). *COVID-19 Overview and Infection Prevention and Control Priorities in non-US Healthcare Settings*. Retrieved February 26, 2021, from https://www.cdc.gov/coronavirus/2019-ncov/hcp/non-us-settings/overview/index.html

Centers for Disease Control and Prevention (CDC). (n.d.-a). *Healthy People 2030*. Retrieved November 11, 2020, from https://health.gov/healthypeople

Centers for Disease Control and Prevention (CDC). (n.d.-b). *Healthy People 2030 Framework*. Retrieved November 11, 2020, from https://health.gov/healthypeople/about/healthy-people-2030-framework

Centers for Disease Control and Prevention (CDC). (n.d.-c). *Mission, Role and Pledge*. Retrieved November 11, 2020, from https://www.cdc.gov/about/organization/mission.htm

Centers for Disease Control and Prevention (CDC). (n.d.-d). *National Health Education Standards*. Retrieved November 12, 2020, from https://www.cdc.gov/healthyschools/sher/standards/index.htm

Centers for Disease Control and Prevention (CDC). (n.d.-e). *National Public Health Performance Standards*. Retrieved November 11, 2020, from https://www.cdc.gov/publichealthgateway/nphps/

Centers for Disease Control and Prevention (CDC). (n.d.-f). *10 Essential Public Health Services*. Retrieved July 1, 2021, from https://www.cdc.gov/publichealthgateway/publichealthservices/essentialhealthservices.html

Centers for Disease Control and Prevention (CDC). (n.d.-g). *Use Healthy People 2030 in Your Work*. Retrieved November 11, 2020, from https://health.gov/healthypeople/tools-action/use-healthy-people-2030-your-work

Centers for Disease Control and Prevention (CDC). (n.d.-h). *Whole School, Whole Community, Whole Child*. Retrieved November 12, 2020, from http://www.cdc.gov/healthyschools/wscc/index.htm

Centers for Disease Control and Prevention (CDC). (n.d.-i). *Youth Risk Behavior Surveillance System*. Retrieved November 12, 2020, from http://www.cdc.gov/healthyyouth/data/yrbs/index.htm

Cipolla, C. M. (1976). *Public health and the medical profession in the Renaissance*. Cambridge, England: Cambridge University Press.

Cortese, P. A. (1993). Accomplishments in comprehensive school health education. *Journal of School Health, 63*(1), 21–23.

De'ath, E. (1995). *The Black Death—1347 AD*. [Film]. (Available from Ambrose Video Publishing Inc., 1290 Avenue of the Americas, Suite 2245, New York, NY 10104).

Donan, C. (1898). *The Dark Ages 476–918*. London: Rivingtons.

Duncan, D. (1988). *Epidemiology: Basis for disease prevention and health promotion*. New York: Macmillan.

Durant, W. (1961). *The Age of Reason begins*. Vol. 7. *The story of civilization*. New York: Simon and Schuster.

Fee, E., & Brown, T. M. (1997). Editorial: Why history? *American Journal of Public Health, 87*(11), 1763–1764.

Gambescia, S. F. (2006). Health education and physical education are core academic subjects. *Health Promotion Practice, 7*(4), 369–371.

Goodnough, A., Abelson, R., Sanger-Katz, M., & Kliff, S. (Nov. 13, 2020). *Obamacare turns 10*. New York Times. Retrieved November 16, 2020, from https://www.nytimes.com/2020/03/23/health/obamacare-aca-coverage-cost-history.html

Goerke, L. S., & Stebbins, E. L. (1968). *Mustard's introduction to public health* (5th ed.). New York: Macmillan.

Gordon, B. (1959). *Medieval and Renaissance medicine*. New York: Philosophical Library.

Green, W. H., & Simons-Morton, B. G. (1990). *Introduction to health education*. Prospect Heights, IL: Waveland Press.

Hansen, M. (1980). *The royal facts of life*. Metuchen, NJ: The Scarecrow Press.

Johns Hopkins University. (2021). *COVID-19 Dashboard by the Center for Systems Science and Engineering (CSEE) at Johns Hopkins University (JHU)*. Retrieved April 1, 2021, from https://coronavirus.jhu.edu/map.html

Johnson, S. (2006). *The ghost map: The story of London's most terrifying epidemic—and how it changed science, cities, and the modern world*. New York: Penguin Books.

Koh, H. K., & Sebelius, K. G. (2010). Promoting prevention through the Affordable Care Act. *The New England Journal of Medicine, 363*, 1296–1299.

Lalonde, M. (1974). *A new perspective on the health of Canadians*. Ottawa: Government of Canada.

Libby, W. (1922). *The history of medicine in its salient features*. Boston: Houghton Mifflin.

Liptak, A. (2021). Biden administration urges Supreme Court to uphold Affordable Care Act. *New York Times*.

Marr, J. J. (1982). Merchants of death: The role of the slave trade in the transmission of disease from Africa to the Americas. *Pharos Alpha Omega Alpha Honor Society, 45*(1), 31–35.

McKenzie, J. F., Pinger, R. R., & Seabert, D. M. (2018). *An introduction to community & public health* (9th Ed.). Burlington, MA: Jones and Bartlett Learning.

Means, R. K. (1962). *A history of health education in the United States*. Philadelphia: Lea & Febiger.

Means, R. K. (1975). *Historical perspectives on school health*. Thorofare, NJ: Charles B. Slack.

Moore, H. H. (1923). *Public health in the United States*. New York: Harper & Brothers.

Musumeci, M., & Kaiser Family Foundation. (2020). Explaining Texas v. U.S.: A Guide to the Case Challenging the ACA. Retrieved November 16, 2020, from http://files.kff.org/attachment/Issue-Brief-Explaining-Texas-v-US-A-Guide-to-the-Case-Challenging-the-ACA

National Board for Professional Teaching Standards. (2020). *National Board Certification Overview*. Retrieved November 12, 2020, from https://www.nbpts.org/national-board-certification/

Newsholme, A. (1936). *The last thirty years in public health*. London: Arno Press & New York Times.

Pickett, G., & Hanlon, J. J. (1990). *Public health administration and practice* (9th ed.). St. Louis: Times Mirror/Mosby.

Rapfogel, N., Gee, E., & Calsyn, M. (2020). 10 ways the ACA has improved health care in the past decade. Center for American Progress. Retrieved April 1, 2021, from https://www.americanprogress.org/issues/healthcare/news/2020/03/23/482012/10-ways-aca-improved-health-care-past-decade/

Ravenel, M. P. (Ed.). (1970). *A half century of public health*. New York: Arno Press & New York Times.

Rogers, J. F. (1936). *Training of elementary teachers for school health work*. U.S. Department of the Interior, Office of Education, Pamphlet No. 67. Washington, DC: U.S. Government Printing Office.

Rosen, G. (1958). *A history of public health*. New York: MD Publications.

Rubinson, L., & Alles, W. F. (1984). *Health education foundations for the future*. St. Louis: Times Mirror/Mosby.

Schouten, J. (1967). *The rod and serpent of Asclepius*. Amsterdam: Elsevier.

SHAPE America. (2020). *About SHAPE America: Our Mission*. Retrieved November 16, 2020, from http://www.shapeamerica.org/about/

Shattuck, L. (1850). *Report of the Sanitary Commission of Massachusetts*. Boston: Dutton and Wentworth.

Sliepcevich, E. M. (1964). *School health education study: A summary report*. Washington, DC: SHES.

Society for Public Health Education (SOPHE). (2011). Physical education and health education in ESEA. Talking points pdf. Available from SOPHE: www.sophe.org

Turner, C. E., Sellery, C. M., & Smith, S. A. (1957). *School health and health education* (3rd ed.). St. Louis: Mosby.

U.S. Department of Health, Education, and Welfare (USDHEW). (1976). *Health in America: 1776–1976*. (DHEW Publication No. (HRA) 76–616). Washington, DC: U.S. Government Printing Office.

U.S. Department of Education (2015). Every Student Succeeds Act (ESSA). Retrieved April 1, 2021, from https://www.ed.gov/essa?src=rn

U.S. Department of Health and Human Services (USDHHS). (1980). *Promoting health/preventing disease: Objectives for the nation*. Washington, DC: U.S. Government Printing Office.

U.S. Department of Health & Human Services (1999). Changes in the Public Health System. *Morbidity and Mortality Weekly Report, 48*(50), 1141.

U.S. National Center for Health Statistics, National Vital Statistics Reports (NVSR). (2009). *Deaths: Final Data for 2006, 57*(14).

U.S. Public Health Service. (1979). *Healthy people: The surgeon general's report on health promotion and disease prevention*. Washington, DC: U.S. Government Printing Office.

U.S. Public Health Service. (2020). *The Mission of the Commissioned Corps*. Retrieved November 11, 2020, from https://www.usphs.gov/about-us

Derryberry, M. (2004). Today's health problems and health education. *American Journal of Public Health, 94*(3), 368–371.

Winslow, C. A. (1944). *The conquest of epidemic disease*. Princeton, NJ: Princeton University Press.

Ziegler, P. (1969). *The Black Death*. New York: Harper & Row.

CHAPTER 3

Philosophical Foundations

CHAPTER OBJECTIVES

After reading this chapter and answering the questions at the end, you should be able to:

- Define the terms *philosophy, wellness, holistic*, and *symmetry*, and identify common elements between them.
- Discuss the importance of developing a personal life philosophy.
- Identify how your personal and occupational philosophy overlap.
- Create your personal philosophy of life and identify the influences on your philosophy.
- Identify and explain the differences between the health education/promotion philosophies.
- Explain how different health education/promotion philosophies would impact the delivery of health education/promotion.
- Tell others your own philosophy of health education/promotion.

Kristy has been exploring health-related careers and is interested in pursuing a major in health education/promotion. Her parents began to lower their cholesterol and increase their exercise by incorporating information and strategies presented by a health education specialist, employed by their physician. The health education specialist worked with Kristy's parents on a regular basis for nearly six months, and they gave rave reviews on that specialist's methodologies. As a result, Kristy's parents were able to reduce or eliminate several of the medications they had been taking. Kristy also had to admit that the entire family's health had benefited from her parents' "new" lifestyle.

In thinking about a career as a health education specialist, Kristy formulated several questions. This inquiry included the philosophies, styles, and methods of practice held or used by health education specialists. Others were related to the profession as a whole and how someone decides whether becoming a health education specialist is a good match for their philosophy of life.

This chapter addresses some of the same questions that Kristy contemplated in relation to the practice of health education/promotion and possibly becoming a health education specialist. To that end, we will explore questions such as

- What is a philosophy?
- Why does a person need a philosophy?
- What are some of the philosophies or philosophical principles associated with the notion of *health*?
- What philosophical viewpoints related to health education/promotion are held by some of the past and current leading health education specialists?
- How is a philosophy developed?
- What are the predominant philosophies used in the practice of health education/promotion today?
- How will adopting any of the health education/promotion philosophies impact the way health education specialists practice in their chosen setting?

The purpose of discussing the development of a health education/promotion philosophy is not to provide a treatise on "the nature of the world," so to speak, but to emphasize the importance of a guiding philosophy to the practice of any profession. (Smith, 2010) notes, "When a health educator identifies and organizes concepts deemed valuable in relation to health outcomes, they can begin to form a philosophical framework for functioning comfortably and effectively" (p. 51). (Gambesia, 2013) adds, "Our philosophy of public health education, therefore, will strongly influence our approach as to what we do as health education specialists" (p. 11).

The term *philosophy* may seem to some to describe an almost ethereal, esoteric academic exercise. In actuality, however, a well-considered philosophy provides the underpinnings that serve to bridge theory and practice. Although various general types of philosophies of health education/promotion are covered later in the chapter, the following example might help you begin to see the importance of how a health education specialist's philosophy helps to determine their

practice approach in working with individuals and communities.

Consider the case of Julieta, a 30-year-old mother of two, who smokes, does not exercise regularly, eats many of her meals at fast-food restaurants, and has a family history of heart disease. Julieta is enrolled in a required personal health course at a local university. She is going back to school to become a bilingual elementary school teacher. Because a health risk appraisal is a required part of the class, she has made an appointment to visit Javier, one of the health education specialists in the health promotion center on campus.

Javier has adopted the philosophy of behavior change. As a proponent of this approach, he believes that all people are capable of changing their health behavior if they can be shown the steps to success. Initially, he would use a behavior change contract method to get Julieta to try to eliminate one or two of her negative health behaviors. As a part of this process, some preliminary analysis would be done in an attempt to identify the triggers that cause her to engage in negative health behaviors. He would help her identify short- and long-term goals. Together they would establish specific and measurable objectives to reach those goals, and strategies to reach the objectives. He would also try to ensure that she receives some appropriate reward for every objective and goal she accomplishes. During the visit, Javier also shares with Julieta that there are other health education specialists at the center who employ different philosophies from his and that she might benefit from also visiting one of them. The results of Julieta's visits to the other health education specialists are covered later in this chapter.

What Is a Philosophy?

The word *philosophy* comes from Greek and literally means "the love of wisdom" or "the love of learning." The term **philosophy** in this chapter means a statement summarizing the attitudes, principles, beliefs, values, and concepts held by an individual or a group. Tountas (2009) points out that the Greeks were the first to connect good health and fighting illness were directly impacted by human behavior and the corresponding social and physical environment. The Greek's view of health was very similar to the tenets of the Ottowa Charter.

In an academic setting, a philosopher studies the topics of ethics, logic, politics, metaphysics, theology, or aesthetics. A person certainly does not need to be an academic philosopher to have a philosophy. All of us have values, convictions, ideas, experiences, and attitudes about one or more of the philosophy topics listed above as they apply to life. These are the building blocks (sometimes known as principles) that make up any philosophy.

A person who has generated their personal philosophy of how life operates for them often is inquisitive about what facts or factors help explain an issue so that the true meaning can help inform both opinion and approach to addressing the issue. Alternative explanations behind issues are explored. Without a philosophy, a person may fall into the trap of thinking that opinion is the same as fact. When opinion is equated with fact (reality), it becomes much more difficult for a person, regardless of occupation, to be open to new ideas or concepts or other ways of looking at the world (see **Figure 3.1**) (Gambescia, 2013) states, "Health education specialists should promote diverse ideas and encourage critical thinking. We should seek a high level of tolerance . . ." (p. 13).

You most likely have already developed certain philosophical viewpoints or notions about what is real and true in the world as you know it. How you chose to act toward other people, the standards you hold yourself to,

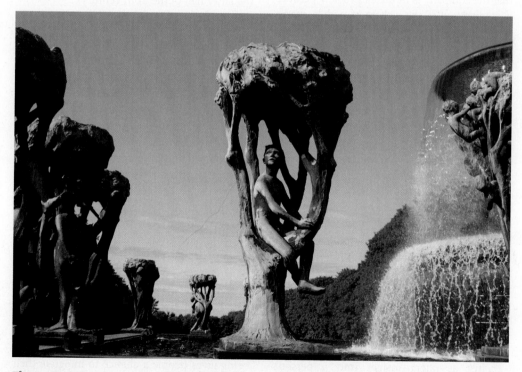

Figure 3.1 Young man contemplating the Tree of Life: What will it hold for me?
Courtesy of Jim Girvan.

and how you decide what is important in your life all reflect your philosophy. We all filter information through what matters most to us. That you are studying to become a health education specialist says something about your philosophical leanings in terms of a career. For example, the profession of health education/promotion is considered a helping profession. (Gambescia, 2007) states that health education "is an enabling good that helps individuals and communities flourish" (p. 722). Those who work in the profession should value helping others.

In today's society, there are many examples of the use of a philosophical position. Corporations, for example, create slogans espousing their purported philosophy, "Just Do It" (Nike). Of course, more than a few of them are also trying to sell a product or service at the same time. The use of caring slogans and catchy phrases is meant to convey to the public that the company is in business solely because it is interested in the welfare of people everywhere and is responsive to their needs. If the company's actions match the slogan, the public is more likely to perceive the slogan as a true representation of the corporate philosophy.

Additionally, many not-for-profit and for-profit agencies and companies have mission statements. A mission statement is meant to convey a philosophy and direction that form a framework for all actions taken by that organization. For example, the mission statement for the Central District Health in Boise, Idaho, is "Healthy People in Healthy Communities."

After reading this statement there is little doubt that the overriding philosophy in this agency is one of promoting prevention for both individuals and communities. For individuals who have a philosophy that emphasizes prevention and early intervention, this is likely to be a place where they might find employment that is personally rewarding and professionally fulfilling.

Just as often, insight into a person's philosophy can be gained by hearing, reading, or analyzing that person's quotes, sayings, or tattoos such as live and let live. Michael J. Fox's (2010) quote embodies his philosophy of life in the face of an incurable disease: "Parkinson's demanded of me that I be a better man, a better husband, father, and citizen. I often refer to it as a gift. With a nod to those who find this hard to believe, especially my fellow patients who are facing great difficulties, I add this qualifier—it's the gift that keeps on taking…but it's a gift" (p. 89). As you will see later and as can be noted from Fox's statement, a philosophy is rarely stagnant, but rather continuous because it is formulated by considering values, beliefs, experiences, and consequences of actions. Composing a philosophy statement allows a person to reflect on what is important to him or her when viewing the world in its many manifestations.

The thoughts stated previously are well summarized by (Bensley, 1993), one of the most influential health education specialists of the latter half of the 20th century:

> Philosophy can be defined as a state of mind based on your values and beliefs. This in turn is based on a variety of factors which include culture, religion, education, morals, environment, experiences, and family. It is also determined by people who have influenced you, how you feel about yourself and others, your spirit, your optimism or pessimism, your independence and your family. It is a synthesis of all learning that makes you who you are and what you believe. In other words, a philosophy reflects your values and beliefs which determine your mission and purpose for being, or basic theory, or viewpoint based on logical reasoning (p. 2).

Please note that a philosophy does not have to be abstract. Pondering the reason for being gives people a chance to integrate their past, present, and future into a coherent whole that guides them through life.

What Is My Philosophy?

The answer to the question "What is your philosophy?" is both simple and complex. Each of us already has a view of the world and what is true for us. This image helps shape the way we experience our surroundings and act toward others in our environment. In other words, our reality is based on our standards and values rooted within our philosophy. Our philosophy is how we answer questions about who we are as individuals, how we see the world, and how we relate to others and the society in which we live.

Of course, some philosophical change is probably inevitable. New experiences, new insights, and new learnings create the possibility that some of the tenets composing the philosophy might need retooling. This is a normal part of growth. Most people's philosophical views are altered somewhat as they study, grow older, and experience the world in different ways. (Gambescia, 2013) concurs when he writes, "experienced health education specialists should seriously think about updating their philosophy statement as it is tangible evidence of one's growth in the field of public health" (p. 110).

Usually, a person's philosophy (e.g., determining how to treat others, what actions are right or wrong, and what is important in life) needs to be synchronous in all aspects of life. This means that a person's philosophical viewpoint holds at home, at school, in the workplace, and at play. If incongruence develops between a person's philosophy and the philosophy of the leaders in the workplace, problems can occur.

As an example, consider the career of a public health education specialist working in HIV/AIDS prevention education who is employed by a state department of education. Assume that this individual has a philosophical view that all human life is sacred and education is the best source of prevention. Also assume that the person's work both on and off the job reflects consistency and a commitment to those ideals. In other words, the person's actions are synchronous with the aforementioned philosophy. As long as the administration in the state department of education and family and friends remain supportive of this health education specialist's role and philosophy, chances are that this person will do well. However, if the state department leadership changes and the new superintendent is opposed to the idea that individuals infected with HIV are worth saving (because they chose their behaviors) or refuses to allow condoms to be mentioned as an age-appropriate secondary source of prevention, the specialist may have a difficult time remaining in that environment. The reason for this statement is that this educator is now not allowed to act according to their beliefs, ideals, and knowledge. There is a disharmony between the philosophical stance and the ability to act in concert with that stance.

Certainly, there are exceptions to this rule. Health education specialists might hold philosophies on how they personally live, yet they might have to educate those who have made choices that are opposed to their belief system. This situation begins to cross the bounds of a general philosophy and get into ethics (right behavior—see Chapter 5). Although a possible moral-philosophical conflict seems apparent in this situation, health education specialists need to remember that their primary concern is to protect and enhance the health of those they serve. The health of any one of us affects the health of all of us in some manner (legally, monetarily, physically, or emotionally). At the very least, the health education specialist should refer this situation to another trained individual who can fulfill the obligation to the public.

The late U.S. Surgeon General C. Everett Koop was confronted with the same dilemma when he was in office during the advent of the AIDS epidemic, 1981–1989. Although he was a strong conservative Christian leader and against the use of drugs and premarital sex, he championed the cause of HIV/AIDS education by stressing that the epidemic was a health problem that required a health-based prevention message. While the action he took may have conflicted with his personal philosophy, he was responsible for protecting and preserving the health of our nation. Through the power of his office, he insisted that HIV/AIDS prevention education include the merits of abstinence, the dissemination of needles to inner-city addicts, and the increased availability of condoms to individuals who choose to be sexually active or have multiple sexual partners.

An additional example that illustrates the impact of a philosophy on the practice of a profession comes from an article by Governali et al. (2005) in which they state, "philosophical thought is central to the delivery of health education. For a profession to stay vital and relevant, it is important to assess its activities, regularly evaluate its goals, and assess its philosophical direction" (p. 211). The emphasis the authors place on the influence of activities and goals related to philosophy is a direct reflection of their personal and professional philosophical foundation formed over the years. A well-reasoned philosophy often plays an important role in the choice of a career path.

A study identifying factors that influence career choices further validates that statement. Tamayose et al. (2004) surveyed public health students enrolled at a west coast university to determine what major influences led them to pursue careers in public health. Researchers found that the top two items mentioned by the students were "enjoyment of the profession/commitment to health improvement" and "provide a health/community service to others." Both of these statements reflect a common philosophical thread that permeates the thinking of a majority of individuals currently practicing in the field of health education/promotion with whom we have come into contact.

In summary, the formation of a philosophy is one of the key determining factors behind the choice of an occupation, a spouse, a religious conviction, a political persuasion, and friends. A firm philosophical foundation serves as a beacon that lights the way and provides guidance for many of the major decisions in life.

Principles and Philosophies Associated with Health

In Chapter 1, the meaning of the term *health* was discussed. Recall that nearly all definitions include the idea of a multidimensional construct that most people value, particularly when health deteriorates. Some see health as an end to itself; others see health as being important in large part because its presence enables the freedom to act as one desires without major physical or mental impediments. Over the past 30 to 50 years, educators have identified several philosophies or philosophical principles that tend to be associated with the establishment and maintenance of health. These philosophies provide a set of guiding principles that help create a framework to better understand the depth of the term *health*.

Rash (1985) mentions that, although health is often not an end in itself, good health does bring a richness and enjoyment to life that will make service to others more possible. He feels that those who seek to enhance the health of others through education should espouse a **philosophy of symmetry**; that is, health has physical, emotional, spiritual, and social components, and each is just as important as the others. Health education specialists should seek to motivate their students or clients toward symmetry (balance) among these components.

Oberteufer (1953) rejected the notions of a dualistic (human = mind + body) or a triune (human = mind + body + spirit) nature for humanity. Instead, he embraced the ideal of a **holistic philosophy** of health when he stated, "The mind and body disappear as recognizable realities and in their stead comes the acknowledgment of a whole being…man is essentially a unified integrated organism" (p. 105). Thomas (1984) is convinced that the holistic view of health produces health professionals who are more passionate about creating a society in which the promotion of good health is seen as a positive goal.

Greenberg (1992), Donatelle (2011), Edlin and Golanty (2004), and Hales (2004), among others, have elevated the construct of wellness to the level of a philosophy. **Wellness**, always a positive quality (as opposed to illness being always a negative quality), is visualized as the integration of the spiritual, intellectual, physical, emotional, environmental, and social dimensions of health to form a whole "healthy person." Those who subscribe to this philosophy believe that all people can achieve some measure of wellness, no matter what limitations they have, and that achieving optimal health is an appropriate journey for everyone. The optimum state of wellness occurs when people have developed all six of the dimensions of health to the maximum of their ability (see **Figure 3.2**).

To be sure, there are those who differ in their philosophical view of health being composed of all of the dimensions of wellness. For example, Balog (2005) believes that health must by nature be seen solely as a physical state because "health must reside in the person" (p. 269), and it is not possible for a person to be truly healthy if the systems of the body are not functioning optimally in the way they were intended to operate. He argues that

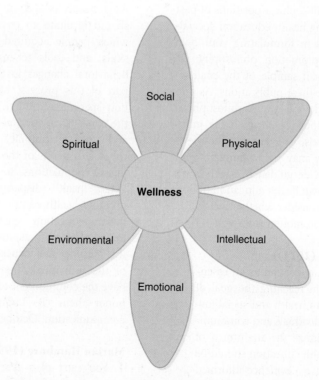

Figure 3.2 The overlapping dimensions of wellness. Optimum health includes each of these components.

any other view of health is really not objective but introduces subjective views of what others value (the good life). In Balog's view, it is important for health education specialists to distinguish that which affects health from that which is health. In other words, he cautions against confusing "good life" with "good health."

The philosophies previously mentioned are not meant to be all inclusive. The purpose of discussing them is to help provide a framework to further assist the reader in developing a philosophy about health and, ultimately, health education/promotion.

Leading Philosophical Viewpoints

Over the past 25 years, several publications and numerous articles have focused on recounting the philosophical positions of past and present leading health education specialists. To assist you in formulating your own health education/promotion philosophy, we present here a small sample of the philosophies expressed in these publications. As previously mentioned, one way a philosophical approach is developed is through the influence of role models, or mentors. The viewpoints that follow may help stimulate your thoughts and provide guidance as you begin developing your own health education philosophy and as you consider whether a career in health education/promotion is for you.

David Birch (2021)

I view health education as an essential strategy in reaching the goal of equal access to health and social justice for all individuals and communities. To maximize the attainment of that goal, health education should be a collaborative, evidence-informed experience that actively engages program participants and community

stakeholders in program planning, implementation, and evaluation. Community assets, priorities, and needs are important considerations throughout these processes. Equity, inclusivity, cultural humility, and cultural responsiveness must be hallmarks of the health educator and the program. Health education should address the social, corporate, and political factors that influence health, and result in individuals who have knowledge and skills that enable them to promote their own health and influence the health of other individuals and the overall health of various populations (D. Birch, personal communication, November 1, 2020).

Raffy Luquis (2021)

As a health education specialist, I should facilitate an environment in which people acquired knowledge, skills, and tools to make positive behavioral changes in their life. As part of this process, health education specialists need to incorporate the concepts of cultural competency and cultural humility to address the health needs of the increasingly diverse populations, to reduce persistent health disparities, and to promote health equity. As such, the health education specialist needs to recognize their own culture; the culture, the values and beliefs of the individuals they serve; and have the commitment to respect and honor them (R. Luquis, personal communication, October 29, 2020).

Marian Hamburg (1993)

1. You can't plan everything. Take advantage of opportunities as they appear. (p. 68)

2. Mentorship is powerful in influencing positive health behaviors. (p. 70)
3. Intersectoral cooperation is essential in effective health programming. Health education specialists can facilitate these collaboratives and unify efforts across school and community. (p. 71)
4. Focus our joint efforts on coalition building. The future of the health education profession depends on the maintenance and expansion of certification. (p. 73)
5. Our practice is based on networking. We bring people with common problems together to seek out solutions by sharing information and listening to each other.

John Seffrin (1993)

Health education specialists enable individuals to achieve a unique level of personal freedom. The unencumbered freedom to make informed choices. Health educators are resourceful and open to change, and the foundation of their work is based on these principles:

1. Appreciate each person's uniqueness
2. Respect ethnic and cultural diversity
3. Protect individual and group autonomy
4. Promote and preserve freedom of choice
5. Use evidence-based interventions. (p. 114).

Philosophies are as individual as the people themselves, yet some common themes (development of individual potential, learning experiences that help in decision making, free choice, and enhancement of individual uniqueness) seem to emerge and hold true regardless of the health education specialist. Let us now examine how these philosophies are actually applied in the practice of health education/promotion.

Developing a Philosophy

Now that it is clear that a philosophy is not some abstraction used only by individuals such as the Dalai Lama or Gandhi, let us explore the ways in which a philosophy is formed. In previous sections, it was noted that most practicing professionals and many organizations have developed certain philosophical stances that serve as their road map and guide for living and working in the world. What provides the basis for forming a philosophy?

Suppose you are searching through the websites of various health education/promotion programs, trying to determine which one might be best for you. In your search, you come across the website for the community health education program at the University of Wisconsin at La Crosse (see the Weblinks section at the end of the chapter for URL references). One of the prominent features of the website is a statement of the mission of this program.

The mission of the BS-CHE (Bachelor of Science—Health Education and Health Promotion) program at the University of Wisconsin-La Crosse (UW-La Crosse) 2021, "To prepare leaders in school and community health through the bridging of competency and standard-based education, scholarship, advocacy, and service-related endeavors, thereby contributing to healthier people and healthier communities."

The process of developing this mission statement most likely involved at least several meetings of faculty, staff, students, and community leaders and administrators. During the meetings, the core beliefs and principles regarding health education/promotion of those in attendance were probably assessed. After coupling the list of beliefs with the required list of core competencies, the mission statement was formulated.

In drafting your own philosophy statement, you should use a similar process (without the committee, of course). Think about what a health education specialist does and what the result of their work should be. Construct lists of your thoughts under headings such as (1) personal values and beliefs (see the Weblinks section for examples of values), (2) what "health" means to you, (3) attributes of people you admire and trust, (4) results of health studies and readings that you find meaningful, and (5) outcomes you would like to see from the process of health education/promotion (e.g., better decision making, more community involvement, promotion of positive behaviors, and healthier communities). From your lists, some common themes will emerge and the identification of these themes is a key to drafting your own health education/promotion philosophy statement. Exploring why you value the topics represented within these themes should enable you to compose your philosophy statement that will reflect a way of thinking, acting, and viewing the world that works for you.

Please note, however, that using this approach to formulate a philosophy is not a guarantee that the philosophy will remain stable. As a matter of fact, there is a strong likelihood that some changes will occur because of new learnings, activities, and experiences (e.g., working in a different culture, experiencing the premature death of a child or spouse, losing a job as a result of downsizing, or encountering a new mentor). A philosophy reflects the sum of knowledge, experience, and principles from which it was formed.

As a further aid to formulating a philosophy statement about health and health education/promotion, we would like to reference a series of questions that Dr. Julie Dietz of Eastern Illinois University gives her students when they are assigned to write their personal philosophy of health education. These questions do a great job of capturing the interface between a personal philosophy of health and a professional philosophy of the profession of health education/promotion. They are

Statement of Personal Health Philosophy

- What does it mean to be *healthy*?
- What are your health-related responsibilities and obligations to yourself?
- What are your health-related responsibilities and obligations to your community or society?
- What do you expect your community and society to do to keep you healthy?

Statement of Professional Health Education and Promotion Philosophy

- What is Health Education/Health Promotion, and what does it mean to be a professional in this field?
- What are your goals for yourself and your profession?
- What are your professional responsibilities to yourself, your community, and to your profession?
- How does community health education fit within these goals?

We conclude this section with a short vignette that illustrates several concepts or principles that need to be considered when formulating a philosophy statement about life, health, and health education/promotion practice.

The story, adapted from the book *The Boy Who Harnessed the Wind* by Kamkwamba and Mealer (2009), is about the amazing accomplishments of William Kamkwamba of the African nation of Malawi. William was curious about how things worked (particularly electricity) and had read a book titled *Using Energy*, which he accessed in a makeshift library in his town; so he was able to construct a functioning windmill from parts of engines and wrecked automobiles he found in a local junkyard. Most people around him said his dream of supplying his family and his community with reliable electricity for lighting homes and pumping water was "crazy." And like many youths in Africa, William's formal education was cut short by the inability of his family to pay the $80 annual tuition. Yet he maintained the initiative to keep on trying and learning despite his family's suffering through famine, disease, and government graft.

Although rudimentary, the windmill he constructed worked well enough to supply power to light four small light bulbs in his home. Eventually, educators and scientists throughout Africa and beyond learned of the accomplishments of this self-taught scholar. As a result, William has been a featured lecturer at several international conferences, he has completed high school at an international school in South Africa (as a result of a grant), he graduated from Dartmouth College in 2014, and he received an ideo.org Global Fellowship. His refusal to abandon his dreams, fueled by his desire to make things better for his village and family, provided a stark contrast to many in his country (and around the world) who take for granted the educational opportunities they have or just give up and settle for the status quo. Given his story, William's philosophy must include values or ideals such as perseverance, ethical conduct, a heart for helping others, and initiative.

All too often, in determining abilities, it is our experience that people set their sights and dreams too low. A personal philosophy needs to incorporate the realization that life sometimes dishes out bumps and bruises. Acknowledging this fact may well prevent any of us from excessively limiting our assessment of our place in the world. In addition, personal philosophy is often a reflection of an individual's perspective of the world and how and why it seems to work that way.

Remember, the formation of a philosophy, whether personal or occupational, requires several steps. First, individuals need to answer the following questions in reference to themselves: What is important to me? What do I value most? What beliefs do I hold? Second, they need to identify ways the answers to the first questions influence the way they believe and act. Third, after carefully considering and writing down the answers to these questions, a philosophy statement can be formulated. The statement reflects and identifies the factors, principles, ideals, values, beliefs, and influences that help shape reality for the person authoring the philosophy statement.

The steps mentioned above can be used to formulate any type of philosophy statement. However, for those who are studying health education/promotion, there is one additional and important question to consider: Is this philosophy statement consistent with being a health education specialist? If the answer is "yes," then for that person, health education/promotion is a profession worthy of further consideration.

Predominant Health Education/Promotion Philosophies

Butler (1997) accurately points out that, even though there are several definitions of the phrase *health education/promotion*, recurring themes in many of the definitions allow for a general agreement as to its meaning. He notes; however, that the methods used to accomplish health education/promotion are less clear. The manner in which a person chooses to conduct health education/promotion can be demonstrated to be a direct reflection of that person's philosophy of health education/promotion. With that in mind, have any predominant philosophies of health education/promotion emerged? If so, what are they?

Welle, Russell, and Kittleson (1995) conducted a study to determine the philosophies favored by health education specialists. As part of the background for their study, they conducted a literature review and identified five dominant philosophies of health education/promotion that have emerged during the last

50 to 60 years. The philosophies identified were behavior change, cognitive-based, decision making, freeing or functioning, and social change.

1. The **behavior change philosophy** involves a health education specialist using behavioral contracts, goal setting, and self-monitoring to try to foster a modification in an unhealthy habit in an individual with whom they are working. The nature of this approach allows for the establishment of easily measurable objectives thus enhancing the ability to evaluate outcomes. Javier from earlier in the chapter uses this approach. (Example: setting up a contract to increase the number of hours of study each week)

2. A health education specialist who uses a **cognitive-based philosophy** focuses on the acquisition of content and factual information. The goal is to increase the knowledge of the individuals or groups so that they are better armed to make decisions about their health. (Example: posting statistics about the number of people killed or injured in automobile accidents who were not wearing seat belts)

3. In using the **decision-making philosophy**, a health education specialist presents simulated problems, case studies, or scenarios to students or clients. Each problem, case, or scenario requires decisions to be made in seeking a "best approach or answer." By creating and analyzing potential solutions, the students develop skills needed to address many health-related decisions they might face. An advantage of this approach is the emphasis on critical thinking and lifelong learning. (Example: using a variety of case study examples of different popular diet programs to see competing perspectives of effectiveness)

4. The **freeing or functioning philosophy** was proposed by Greenberg (1978) as a reaction to traditional approaches of health education/promotion that he felt ran the risk of blaming victims for practicing health behaviors that were often either out of their control or not considered in their best interests. The health education specialist who uses this philosophical approach has the ultimate goal of freeing people to make the best health decisions possible based on their needs and interests—not necessarily the interests of society. Some health education specialists classify this as a subset of the decision-making philosophy discussed previously. (Example: lessons on the responsible use of alcohol)

5. The **social change philosophy** emphasizes the role of health education specialists in creating social, economic, and political change that benefits the health of individuals and groups. Health education specialists espousing this philosophy are often at the forefront of the adoption of policies or laws that will enhance the health of all. (Example: no smoking allowed in restaurants, or new housing developments with pedestrian-friendly areas such as sidewalks and parks)

The previously listed philosophies of health education/promotion are the products of more than 50 years of study, experimentation, and dialogue within the profession. The research conducted by Welle et al. (1995) found that the philosophy most preferred by both health education/promotion practitioners and academicians was decision making. Both groups listed behavior change as a second choice, and both agreed that their least favorite was cognitive based. Ratnapradipa and Abrams (2012) report that crafting a philosophy of health promotion statement may well move a health education specialist away from the use of only cognitive-based strategies (lecture) to incorporate more problem-based approaches to learning (decision-making) for their clients and communities. The fact that health education specialists who are employed in the academic setting and those who are employed as practitioners in the field agreed on these choices as predominant philosophies speaks well for the interface between preparation programs and practice.

Another interesting finding from the study occurred when, as a part of the survey, the health education specialists were given health education/promotion vignettes to address or solve. In many cases, the respondents changed the philosophical approach they used depending on the setting (school, community, worksite, or medical). The responding health education specialists had earlier identified a specific health education/promotion philosophy they favored. These results indicate that health education specialists are adaptable and resourceful, and they will use any health education/promotion approach that seems appropriate to the situation, that is, an **eclectic health education/promotion philosophy** (see Practitioner's Perspective).

In a thought-provoking essay, Buchanan (2006) introduced a different philosophical paradigm calling for health education specialists to "return to their roots" and reconsider the meaning of the word *education* in the practice of health education/promotion. He feels that the practice of health education/promotion buys into the medical model so often that health education specialists have lost their bearings and are now more often

purveyors who almost demand that persons or the public adopt behaviors that "we know" will lead to a healthier life.

Instead, he suggests that health education specialists should be "disseminators of factual information and facilitators of rational choice" (p. 301). Using this philosophy, our profession should not strictly focus on the outcome of changing peoples "behavior but did the strategies enable people to think specifically and broadly about their life goals, how their health behaviors impact those goals and what environmental factors within the community will support everyone living healthy and fulfilling lives." (p. 301).

In actuality, Buchanan's views seem to incorporate the use of the cognitive-based, the decision making, and the freeing or functioning health education/promotion philosophies outlined previously. This is not surprising because in any list of philosophies, there is always the possibility of one philosophy overlapping with another, so in practice, not all is as clean as it might seem. In making a similar argument as Buchanan, Governali et al. (2005), call for an integrated behavioral ecological philosophy so that health education specialists use the multidimensional nature of the interaction of the individual and the environment. This approach also resembles the eclectic philosophical model.

Practitioner's Perspective

Philosophy of Health Education Promotion: Travis C. Leyva

CURRENT POSITION/TITLE: Disease Prevention Program Manager

EMPLOYER: New Mexico Department of Health

DEGREE/INSTITUTION/YEAR: Bachelor in Community Health, New Mexico State University, 2004

MAJOR: Community Health

MINOR: Environmental Health

Describe your past and current professional positions and how you came to hold the job you now hold (How did you obtain the position?):
A week prior to graduating with my Bachelor's in Community Health,

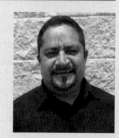
Courtesy of Travis C. Leyva.

(continues)

Practitioner's Perspective **(continued)**

Philosophy of Health Education Promotion: Travis C. Leyva

I had come across a job posting online for a Disease Prevention Specialist (DPS)—Health Educator position that caught my interest. It was a position that would conduct surveillance and field investigations for all reportable sexually transmitted diseases (STDs) in the region. I applied, interviewed, and three months later, I started my journey as a health educator.

After a year as a DPS, I was promoted to Regional Emergency Preparedness Specialist where I coordinated responses to public health emergencies and bioterrorism threats. After one year in that position, I was promoted as the Border Infectious Disease Surveillance (BIDS) Officer Epidemiologist, where I coordinated with Mexican health officials on Border Health Infectious Disease issues. Following two years in that position, I was promoted to Program Manager of Disease Prevention, where I now supervise all of the positions I was in and more! I must say that all of my promotions started with a supervisor who encouraged and motivated me to work hard and promote myself to where I am today.

Describe the duties of your current position: I oversee six different program areas in my current position. They include STD & TB Surveillance and Field Investigation, Hepatitis Surveillance and Field Investigation, HIV Prevention, HIV Medical Case Management, Harm Reduction Program, and Emergency Preparedness Program.

My job is to ensure that all deliverables are obtained by setting goals and objectives for our staff to follow. In separate intervals, I strategize, implement, and evaluate certain activities conducted by our staff to optimize the output of our services. An activity that I am most proud of is the creation of a small group, video-based intervention titled "iHEAL—Integrated Health Education for Addictive Lifestyles." This intervention educates and creates risk-reduction plans for those who may be infected and/or affected by HIV, hepatitis C, STDs, or injection drug use. iHEAL is currently being presented at detention centers, state prisons, drug rehabilitation centers, probation and parole workshops, teen drug court programs, and some high schools. The intervention has now been requested to be presented throughout the state, and a DVD of the presentation is currently being made to distribute to health educators in the Disease Prevention field.

Describe what you like most about this position: The best thing about my position is the staff and clients I work with on a daily basis. All the staff that I work with have a unique, nonjudgmental attitude that focuses on helping people who may be infected or affected by a disease. Usually clients who we serve are unaware of how they became infected with a disease or how they could transmit a disease to others, and after we as health educators work with them, it is quite rewarding that we have made a difference in one person's life, sometimes even saving it.

Describe what you like least about this position: There is always change in public health. Although it can be a good thing at times, sometimes change can be difficult and uncertain. Working with grant-funded programs, there are always new deliverables that need to be met and at times it means stopping the processes that are in place and creating new ones, usually without any new new resources. Also, there is always a change in administration, which means there may be new directives and new priorities.

How do you use your philosophy of health education/promotion in your position? My philosophy among my staff is to educate and promote healthy lifestyle choices to every individual as you would like for it to be done to you. Being nonjudgmental and courteous is key to being a successful health educator. A major component to my philosophy is that we as health educators cannot direct an individual to make healthier lifestyle choices, but rather we can provide them with options for them to choose how to make healthier lifestyle choices for themselves. Those who choose to make a change or difference usually succeed and maintain those choices.

What recommendations/advice do you have for current health education students? My advice to current health education students is to first find a niche in public health. Whether it be STDs, Children Medical Services, Family Planning, or Harm Reduction, once you find a niche, my best recommendation is to integrate all public health programs into your health education deliveries. Some of the best health educators I have seen and worked with are those who can educate on a topic and also refer to other areas that can only benefit and support the topic area they are presenting on. People recognize when a health educator is an integrated subject matter expert.

Impacting the Delivery of Health Education/Promotion

This section uses scenarios to help focus on the methods that health education specialists might use, depending on their philosophical stance. The decision to use any philosophy involves understanding and accepting the foundation that helped create the philosophy in the first place. To this end, Welle et al. (1995) state, part of our professional development process includes delving into the different philosophical approaches and determining both our personal and professional philosophy. An important question for each professional to answer is what guiding principles for their work. The answers and resulting philosophy determine how professionals approach their work, the methods and interventions they choose and how they interact with individual and community members. These choices all reflect on the philosophical assumptions about the roles of health education and promotion, the health education specialist, and the intended audience. A philosophy like the selected interventions may be impacted by different work settings. Every health education specialist should be cognizant of the aspects of their individual philosophies they are willing to alter depending on the presenting circumstances.

At the outset, it is important to remember that one of the overriding goals of any health education/promotion intervention is the betterment of health for the person or the group involved. All the philosophies have that goal. They differ, however, in how to approach that objective.

Remember the case of Julieta discussed early in this chapter. The encounter with Javier, a university-based health education specialist who used a behavior change philosophical approach, was also described earlier. We now continue this scenario with Julieta visiting the other university health education specialists.

Javier had referred Julieta to Nokomis, a health education specialist who advocates for a decision-making philosophy. This means that Nokomis believes in equipping clients with problem-solving and coping skills, so that they make the best possible health choices. Initially, Nokomis might sit down with Julieta and hypothesize some situations that would necessitate Julieta thinking through the rationale behind the negative health behaviors. Nokomis also would most likely try to encourage Julieta to see that some of the behaviors affect others too. The main goal is to move Julieta to a point of admitting that some of the health behaviors need to be changed and to help identify the reasons that changing them would improve one's life.

In the third and final visit, Julieta visits health education specialist Li Ming, an advocate of a freeing or functioning philosophy of health education/promotion. Li Ming feels that, too often, health education specialists fail to find out the needs and desires of the client. They simply "barge in" and either overtly or covertly blame the client for any negative health behaviors. Li Ming would advocate change only if the behavior were infringing on the rights of others. In the beginning, Li Ming would confer with Julieta and find out "how their life was going." Li would ask Julieta to identify any behaviors they wanted to change, making certain that Julieta had all the information necessary to make an informed decision. Although Li Ming might believe that Julieta should stop smoking and start exercising, Li would help Julieta change only those behaviors Julieta wanted to change.

One caveat needs to be mentioned at this time. The fact that Julieta was required to take a personal health course in the teacher preparation program and that the instructor required a health risk assessment illustrates the social change philosophy at work at a microlevel. If health were not a state requirement (legislation) in the first place, Julieta might not have considered changing any negative health behaviors.

Julieta's situation demonstrates a point made previously—in practice, there often is a natural mixing of some of the philosophies. For example, all the approaches mentioned used portions of the cognitive-based health education/promotion philosophy. To reiterate, this philosophy is based on the premise that persons need to be provided with the most current information that impacts their health behaviors, and the acquisition of that information should create a dissonance and cause change.

The fifth philosophy, social change, is probably not as well suited to addressing the health behaviors of individuals. Proponents stress changes in social, economic, and political arenas to impact the health of populations. Of course, populations are made up of individuals, so changing the environment of a disadvantaged neighborhood to be healthier (e.g., creating jobs, ensuring adequate and safe housing and high-quality schools, and providing healthcare coverage for all) ultimately impacts the health of people at the individual level as well.

Summary

The term *philosophy* means a statement summarizing the attitudes, principles, beliefs, and concepts held by an individual or a group. Forming both a personal and an occupational philosophy requires reflection and the ability to identify the factors, principles, ideals, and influences that help shape your reality. The decision to use any philosophy involves understanding and accepting the foundation that helped create the philosophy in the first place. A sound philosophical foundation serves as a guidepost for many of the major decisions in life.

The five predominant philosophies of health education/promotion that were identified in the chapter are (1) behavior change, (2) cognitive-based, (3) decision making, (4) freeing or functioning, and (5) social change. Health education specialists might disagree on which philosophy works best. They might even use an eclectic or multidimensional philosophical approach, depending on the setting or situation. However, it is important to remember that one of the overriding goals of any health education/promotion intervention is the betterment of health for the person or community involved. All the philosophies have that goal. They simply differ in how to attain it.

Review Questions

1. Define each of the following and explain their relationship to one another.
   - Philosophy
   - Wellness
   - Holistic
   - Symmetry
2. Why is it important to have a personal life philosophy?
3. Compare and contrast the value of having a personal life philosophy and a personal work philosophy that are similar.
4. Define and explain the differences between:
   - A behavior change philosophy and a cognitive-based philosophy
   - A decision-making philosophy and a social change philosophy
   - A freeing or functioning philosophy and an eclectic health education/ promotion philosophy
5. Explain how a person might use each of the five major health education/ promotion philosophies and the eclectic philosophy to address a societal problem that can be addressed by health education/promotion (e.g., smoking, seat belt use, air pollution, exercise, diet, medication compliance, and cancer risk reduction).

Case Study

You are entering the final semester of your senior year of study with a major in public health education. The health education/ promotion program at your university requires seniors in their last semester to intern a minimum of 25 hours per week at a state or nonprofit agency. For this capstone experience, you have been assigned to the mayor's office in a medium-size city near the campus.

During an orientation on the first day, you overhear that one of the tasks you will be assigned will involve meeting with the leaders of several community groups with the goal of creating smoke-free public parks in the city. The smoke-free park concept represents one of the mayor's main objectives in her second term in office. You also hear that the mayor is excited to have a health education student intern because she greatly respects the skills that a health education specialist possesses.

On the second day, you have the opportunity to meet with the mayor, and, in fact, she does introduce to you the idea of a smoke-free public park system. During this meeting, you discover that she is quite knowledgeable about the negative health effects of second- and third-hand smoke in part because her son, a lifetime nonsmoker who worked in a pub in town (smoking was allowed in pubs), died last year from lung cancer at the age of 36. At the close of the meeting, the mayor asks you to submit to her your philosophy of health education/ promotion so that she can see what approach you might take with the community groups.

Using the model outlined in this chapter, write out your health education/promotion philosophy. Based on your philosophy statement and given the project that you will be assigned, is the mayor's office a good place for you to intern to hone your skills? Why or why not?

Critical Thinking Questions

1. Of the five basic health education/ promotion philosophies identified by Welle et al. (1995), why do you think that the least favorite among health

education specialists was the cognitive philosophy? Why do you think decision making was viewed as most popular?

2. What is the purpose of health education/promotion? How might the formulation of a purpose statement be reflected in your philosophy of health education/promotion?

3. You have been hired by a local pharmacy to provide health education/promotion services to customers and employees. Shortly after you begin work; however, you discover that much of your job is marketing nutritional supplements and nonpharmaceutical health-related services provided by the pharmacy and not the health education/promotion you had envisioned. How might this apparent conflict of interest have been avoided?

4. Suppose that you are a proponent of the social change philosophy. How might this philosophy be employed by a health education specialist to reduce or eliminate exposure to the COVID-19? Defend your answer to a group that advocates for use of the cognitive philosophy as the best approach to address this problem.

5. An article by Bruess (2003) in the *American Journal of Health Education* discusses the notion of "role modeling" for health education specialists. (The reference for the article can be found at the end of this chapter.) After reading the article, summarize Dr. Bruess's main points and use your answer to determine which philosophical viewpoint(s) a health education specialist must hold to feel as Dr. Bruess does on the issue of role modeling. Finally, assess how you feel about the issue. Do you agree or disagree with him? Provide a rationale for your answer.

Activities

1. Do an Internet search for "health education philosophy examples" then compare and contrast your philosophy to those written by three other individuals. What are the differences and similarities?

2. After reexamining the philosophies of health, write a paragraph that could be used to explain your philosophy of health to a potential employer or colleague.

3. Interview a health education specialist. Ask what their philosophy of health education/promotion is. Then ask about the influences that helped the educator form their philosophy. Summarize the interview in a one-page paper.

4. Use any three of the five philosophical approaches to health education/promotion discussed in the chapter and address the following situation: In the past week in your community, two teenagers have been killed in separate incidents while riding scooters. In neither case was the teenager wearing a helmet. A local citizens group has asked you and two of your health education specialist colleagues to attend a meeting concerning what to do about this issue.

5. Have students listen or read Dr. Anthony Fauci's 2005 This I Believe Essay on NPR (Alexanian, 2005). How does his personal philosophy reflect his professional life and handling of COVID in 2020?

Weblinks

1. **https://www.uwlax.edu/health -education-and-health-promotion/**

   Mission statement of the Department of Health Education and Health Promotion program at the University of Wisconsin, La Crosse.

   The program description provides a fine example of a mission and philosophy statement for health education and health promotion based on the eight responsibilities of health education specialists.

2. **https://casaa.unm.edu/inst/Personal %20Values%20Card%20Sort.pdf**

   Download the Personal Values Card Sort activity and have students identify which values are important, very important, or not important. The student then identifies their top three most important values. This helps students identify possible values or beliefs they might hold. Having these terms delineated helps in the initial stages of the development of both a personal and a professional philosophy. Students can also find app versions of this activity online.

3. Log on to your university library and find the online version of Dr. Stephen Gambescia's Presidential keynote address to the 2007 Society for Public Health Education (SOPHE) convention (see below in reference list). It provides an excellent "tour" through the thought processes of the rationale for forming a philosophy of health education for the profession of health education.

References

Alexanian, N. (2005) This I believe: A goal of service to humankind [Radio broadcast]. NPR. https://www.npr.org/templates/story/story.php?storyId=4761448

Balog, J. E. (2005). The meaning of health. *American Journal of Health Education, 36*(5), 266–273.

Bensley, L. B. (1993). This I believe: A philosophy of health education. *The Eta Sigma Gamma Monograph Series, 11*(2), 1–7.

Bruess, C. E. (2003). This I believe: A philosophy of health education. *American Journal of Health Education, 34*(4), 237–239.

Buchanan, D. R. (2006). Perspective: A new ethic for health promotion: Reflections on a philosophy of health education for the 21st century. *Health Education & Behavior, 33*(3), 290–304.

Butler, J. T. (1997). *The principles and practices of health education and health promotion.* Englewood, CO: Morton.

Donatelle, R. J. (2011). *Health: The basics, green edition.* San Francisco: Pearson Education.

Edlin, G., & Golanty, E. (2004). *Health and wellness* (8th ed.). Sudbury, MA: Jones and Bartlett.

Fox, M. J. (2010). *A funny thing happened on the way to the future: Twists and turns and lessons learned.* New York: Harper-Collins.

Gambescia, S. F. (2007). 2007 SOPHE presidential address: Discovering a philosophy of health education. *Health Education & Behavior, 34*(5), 718–722.

Gambescia, S. F. (2013). A process for updating a philosophy of education statement. *Health Promotion Practice, 14*(1), 10–14.

Governali, J. F., Hodges, B. C., & Videto, D. M. (2005). Health education and behavior: Are school health educators in denial? *American Journal of Health Education, 36*(4), 210–214.

Greenberg, J. S. (1978). Health education as freeing. *Health Education, 9*(2), 20–21.

Greenberg, J. S. (1992). *Health education: Learner centered instructional strategies* (2nd ed.). Dubuque, IA: William C. Brown.

Hales, D. (2004). *An invitation to health* (3rd ed.). Belmont, CA: Thomson-Wadsworth.

Hamburg, M. V. (1993). Would I do it all over! *The Eta Sigma Gamma Monograph Series, 11*(2), 67–74.

Kamkwamba, W., & Mealer, B. (2009). *The boy who harnessed the wind.* New York: Harper-Collins.

Miller, W., C'de Baca, J., Matthews, D., & Wilbourne, P. (2001). Personal Values Card Sort. Retrieved April 12, 2021, from https://motivationalinterviewing.org/personal-values-card-sort

Oberteufer, D. (1953). Philosophy and principles of school health education. *Journal of School Health, 23*(4), 103–109.

Rash, J. K. (1985). Philosophical bases for health education. *Health Education, 16*(2), 48–49.

Ratnapradipa, D., & Abrams, T. (2012). Framing the teaching philosophy statement for health educators: What it includes and how it can inform professional development. *The Health Educator, 44*(1), 37–42.

Seffrin, J. R. (1993). Health education and the pursuit of personal freedom. *The Eta Sigma Gamma Monograph Series, 11*(2), 109–118.

Tamayose, T. S., Madjidi, F., Schmieder-Ramirez, J., & Rice, G. T. (2004). Important issues when choosing a career in public health. *Californian Journal of Health Promotion, 2*(1), 65–73.

Thomas, S. B. (1984). The holistic philosophy and perspective of selected health educators. *Health Education, 15*(1), 16–20.

Tountas, Y. (2009). The historical origins of the basic concepts of health promotion and education: The role of ancient Greek philosophy and medicine. *Health Promotion International, 24*(2), 185–192.

University of Wisconsin La Crosse. (2021). Mission statement from Health Education and Health Promotion. Retrieved January 17, 2021, from https://www.uwlax.edu/health-education-and-health-promotion/

Welle, H. M., Russell, R. D., & Kittleson, M. J. (1995). Philosophical trends in health education: Implications for the 21st century. *Journal of Health Education, 26*(6), 326–332.

CHAPTER 4

Theories and Planning Models

CHAPTER OBJECTIVES

After reading this chapter and answering the questions at the end, you should be able to:

- Define and explain the difference among *theory*, *concept*, *construct*, *variable*, and *model*.
- Explain the importance of theory to health education/promotion.
- Explain what is meant by behavior change theories and planning models.
- Describe how the concept of socio-ecological approach applies to using theories.
- Explain the difference between continuum theories and stage theories.
- Identify and briefly explain the behavior change theories and their components used in health education/promotion:
  - Health Belief Model
  - Theory of Planned Behavior
  - Elaboration Likelihood Model of Persuasion
  - Information-Motivation-Behavioral Skills Model
  - Transtheoretical Model of Change
  - Precaution Adoption Process Model
  - Social Cognitive Theory
  - Social Network Theory
  - Social Capital Theory
  - Diffusion Theory
  - Community Readiness Model
- Identify and briefly explain the planning models and their components used in health education/ promotion:
  - PRECEDE-PROCEED
  - Multilevel Approach to Community Health (MATCH)
  - Intervention Mapping
  - Social Marketing Assessment and Response Tool (SMART)
  - Mobilizing for Action through Planning and Partnerships (MAPP)
  - Generalized Model (GM)

As noted in Chapter 1, the profession of health education/promotion evolved from other biological, behavioral, psychological, sociological, and health science disciplines. As this profession has grown, so has the number of theories and models used by health education specialists in their work. This chapter introduces the terms *theory, concept, construct, variable*, and *model* and explains why theory is used in health education/promotion. The chapter also presents an overview of theories that focus on behavior change, as well as the models associated with program planning. However, space does not permit comprehensive coverage of all theories and models used by health education specialists. For example, theories and models associated with implementation and evaluation processes are not covered in this chapter.

Because theories and models are dynamic, they change and evolve (Crosby et al., 2009). To that end, we will not attempt to introduce every possible theory or planning model in this chapter. Health education specialists continually deal with both revised and new theories and models. Future courses and the books, articles, and associated materials in those courses will likely expose you to more complete coverage of health education/promotion's theoretical base (e.g., DiClemente et al., 2009; DiClemente et al., 2013; Edberg, 2020; Glanz et al., 2015a; Goodson, 2010; Green & Kreuter, 2005; Hayden, 2019; Institute of Medicine [IOM], 2001; Sharma, 2017; Simons-Morton et al., 2012).

Definitions

To understand the theoretical foundations presented in this chapter, you must be familiar with some key related terms. Let us begin with **theory**. One of the most frequently quoted definitions of this term was provided by Glanz et al. (2015b), who modified a previous definition by Kerlinger (1986). It states: "A *theory* is a set of interrelated concepts, definitions, and propositions that presents a *systematic* view of events or situations by specifying relations among variables in order to *explain* and *predict* the events of the situations" (p. 26). Stated a little differently, "a theory is a systematic arrangement of fundamental principles that provide a basis for explaining certain happenings of life" (McKenzie et al., 2013, p. 163). Thus, "the role of theory is to untangle and simplify for human comprehension the complexities of nature" (Green et al., 1994, p. 398).

As applied to the profession of health education/promotion, a theory is a general explanation of why people act, or do not act, to maintain and/or promote the health of themselves, their families, organizations, and communities. The primary elements of theories are known as **concepts** (Glanz et al., 2015b). When a concept has been developed, created, or adopted for use with a specific theory, it is referred to as a **construct** (Kerlinger, 1986). In other words, "the key concepts of a theory are its constructs" (Rimer & Glanz, 2005, p. 4). The operational form (practical use) of a construct is known as a **variable**. A variable is a quantitative measurement of a construct.

A **model** "is a composite, a mixture of ideas or concepts taken from any number of theories and used together" (Hayden, 2019, p. 1). Stated a bit differently, "Models draw on a number of theories to help people understand a specific problem in a particular setting or context. They are not always as specific as theory" (Rimer & Glanz, 2005, p. 4). Unlike theories, models do "not attempt to explain the processes underlying learning, but only to represent them" (Chaplin & Krawiec, 1979, p. 68).

Consider how these terms are used in practical application. A personal belief is a *concept* related to various health behaviors. For example, people are more likely to behave in a healthy way—such as exercise regularly—if they feel confident in their ability to actually engage in a healthy form of exercise. Such a concept is captured in a *construct* of the Social Cognitive Theory (SCT) called *self-efficacy*. (See the discussion of the SCT later in this chapter.) If health education specialists want to develop an intervention to assist people in exercising, the ability to measure the peoples' self-efficacy toward exercise will help create the intervention. The measurement may consist of a few questions that ask people to rate their confidence in their ability to exercise. This measurement, or operational form, of the self-efficacy construct is a *variable*. However, because of the complexity of getting a nonexerciser to become an exerciser, the health education specialist may need to use constructs from several theories (a *model*) to plan the intervention. In our example, it is possible that no one theory may work perfectly to assist the nonexerciser to begin and sustain a habit of exercising.

In the health education/promotion profession, the adjective *theory-based* (as in theory-based planning, theory-based practice, or theory-based research) commonly refers to both theories and models. In fact, some of the best-known and often used theories use "model" in their title (e.g., Health Belief Model). Goodson (2010) explains why "model" and "theory" are used inconsistently. She indicates that when some models were created, they were properly titled as models. They were created using constructs from several theories to explain specific phenomena. They had little empirical testing to prove their worth. Over time, these models were tested and refined, gaining theory status. Goodson (2010) concludes, "because we tend to borrow the theories we employ from other disciplines and fields and because our concern usually centers in applying these theories (or models) to practice or research, it seems to matter little to us whether we deal with theories or with models; it seems to matter even less what labels we attach to them" (p. 228).

The Importance of Using Theory in Health Education/ Promotion

Using theory is important in all professions, not just in health education/promotion. Theory helps organize various forms of knowledge (e.g., data, facts, and information) so that they take on meaning that would not occur if the pieces of knowledge were presented in isolation. Such meaning helps to guide the work of a practitioner (Timmreck et al., 2010).

Theory helps health education specialists plan, implement, and evaluate programs. More specifically, theory (1) indicates reasons why people are not behaving in healthy ways, (2) identifies information needed before developing an intervention, (3) provides a conceptual framework for selecting constructs to develop the intervention, (4) gives insights into how best to deliver the intervention, and (5) identifies measurements needed to evaluate the intervention's impact (Crosby et al., 2009; Glanz et al., 2015b; Salazar et al., 2013). Theory also "provides a useful reference point to help keep research and implementation activities clearly focused" (Crosby et al., 2009, p. 11), and it infuses ethics and social justice into practice (Goodson, 2010). In addition, "using theory as a foundation for program planning and development is consistent with the current emphasis on using evidence-based interventions in public health, behavioral medicine, and medicine" (Rimer & Glanz, 2005, p. 5).

In the rest of this chapter, some of the theories and models used by health education specialists are presented in two main groups. The first group contains theories that focus on behavior change. Through their constructs, these theories help explain how change might take place. The second group contains planning models, which give structure and organization to the program planning process. These models provide health education specialists with step-by-step procedures, "integrating multiple theories to explain and address health problems," (Rimer & Glanz, 2005, p. 36), as they plan, implement, and evaluate health education/promotion programs.

There is not enough space in this chapter to adequately describe all the theories that have been developed to explain how behavior change occurs. Several of the theories that are not explained in detail in this chapter and are used less frequently in the health education/promotion setting but are nevertheless important are listed in **Box 4.1**.

Box 4.1 Other Behavior Change Theories

Community Organization Theory (Minkler et al., 2001)

Extended Parallel Processing Model (Gore & Bracker, 2005)

Protection Motivation Theory (PMT) (Rogers, 1983)

Public Health Model (PHM) (Street, Hopkins, & Olson, 2002)

Resilience Theory (Ungar, 2008)

Behavior Change Theories

There are a number of behavior change theories that can be used by health education specialists to design interventions to encourage behavior change. Each theory provides a distinct process for helping to explain and change health behavior (Crosby et al., 2013a), and each works better in some situations than in others, depending on which level of influence is used to plan a health education/promotion program.

"Levels of influence" are at the heart of the **socio-ecological approach** (also called the *ecological perspective*). This multilevel, interactive approach examines how physical, social, political, economic, and cultural dimensions influence behaviors and conditions. The socio-ecological approach "emphasizes the interaction between, and the interdependence of, factors within and across all levels of a health problem" (Rimer & Glanz, 2005, p. 10). In other words, changes in health behavior do not take place in a vacuum. "Individuals influence and are influenced by their families, social networks, the organizations in which they participate (workplaces, schools, religious organizations), the communities of which they are a part, and the society in which they live" (IOM, 2001, p. 26).

The concept of the socio-ecological approach comes from Bronfenbrenner's (1974, 1979) ecological paradigm, which was created to understand human development. Several authors applied his work to health promotion/education. Those most often cited in the literature are McLeroy et al. (1988), who identified five levels of influence: "(1) the individual and individual's characteristics, such as knowledge, attitudes, values, and skills; (2) social relationships, including family and friendship ties and connections; (3) organizational influences and factors; (4) community characteristics; and (5) public policy"; and two additional levels "(6) the physical environment and (7) culture" were added (Simons-Morton et al., 2012, p. 45). **Table 4.1** lists and defines each of the seven levels. **Figure 4.1** provides a visual representation of the socio-ecological framework. By examining a health problem using this multilevel approach, health education specialists can get a better understanding of how to "attack" the problem.

Consider how the levels of influence can be applied to cigarette smoking in the United States. At the *intrapersonal* (or *individual*) *level,* a large majority of smokers know that smoking is bad for them, and a slightly smaller majority have indicated they would like to quit. Many have tried to quit—some have tried on many occasions. At the *interpersonal level (or within groups)*, many smokers are encouraged to quit by those in their social networks, such as their

Table 4.1 **An Ecological Perspective: Levels of Influence**

Ecological Level	Definition
Intrapersonal	Individual characteristics that influence behavior, such as knowledge, attitudes, beliefs, and personality traits
Interpersonal	Interpersonal processes and primary groups, including family, friends, and peers that provide social identity, support, and role definition
Organizational	Rules, regulations, policies, and informal structures, which may constrain or promote recommended behaviors
Community	Social networks and norms, or standards, which exist as formal or informal among individuals, groups, and organizations
Public Policy	Local, state, and federal policies and laws that regulate or support healthy actions and practices for disease prevention, early detection, control, and management
Physical Environment	Natural and built environment
Culture	Shared beliefs, values, behaviors, and practices of a population

Reproduced from Rimer, B. K., & Glanz, K. (2005). *Theory at a glance: A guide for health promotion practice* (2ed ed., NIH Pub. No. 05-3896). National Cancer Institute.

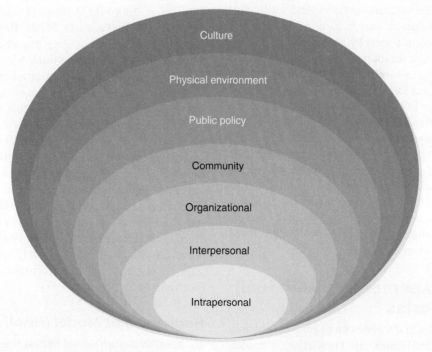

Figure 4.1 The socio-ecological model.

Reproduced from Simons-Morton, B. G., McLeroy, K. R., & Wendel, M. L. (2012). *Behavior theory in health promotion practice and research* (p. 45). Jones & Bartlett Learning.

physician and/or family and friends. Some smokers may attempt to quit on their own, or they may join a formal smoking cessation group.

At the *institutional* (or *organizational*) *level,* institutions, such as churches and businesses, often have policies that regulate smoking. These institutions may offer smoking cessation classes or support groups to assist those who "belong" to the organization, to quit smoking. At the *community level,* some towns, cities, and counties have ordinances that prohibit smoking in public places. At the *public policy* or *population level,* many states have high cigarette taxes and/or laws that limit smoking. Also at this level, the federal government spends many dollars for public service announcements (PSAs) and other forms of media advertising the dangers of tobacco use.

The *physical environment* can also impact smoking behavior. Some of the laws that are written to prohibit indoor smoking are written in such a way that people are permitted to smoke in certain areas of a building if it has a separate ventilation system. And finally, culture can play a part in nicotine addiction as most recently seen by the invention of electronic cigarette devices, which allow individuals to get a nicotine fix without the irritating effects and social stigma of cigarette smoke.

The following sections describe some of the theories and models that focus on behavior change. These theories/models are grouped according to the levels of influence where they may be most effective. To simplify the presentation of the socio-ecological model, Glanz & Rimer (1995) combined the levels of institutional, community, and public policy factors into a single "community" level. We have used it here as well.

Intrapersonal (Individual) Theories

Intrapersonal theories focus on factors within individuals such as knowledge, attitudes, beliefs, self-concept, developmental history, past experiences, motivation, skills, and

behavior (Rimer & Glanz, 2005). Several of the theories used by health education specialists to develop interventions at the intrapersonal level are the Health Belief Model (HBM), the Protection Motivation Theory (PMT), the Theory of Planned Behavior (TPB), the Elaboration Likelihood Model of Persuasion (ELM), the Information-Motivation-Behavioral Skills Model (IMB), the Transtheoretical Model of Change (TMC), and the Precaution Adoption Process Model (PAPM).

Although all of the theories listed above fall into the intrapersonal category, they can be divided further into continuum theories, or stage theories. A **continuum theory** identifies variables that influence actions (i.e., beliefs, attitudes), quantifies the variables, and combines those variables into a single equation that predicts the likelihood of action (Weinstein et al., 1998; Weinstein et al., 2008). Thus, people can be "placed along a continuum of action likelihood" (Weinstein et al., 1998, p. 291). The HBM (Rosenstock, 1966), PMT (Rogers, 1975), TPB (Ajzen, 2006), ELM (Petty & Cacioppo, 1986), and IMB (Fisher & Fisher, 1992) are examples of continuum theories that are appropriate for use at the intrapersonal level.

A **stage theory** consists of an ordered set of categories into which people can be classified. It identifies factors that could induce movement from one category to the next (Weinstein & Sandman, 2002). More specifically, stage theories have four principal elements: (1) a category system to define the stages, (2) an ordering of stages, (3) barriers to change that are common to people in the same stage, and (4) different barriers to change, facing people in different stages (Weinstein et al., 1998). The most commonly reported stage theory is the TMC (Prochaska, 1979; Prochaska & DiClemente, 1983).

Health Belief Model (HBM)

The **Health Belief Model (HBM)** was developed in the 1950s by a group of psychologists to help explain why people would or would not use health services such as tuberculosis screenings (Rosenstock, 1966). The HBM "addresses the individual's perceptions of the threat posed by a health problem (susceptibility, severity), the benefits of avoiding the threat, and factors influencing the decision to act (barriers, cues to action, and self-efficacy)" (Rimer & Glanz, 2005, p. 12). As you read the following example of why a person may or may not choose to enroll in a weight loss program, refer to the graphic representation of the HBM in **Figure 4.2**.

Suppose a person sees an advertisement about a weight loss program while scrolling through Facebook. This is a **cue to action**

that gets the individual thinking about the possibility of losing weight. There may be some variables (demographic, socio-psychological, and structural) that cause the individual to think about it a little more. They remember their college health course, which included information about weight gain and heart disease. This individual knows they are at a higher than normal risk for heart disease because of family history, age, and less-than-desirable food and exercise choices. Therefore, they come to the conclusion that they are susceptible to heart disease (**perceived susceptibility**). The individual also believes that if they develop a heart or

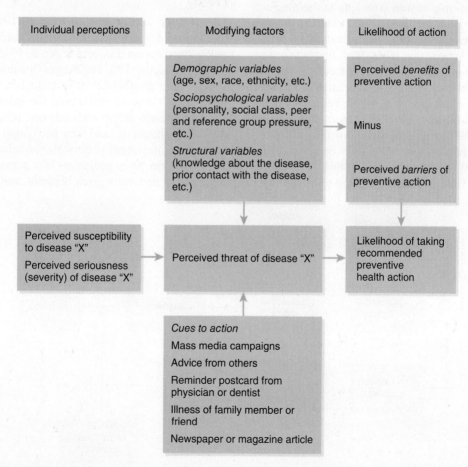

Figure 4.2 Health Belief Model as a predictor of preventive health behavior.

Reproduced from Becker, M. H., Drachman, R. H., & Kirscht, J. P. (1974, March). A new approach to explaining sick-role behavior in low income populations. *American Journal of Public Health, 64*(3), 205–216. https://doi.org/10.2105/AJPH.64.3.205

vascular condition, it can be serious (**perceived seriousness/severity**).

Based on these factors, the individual thinks that there is reason to be concerned about heart disease (**perceived threat**). They know that reducing their weight reduces the chances of a heart attack or stroke (**perceived benefits**). But continuing on a weight loss program takes time and effort, and this individual does not always remember and is not always motivated to do it (**perceived barriers**). They must now analyze the difference between the benefits of and the barriers to enrolling in a weight loss program (**reduction of threat**). For this individual, the **likelihood of taking action** (enrolling in the program) will be determined by considering the perceived threat against the reduction of threat.

When the HBM was first conceived, **self-efficacy** (confidence in one's own ability to perform a certain task or function) was not part of the model. However, because evidence showed self-efficacy was a meaningful concept in the perceived barriers construct, it was recommended that self-efficacy be added to the HBM (Rosenstock et al., 1988). According to the HBM, if people are going to be successful in changing a behavior, they must feel threatened by their current behavior (i.e., perceived susceptibility and severity), feel that a change in the behavior will result in an outcome they value (perceived benefit), and believe that they are competent (self-efficacy) to overcome perceived barriers (perceived cost) to engage in the new behavior (Champion & Skinner, 2008). Because dieting has a high failure rate, support groups such as Weight Watchers can increase a person's self-efficacy because it can help them feel competent in adopting a new lifestyle (Mann et al., 2007).

Theory of Planned Behavior (TPB)

The **Theory of Planned Behavior (TPB)** (see **Figure 4.3**) is an extension of the Theory of Reasoned Action (Fishbein & Ajzen, 1975). According to the TPB, individuals' intention to perform a given behavior is a function of their attitude toward performing the behavior, their beliefs about what relevant others think they should do, and their perception of the ease or difficulty of performing the behavior. **Intention** "is an indication of a person's readiness to perform a given behavior, and it

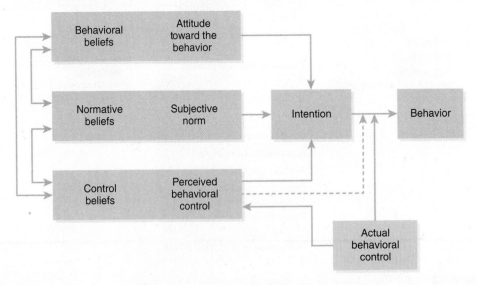

Figure 4.3 Theory of Planned Behavior (TPB).

is considered to be the immediate antecedent of behavior" (Ajzen, 2006). Unlike the Theory of Reasoned Action, the TPB was not only developed to explain health behaviors but also all voluntary behaviors. Using the example of the use of marijuana as a behavior not fully under voluntary control, the TPB predicts that people intend to give up its use if they:

- Have a positive attitude toward quitting (**attitude toward the behavior**).
- Think that others whom they value believe it would be good for them to quit (**subjective norm**) (see **Figure 4.4**).
- Perceive that they have control over whether or not they quit (**perceived behavioral control**).
- Have the skills, resources, and other prerequisites needed to quit (**actual behavioral control**).

Elaboration Likelihood Model of Persuasion (ELM)

The **Elaboration Likelihood Model of Persuasion (ELM)** or the Elaboration Likelihood Model for short, was initially developed

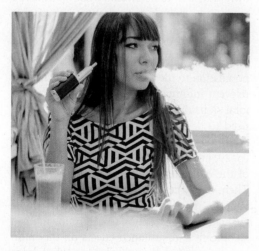

Figure 4.4 Subjective norm is an important construct to be considered when planning programs for adolescents and young adults.

© prostooleh/iStock/Getty Images Plus.

to help explain inconsistencies in research results from the study of attitudes (Petty et al., 2009). Specifically, the ELM was designed to help explain how persuasion messages (communication), aimed at changing attitudes, are received and processed by people. Although not created specifically for health communication, the ELM has been used to interpret and predict the impact of health messages.

The ELM does three things. First, it proposes that attitudes can be formed via two different types of routes to persuasion: peripheral routes and central routes (Petty et al., 2009). The distinction between the two routes is the amount of elaboration. **Elaboration** refers to the amount of cognitive processing (i.e., thought) that a person puts into receiving messages. Peripheral route processing involves minimal thought and relies on superficial cues, or mental shortcuts (called *heuristics*), about issue-relevant information as the primary means for attitude change (Petty et al., 2009). For example, people may form an attitude after hearing a persuasive message simply because the person delivering the message is someone they admire.

On the other hand, central route processing involves thoughtful consideration (or effortful cognitive elaboration) of issue-relevant information and one's own cognitive responses as the primary bases for attitude change: "Two conditions are necessary for effortful processing to occur—the recipient of the message must be both *motivated* and *able* to think carefully" (Petty et al., 2009, p. 188). An example of central route processing is a motorcyclist's formation of an attitude about wearing a helmet. Processing is based on thoughtful consideration of a message about the pros and cons of helmet use, recalling knowledge learned in a motorcycle safety class, and possibly the outcomes of a motorcycle crash in which a relative was involved.

Second, when using the ELM, the results of the two routes can be similar. However, the two routes usually lead to attitudes with different consequences. "Attitudes changed through central route processing are more enduring and have different effects on behavior than attitude change achieved through more peripheral processing, which is less resilient to counterarguments" (Simons-Morton et al., 2012, p. 285).

Third, "the model specifies how variables have an impact on persuasion" (Petty et al., 2009, p. 197). The variable can have an influence on people's motivation to think or ability to think, as well as the valence of people's thought or the confidence in the thoughts generated (Petty et al., 2009). For example, variables that have an impact on how a message is processed include the source of the message (e.g., friend, expert), the message itself (e.g., funny, serious), the context (e.g., delivered person-to-person, on the Internet), and various characteristics of the recipient (e.g., intelligence, age, attentiveness).

Utilizing the routes to processing that the ELM provides, health education specialists can create health messages that are more meaningful to a priority population, and in turn, can be more successful in reaching program goals. **Figure 4.5** provides a diagram of the ELM as presented by Petty and colleagues (2009).

Information-Motivation-Behavioral Skills Model (IMB)

The Information-Motivation-Behavioral Skills Model (IMB) (see **Figure 4.6**) was initially created to address the critical need for a strong theoretical basis for HIV/AIDS prevention efforts (Fisher & Fisher, 1992). Because of its success in dealing with HIV/AIDS prevention behavior, the IMB model has been applied to a number of other risk reduction behaviors (Fisher et al., 2009). According to this model, the constructs of information, motivation, and behavioral skills are the fundamental determinants of preventive behavior. The information provided needs to be relevant, easily enacted based on the specific circumstances, and serve as a guide to personal preventive behavior. "In addition to facts that are easy to translate into

behavior, the IMB model recognizes additional cognitive processes and content categories that significantly influence performance of preventive behavior" (Fisher et al., 2009, p. 27). An example is the following guideline that someone may use to make a decision: "If my best friend is willing to ride a motorcycle without a helmet, it must be okay."

Even though people are well informed about a particular health issue, they may not be motivated to act. According to the IMB model, prevention motivation includes both personal motivation to act (i.e., one's attitude toward a specific behavior) and social motivation to act (social support for the preventive behavior) (Fisher et al., 2009). Both types of motivation are necessary to act.

In addition to being well informed and motivated to act, the IMB model also indicates that people must possess behavioral skills to engage in the preventive behavior. The behavioral skills component of the IMB model includes an individual's objective ability and their perceived self-efficacy to perform the preventive behavior.

When applying the IMB model, health education specialists cannot just use their own judgment to determine what information to provide, how best to motivate, and what behavioral skills to teach to a given population. The process should begin by eliciting information from a subsample of the priority population to identify deficits in their health-relevant information, motivation, and behavioral skills. Next, health education specialists need to design and implement "*conceptually-based, empirically-targeted, population-specific*" (p. 29) interventions, constructed on the bases of the elicited findings (Fisher et al., 2009). Then, after the implementation of the intervention, health education specialists must evaluate the intervention to determine if it had significant and sustained effects on the information, motivation, and behavioral skill determinants of the preventive behavior and on the preventive behavior itself (Fisher et al., 2009).

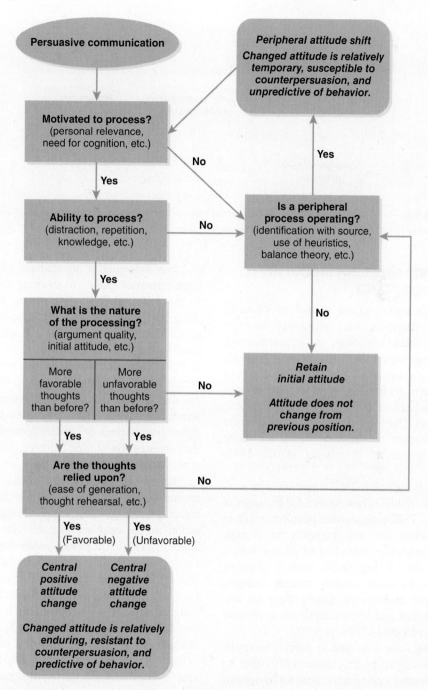

Figure 4.5 The Elaboration Likelihood Model of Persuasion (ELM).

Reproduced from Petty, R. E., Barden, J., & Wheeler, S. C. (2009). The elaboration likelihood model of persuasion: Developing health promotions for sustained behavioral change. In R. J. DiClemente, R. A. Crosby, & M. Kegler (Eds.), *Emerging theories in health promotion practice and research* (2nd ed., p. 196). John Wiley & Sons, Inc.

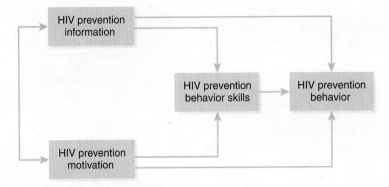

Figure 4.6 The Information-Motivation-Behavioral Skills Model of HIV prevention health behavior.

Reproduced from Fisher, J. D., & Fisher, W. A. (1992). Changing AIDS risk behavior. *Psychological Bulletin, 111*(3), 455–474.

Transtheoretical Model of Change (TMC)

The **Transtheoretical Model of Change (TMC)** proposes that intentional behavior change "occurs in stages. As people attempt to change their behavior, they move through different stages using a variety of processes to help them get from one stage to the next until a desired behavior is attained" (Hayden, 2019, pp. 112). The TMC draws from the constructs of a number of theories, "hence the name 'Transtheoretical'" (Prochaska et al., 1998, p. 59).

Although each TMC construct is important, this model is best known for its stages of change. TMC suggests that "people move from *precontemplation*, not intending to change, to *contemplation*, intending to change within 6 months, to *preparation*, actively planning change, to *action*, overtly making changes, and into *maintenance*, taking steps to sustain change and resist temptation to relapse" (Prochaska et al., 1994, p. 473).

TMC was first used in psychotherapy. It was developed by Prochaska (1979) after he completed a comparative analysis of various therapy systems and many therapy studies. Since then, program planners have used TMC with a wide variety of topics ranging from alcohol abuse to weight control (Prochaska et al., 2008; Spencer et al., 2006).

The following is an example of TMC's stage construct applied to smoking cessation. In the **precontemplation stage**, smokers "have no intention to take action in the foreseeable future (usually defined as within the next 6 months)" (DiClemente et al., 2013, p. 109). There are a number of reasons why people are in this stage. It may be that they are discouraged from previous unsuccessful attempts at changing, or it may be that they are either uninformed or underinformed about the consequences of their behavior (Prochaska et al., 2008).

In the **contemplation stage**, smokers know that smoking is bad for them and consider quitting. They "are intending to take action in the next six months" (Prochaska, 2005, p. 111). In the **preparation stage**, the smokers have combined intention and behavioral criteria. Often, during the past year, they have already taken a step toward changing their behavior. For example, they may have enrolled in an organized class to help them change, had a conversation with a physician or counselor, or purchased a self-help book or app for their smartphone to help guide their change (Prochaska et al., 2008).

In the **action stage**, smokers have overtly made changes in their behavior, experiences, or environment to stop smoking in the past six months, yet not all modifications count as action (Prochaska et al., 2008). To be considered in this stage, people need to meet a level of behavior that scientists and professionals agree is sufficient to reduce the risk of disease. In our example, reducing the number of cigarettes smoked per day does not meet the necessary level for action; only total abstinence qualifies (Prochaska et al., 2008). As smokers make these changes, they are moving toward the next stage, maintenance.

The focus of the **maintenance stage** is to prevent relapse. Thus, individuals who have quit smoking are working not to smoke again. People in this stage have changed their problem behavior for at least six months and are increasingly more confident that they can continue their change (Prochaska et al., 1998; Redding et al., 1999). In other words, their change is more of a habit, and their chance of relapse is lower, but their new behavior still requires some attention (Redding et al., 1999).

The final stage is **termination**. This stage is defined as the time when individuals who made a change now have zero temptation to return to their old behavior. They have 100% self-efficacy (a lifetime of maintenance). In our example, smokers have become nonsmokers. No matter what their mood, they will not return to their old behavior (Prochaska et al., 2008). This is a stage that few people reach with certain behaviors (e.g., alcoholism).

Precaution Adoption Process Model (PAPM)

The Precaution Adoption Process Model (PAPM) tries to explain how people get to the point of making a decision about taking action and how they apply their decision to taking action (Weinstein et al., 2008). Although the previously discussed TMC and the PAPM are both stage models that appear similar, they are applied quite differently. The PAPM is most applicable for the adoption of a new precaution (e.g., getting a mammogram or a COVID-19 vaccination), or the abandonment of a risky behavior that requires a deliberate action (e.g.,

not wearing a safety belt). It can also be used to explain why and how people make deliberate changes in habitual patterns (e.g., flossing one's teeth two times a day instead of one). The PAPM is not applicable for actions that require the gradual development of habitual patterns of behavior, such as exercise and diet (Weinstein et al., 2008).

In the following example, the seven stages of the PAPM (see **Table 4.2**) are applied to participating in a colon cancer screening program. In Stage 1, Unaware of Issue, people are totally unaware of the need to be screened. When people first learn something about the screening, they are no longer unaware, but they are not necessarily engaged by it, either. This is Stage 2, Unengaged.

In Stage 3, Deciding about Acting, people have become engaged in thinking about the screening, and they are considering participation. Once people have reached this stage, one of three things happen: (1) they suspend judgment and stay in this Stage, (2) they decide to act and move to Stages 5–7, or (3) they decide not to act (Stage 4) (Weinstein et al., 2008).

Once the people participate in the screening, they have initiated the behavior, and they are in Stage 6, Acting. Finally, if the people participate in the screening at the medically recommended intervals, they are in Stage 7, Maintenance. Note that this last stage of the PAPM is not applicable to some decision-making processes, for example, actions required only once in a lifetime, such as a vaccination that immunizes a person for life (Weinstein et al., 2008).

Interpersonal Theories

The category of interpersonal theories contains theories that "assume individuals exist within, and are influenced by, a social environment. The opinions, thoughts, behavior, advice, and support of the people surrounding an individual influence his or her feelings and behavior, and the individual has a reciprocal effect on those people" (Rimer & Glanz, 2005, p. 19). Research shows that social

Table 4.2 **Stages of the Precaution Adoption Process Model (PAPM) Applied to the COVID-19 Vaccine**

PAPM Stage	Process in Adoption of COVID Vaccine
1. Unaware of the potential issue	People are unaware there is a COVID-19 vaccine; they do not have formed opinions about getting the vaccine
2. Unengaged by issue	People are aware about COVID and the vaccine, but have not considered whether they need to do anything about it
3. Undecided about acting	The decision-making stage; people are reading and learning about the COVID vaccine and are considering whether or not to get the injection
4. Decided not to act	Halting the adoption/behavior change process; decided not to get the COVID vaccine
5. Decided to act	Deciding to get the vaccine and in the process of making an appointment for the injection
6. Acting	Arrived at the appointment time and place to receive the injection; planning to get second dose if required
7. Maintenance	Fully vaccinated; following news to determine if a booster will be needed in the future

relationships can be a powerful influence on health and health behaviors (Heaney & Israel, 2008). As such, a number of theories have been created to explain concepts such as

- *Social norms*—"*what are perceived to be true and acceptable*" (Simons-Morton et al., 2012, p. 158)
- *Social learning*—learning that occurs in a social context
- *Social power*—ability to influence others or resist activities of others
- *Social integration*—structure and quality of relationships
- *Social networks*—"person-centered webs of social relationships or all the relationships that an individual has in his or her life" (Sharma, 2017, p. 120)
- *Social support*—"help obtained through social relationships and interpersonal exchanges" (Sharma, 2017, p. 119)
- *Social capital*—"the relationships and structures within a community, such as civic participation, networks, norms of reciprocity, and trust, that promote

cooperation of mutual benefit" (Putnam, 1995, p. 66)

- *Interpersonal communication*

Because of space limitations, only three interpersonal theories are overviewed in this chapter, one that is well-established (Social Cognitive Theory) and two newer theories (Social Network Theory and Social Capital Theory). The latter two may be theories in name only. As stated previously in this chapter, some theories have the term *model* in their title because that is the way they were initially identified. Even though there is now empirical evidence to call them theories, the model title has remained. The social network and social capital theories may have been called theories prematurely; they are probably more in the model stage. However, you should be aware of the main concepts in each one.

Social Cognitive Theory (SCT)

The Social Cognitive Theory (SCT) (Bandura, 1986) dates back to the 1950s (Bandura, 1977; Rotter, 1954), when it was known as the

Social Learning Theory (SLT). When studying about theories, you may yet hear a reference to SLT. In brief, the SCT asserts "that the social environment, the personal characteristics of the individual, and behavior interact and influence each other" (Crosby et al., 2013b, p. 164). Those who advocate for the SCT believe that reinforcement contributes to learning. However, the combination of reinforcement with an individual's expectations of the behavior's consequences is what determines the behavior. The SCT explains learning through its constructs. Unlike the other theories presented so far in this chapter, there is no diagram for the SCT nor is the interrelationship of its constructs specific in nature. Those constructs most often used in health education/promotion are presented in **Table 4.3**, along with an example of each.

Social Network Theory (SNT)

The term **social network** refers to the "person-centered web of social relationships" (Sharma, 2017, p. 120). Barnes, a sociologist who studied Norwegian villages (Barnes, 1954), created the term in the 1950s. He used it to describe villagers' social relationships and characteristics that were not traditional social units like families (Edberg, 2020; Heaney & Israel, 2008). Since that time, sociologists and professionals in various disciplines, including health education/promotion, have continued to study and use the social network concept.

Social epidemiological observational studies clearly document the beneficial effects of supportive networks on health status (Heaney & Israel, 2008). But some people question whether there is enough evidence to suggest a Social Network Theory (SNT). Heaney and Israel (2008) feel that the social network concept, and the closely related one of social support, are really not theories but rather are concepts that describe social relationships. They feel that intervention studies are "needed to identify the most potent causal agents and critical time periods for social network enhancement" (p. 197). For example, it is not known how much social networking is needed to enhance health, or how much is too much. Also unknown are the characteristics of "good networks" that result in positive health behavior (i.e., regular exercise) versus characteristics of "bad networks" that lead to negative health behavior (i.e., binge drinking). We do know, however, that people who are part of social networks are healthier, as a whole, than those who are not involved in social networks.

Edberg (2020) described different types of social networks such as ego-centered networks and full relational networks (see **Figure 4.7**). He indicated that the key component to SNT is the relationships between and among individuals, including how those relationships influence beliefs and behaviors. He further stated that those using SNT need to consider the following items when assessing a network's role on the health behavior of individuals who are part of the network (Edberg, 2020):

- Centrality versus marginality of individuals in the network: How involved is the person in the network?
- Reciprocity of relationships: Are relationships one way or two ways?
- Complexity or intensity of relationships in the network: Do the relationships exist between two people, or are they multiplexed?
- Homogeneity or diversity of people in the network: Do all members of the network have similar characteristics, or are they different from one another?
- Subgroups, cliques, and linkages: Are there concentrations of interactions among some members? If so, do they interact with others, or are they isolated from others?
- Communication patterns in the network: How does information pass between the members in the network?

In summary, we know that social networks can impact health, but the specifics of who is most affected and how best to set up and use social networks are unknown. Even so,

Table 4.3 Often-Used Constructs of the Social Cognitive Theory and Examples of Their Application

Construct	Definition	Example
Behavioral capability	Knowledge and skills necessary to perform a behavior	If a woman is going to perform a breast self-exam, she needs to know the proper way to do it.
Expectations	Beliefs about the likely outcomes of certain behaviors	If a woman performs BSE or receives a mammogram, she expects the process to find cancer at an early vs. late stage.
Expectancies	Values people place on expected outcomes	Does the woman value early detection?
Locus of control	Perception of the center of control over reinforcement	Women who feel they have control over reinforcement are said to have internal locus of control and feel participating in screening provides them the ability to detect cancer early. Those who perceive reinforcement under the control of an external force are said to have external locus of control. These women practicing BSE or having a mammogram won't help because if they are going to get cancer; it is their fate.
Reciprocal determinism	"Environmental factors influence individuals and groups, but individuals and groups can also influence their environments and regulate their own behavior" (McAlister et al., 2008, p. 171)	If women are not utilizing mammograms because of time off from work, employers can schedule a mobile mammogram unit to come to the worksite.
Observational learning	Learning by watching others	Provide women with the opportunity to watch others (in person or on a video) properly performing BSE on a breast model.
Reinforcement (directly, vicariously, self-management)	Responses to behaviors that increase the chances of recurrence	Giving verbal encouragement to those women who have completed their mammogram or correctly performed BSE.

Self-control, or self-regulation	Gaining control over own behavior through monitoring and adjusting it	If want to increase BSE, have women track how often they perform it.
Self-efficacy	People's confidence in their ability to perform a certain desired task or function	If women are going to properly perform BSE, they must feel they can do it.
Collective efficacy	Beliefs about the ability of the group to perform concerted actions that bring desired outcomes (McAlister et al., 2008, p. 171)	If a group of women is going to work to change a community's culture toward mammograms, they must feel that they can do it.
Emotional-coping response	For people to learn, they must be able to deal with the sources of anxiety that surround a behavior	Fear is an emotion that can be involved in learning, and people would have to deal with it before they could learn a behavior. If the women feel scared they will find a lump, or if they do, it is fatal, that fear can prevent them from doing screenings.

Data from Baranowski, T., Perry, C. L., & Parcel, G. S. (2002). How individuals, environments, and health behavior interact: Social cognitive theory. In K. Glanz, B. K. Rimer, & F. M. Lewis (Eds.), *Health behavior and health education: Theory, research, and practice* (3rd ed., pp. 165–184); McAlister, A. L., Perry, C. L. & Parcel, G. S. (2008). How individuals, environments, and health behavior interact: Social cognitive theory. In K. Glanz, B. K. Rimer, & K. Viswanath (Eds.), *Health behavior and health education: Theory, research, and practice* (4th ed., pp. 169–188); McKenzie, J. F., Neiger, B. L., & Thackery, R. (2013). *Planning, implementing, and evaluating health promotion programs: A primer* (6th ed.). Pearson; Simons-Morton, B. G., McLeroy, K. R., & Wendel, M. L. (2012). *Behavior theory in health promotion practice and research.* Jones & Bartlett Learning.

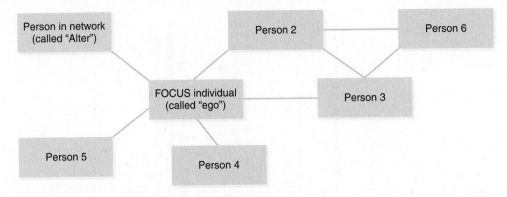

Figure 4.7 A simple sociogram, centered on a "focus individual" or ego.

Reproduced from Edberg, M. (2019). *Essentials of health behavior: Social and behavioral theory in public health* (3rd ed., Fig. 5-1, p. 56). Jones & Bartlett Learning.

health education specialists who are planning interventions need to consider whether social networks should be a part of their strategy to bring about change. With the power of the Internet, the impact of social networks in the work of health education specialists continues to grow.

Social Capital Theory

The term **social capital** got its start in political science and has been used in health education/promotion since the mid-1990s. An often-quoted definition is "the relationships and structures within a community, such as civic participation, networks, norms of reciprocity, and trust that promote cooperation of mutual benefit" (Putnam, 1995, p. 66). "Social capital is a collective asset, a feature of communities rather than the property of individuals. As such, individuals both contribute to it and use it, but they cannot own it" (Warren et al., 2001, p. 1).

"The influence of social capital is well documented" (Crosby et al., 2009). There are epidemiological studies that show that greater social capital is linked to several different positive outcomes (i.e., reduced mortality). There are also correlational studies that show a lack of social capital is related to poorer health outcomes (e.g., Kawachi et al., 1997). But as with social networks, a cause-effect

relationship has not been established between social capital and better health. "Social capital does not provide theories of change, tools, or time lines for change; nor does it necessarily guarantee improved outcomes if social capital is improved" (Minkler & Wallerstein, 2005, p. 38). However, it does seem to have an impact on health.

Figure 4.8 provides a graphic representation of social capital. This particular figure includes the key concepts of Putman's (1995) definition of social capital and three different types of network resources: bonding, bridging, and linking social capital. These three types are differentiated based on the strength of the relationships between/among those people in the social network (Hayden, 2019). Originally, *bonding social capital*, sometimes referred to as exclusive social capital, was defined as "the type that brings closer together people who already know each other" (Gittell & Vidal, 1998, p. 15). More recently, this concept was expanded to include people who are similar or people who are members of the same group. Examples of bonding social capital include those who may be members in a service organization (e.g., Kiwanis, Rotary International) or religious community.

Bridging social capital, sometimes referred to as inclusive social capital, was originally defined as "the type that brings together people

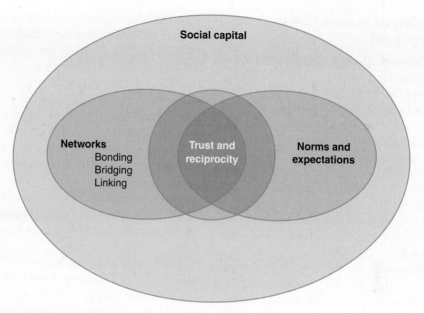

Figure 4.8 Social capital.

Reproduced from Hayden, J. (2019). *Introduction to health behavior theory* (3rd ed., Fig. 11.4, p. 259). Jones & Bartlett Learning.

or groups who previously did not know each other" (Gittell & Vidal, 1998, p. 15). Bridging social capital is now seen more as the resources people obtain from their interaction with others outside their group, who often are people with different demographic characteristics. An example is people from different parts of a community who come together to create a community park.

The most recently recognized and weakest (Hayden, 2019) network resource is *linking social capital*. This type of network resource comes from relationships between or among "individuals and groups in different social strata in a hierarchy where power, social status, and wealth are accessed by different groups" (U.K. Office of National Statistics, 2001, p. 11). An example may be when a boss and an employee are working together on a project.

As with social networks, it is important that health education specialists think about the concept of social capital when planning interventions. Although it is not an intervention, it is a concept that needs to be considered and monitored.

Community Theories

This group of theories includes three categories of factors from the socio-ecological approach—organizational, community, and public policy. Organizational factors include rules, regulations, and policies of an organization that can impact health behavior. Community factors include social norms (e.g., what is deemed a desirable behavior within a particular community) whereas public policy includes legislation that can impact health behavior such as antismoking laws or motorcycle helmet laws. Theories associated with these three factors include theories of community organizing and community building (see Chapter 1), organizational change, the Diffusion Theory, and the Community Readiness Model (a stage model). The latter two are described in the following sections.

Diffusion of Innovations Theory (DIF)

The **Diffusion Theory (DIF)** provides an explanation for how new products, ideas, techniques, behaviors, or services (known as innovations) are adopted within populations. When people become "consumers" of an innovation, they are referred to as adopters. Rogers (2003) categorized adopters on the basis of when they adopt innovations. These categories include innovators, early adopters, early or late majority, and laggards. The rate at which people become adopters can be represented by the bell-shaped curve (see **Figure 4.9**).

Innovators are the first to adopt an innovation. They are venturesome, independent, risky, and daring. They want to be the first to do something. **Early adopters** are very interested in innovation, but they do not want to be the first involved. Early adopters are respected by others in the social system and looked at as opinion leaders.

Following the early adopters is the **early majority**. This group of people may be interested in the innovation but need some external motivation to get involved. These people, along with those in the late majority, make up the largest groups. The **late majority** comprises people who are skeptical. They will not adopt an innovation until most people in the social system have done so. The **laggards** are the last ones to get involved in an innovation, if they get involved at all.

Following is an application of the Diffusion Theory. The health education staff at the Family Medicine Residency (FMR) is beginning a new series of classes designed to

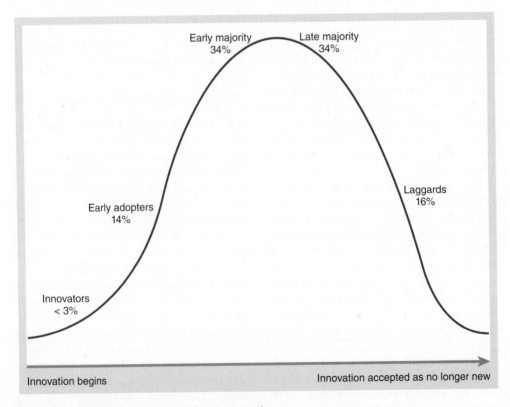

Figure 4.9 Bell-shaped curve and adopter categories.

assist adults in patient families make healthier choices when shopping for food. Approximately 3% of the patients (the innovators) will sign up and attend the classes as soon as they hear about the series. Shortly thereafter, another 14% (early adopters) will probably get involved, possibly after reading about the program's merits. At this point, the health education staff must work harder to attract others to the program. It will take constant reminders to get the early majority (~34%) involved. Buddy, peer, or mentoring programs might be needed to get the late majority (~34%) involved. The laggards (~16%) probably will not attend the food shopping sessions at all.

Community Readiness Model (CRM)

The Community Readiness Model (CRM) is a stage theory for communities. Communities, like individuals, are in various stages of readiness for change. Yet, the stages of change for communities are not the same as for individuals. "The stages of readiness in a community have to deal with group processes and group organization, characteristics that are not relevant to personal readiness" (Edwards et al., 2000, pp. 296–297). Although the CRM was developed initially to deal with alcohol and drug abuse, it also has been used in a variety of health and nutrition areas, environmental issues, and social programs (Edwards et al., 2000). The CRM has nine stages (Edwards et al., 2000):

1. *No Awareness.* The problem is not generally recognized by the community or leaders.
2. *Denial.* There is little or no recognition in the community that there is a problem. If recognition exists, there is a feeling that nothing can be done about the problem.
3. *Vague Awareness.* Some people in the community feel there is a problem and

something should be done, but there is no motivation or leadership to do so.
4. *Preplanning.* There is a clear recognition by some that a problem exists and something should be done. There are leaders, but no focused or detailed planning.
5. *Preparation.* Planning is taking place but it is not based on collected data. There is leadership and modest support for efforts. Resources are being sought.
6. *Initiation.* Information is available to justify and begin efforts. Staff is either in training or has just completed training. Leaders are enthusiastic. There is usually little resistance and involvement from the community members.
7. *Stabilization.* The program is running, staffed, and supported by the community and decision makers. The program is perceived as stable with no need for change. This stage may include routine tracking, but no in-depth evaluation.
8. *Confirmation/Expansion.* Standard efforts are in place, which are supported by the community and decision makers. The program has been evaluated and modified, and efforts are in place to seek resources for new efforts. There is ongoing data collection to link risk factors and problems.
9. *Professionalism.* Much is known about prevalence, risk factors, and cause of problems. Highly trained staff members run effective programs aimed at the general population and appropriate subgroups. Programs have been evaluated and modified. The community is supportive but should hold programs accountable.

A community's readiness can be assessed through interviews with key informants. As with other stage theories, once the stage of readiness is known, there are suggested processes for moving a community from one stage to the next. **Table 4.4** presents the nine stages and the goal for each stage.

Table 4.4 Stages of the Community Readiness Model as Applied to Suicide Prevention

Stages of Readiness	Description
1. No Awareness	SUICIDE PREVENTION is not generally recognized by the community or leaders as a problem (or it may truly not be an issue).
2. Denial/Resistance	At least some community members recognize that SUICIDE is a concern, but there is little recognition that it might be occurring locally.
3. Vague Awareness	Most feel that there is local concern, but there is no immediate motivation to do anything about it.
4. Preplanning	There is clear recognition that something must be done, and there may even be a group addressing it. However, efforts are not focused or detailed.
5. Preparation	Active leaders begin planning in earnest. Community offers modest support of efforts.
6. Initiation	Enough information is available to justify efforts. Activities are underway.
7. Stabilization	Activities are supported by administrators or community decision makers. Staff are trained and experienced.
8. Confirmation/Expansion	Efforts are in place. Community members feel comfortable using services, and they support expansions. Local data are regularly obtained.
9. High Level of Community Ownership	Detailed and sophisticated knowledge exists about SUICIDE and SUICIDE PREVENTION prevalence and consequences. Effective evaluation guides new directions. Model is applied to other issues.

Reproduced from Plested, B. A., Jumper-Thurman, P., & Edwards, R. W. (2014). *Community readiness manual on suicide prevention in native communities.* Substance Abuse and Mental Health Services Administration Tribal Training and Technical Assistance Center https://www.samhsa.gov/sites/default/files /tribal_tta_center_2.3.b_commreadinessmanual_final_3.6.14.pdf. (Original work published 2006).

Planning Models

Good health education/promotion programs are not created by chance. Well-thought-out and well-conceived models provide health education specialists with "frames" on which to build plans (see Practitioner's Perspective). Although many planning models have similar principles and common elements, those elements may have different labels. In fact, "there are important differences in sequence, emphasis, and the conceptualization of the major components that make certain models more appealing than others to

individual practitioners" (Simons-Morton, et al., 1995, pp. 126–127).

The following sections provide an overview of seven models used for planning health education/promotion programs. Although many more models exist, these seven have been used successfully, and they represent a wide range of planning approaches. **Box 4.2** lists other planning models that may be just as sound from a theoretical perspective, but currently they are not used as frequently in health promotion research. For more detailed explanations, see the original publications of the models.

Practitioner's Perspective

Theories and Planning Models: Trevor W. Newby

CURRENT POSITION/TITLE: Public Health Advisor / Project Officer

EMPLOYER: Centers for Disease Control and Prevention (CDC)

MAJOR: Health Promotion

DEGREES: Master of Health Science in Health Promotion and Bachelor of Science in Health Promotion

INSTITUTION: Boise State University

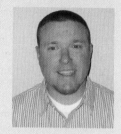

Courtesy of Trevor W. Newby.

How I obtained my job: Obtaining my current job started in college with my graduate assistantships, where I was able to align myself with supervisors and professors at Boise State University, which made me more marketable upon graduation. Following a lead from a professor, I applied for a position as a Health Education Specialist with the Idaho State Respiratory Health Program. This experience allowed me to work with a number of statewide programs and a variety of different organizations while taking part in a number of collaboration efforts related to that position. Most notably, I was able to work with our project officer, as well as others from the CDC, who mentored me with technical assistance and programmatic directives related to the grant I was working on. This not only increased my knowledge in public health but also allowed me to gain the networking I needed to take the next step in my professional career.

How I use theory in my job: At CDC, I have the opportunity to provide technical assistance for tobacco prevention and control efforts taking place on a nationwide level. This involves knowing a wide variety of theories including stages of change that is commonly used to assist smokers quit tobacco from the precontemplation stage through the maintenance stage of their behavior change process. Social norm changes are implemented with policies from the local and state levels, which are supported by CDC providing written testimony, evidence-based science, and supporting data. In addition to this, public health–related theories are also commonly used and supported by CDC to maintain and enhance programmatic and policy-driven efforts. These include states collaborating with partners to implement clean indoor air laws, point of sale restrictions to prevent minors from purchasing tobacco, and other environmental change strategies that promote smoking cessation and decrease exposure to secondhand smoke.

Programmatic efforts are organized using logic models, work plans, and budgets that are implemented and evaluated at the state level. These plans are approved by CDC project officers. In addition to this, monthly technical assistance calls are used to verify the progression and challenges being faced concerning work plan efforts. Evaluation efforts are also monitored on a monthly basis, and data collected from the states are used to formulate state-specific data, as well as comparisons on a nationwide basis in relation to tobacco.

Recommendations for health education specialists: First, secure internship opportunities. Internship settings will not only provide valuable work experience that will put you ahead of other potential job seekers but will also allow you to apply classroom learning while offering networking opportunities at the same time. The more internships you secure, the more diverse and enticing your portfolio will become for potential employers. Never base your internships on a lack of knowledge or the amount of pay it offers, if any. Second, be proficient in grant writing and managing a budget. These are valuable skills that are necessary in the public health profession. Third, take a number of marketing classes. Marketing plays an imperative role in public health. A public health program could have the most dynamic program or resource available, but it won't provide any benefit unless it is effectively marketed to its intended

(continues)

Practitioner's Perspective *(continued)*

Theories and Planning Models: Trevor W. Newby

audience. Fourth, be your own advocate. Take every opportunity to network within a wide variety of public health topics. Do not limit your networking opportunities to the public health topic you are currently assigned. Knowledge is important, but knowing the individuals that can help you open doors to career opportunities or new innovative ideas is paramount to your success. Networking will play a vital role in helping you achieve these goals. Lastly, don't be afraid to learn. Public health is a constantly evolving field with a wide variety of topics. In order to be a proficient educator, constant research and information gathering are critical.

Future of the health education/promotion profession: I consider the future of health education specialists in public health to be very positive. It has taken many years for businesses, lawmakers, and policy makers to realize the worth of proper prevention methods provided by public health professionals, but now the dynamic is changing. Prevention practices have already been proven to be effective with research surrounding tobacco. Prevention strategies, such as those found in CDC's *Best Practices*, have saved millions of dollars in healthcare costs to taxpayers in relation to tobacco use and have begun to change the social norm of tobacco use as a whole. I am certain prevention practices will play a vital role in the Affordable Care Act with tobacco cessation being a utilized strategy, along with a host of other prevention strategies pertaining to public health. As more emphasis is placed on prevention practices, the government, as well as businesses, will save millions of dollars on secondary and tertiary clinical care by implementing effective prevention practices provided by public health professionals. This will provide many jobs to health education specialists in an increasingly changing and meaningful profession.

PRECEDE-PROCEED

Currently, the best known planning model is **PRECEDE-PROCEED**. As its name implies, this model has two components. PRECEDE is an acronym that stands for predisposing, reinforcing, and enabling constructs in educational/ecological diagnosis and evaluation. PROCEED stands for policy, regulatory, and organizational constructs in educational and environmental development (Green & Kreuter, 2005).

The PRECEDE-PROCEED model was developed over a period of 15 to 20 years.

Box 4.2 Other Planning Models

- *Comprehensive Health Education Model* (Sullivan, 1973)
- *Model for Health Education Planning* (Ross & Mico, 1980)
- *Model for Health Education Planning and Resource Development* (Bates & Winder, 1984)
- *Planned Approach To Community Health (PATCH)* (CDC & USDHHS, n.d.)
- *Generic Health/Fitness Delivery System* (Patton, Corry, Gettman, & Graff, 1986)
  - *Community Health Assessment and Group Evaluation (CHANGE) Tool* (CDC, 2019)

- *Assessment Protocol for Excellence in Public Health (APEX/PH)* (National Association of County and City Health Officials [NACCHO], 1991)
  - *Logic Model* (W.K. Kellogg Foundation, 2004 and Weiss, C., & Wholey, J., n.d.).
- *Healthy People in Healthy Communities* (U.S. Department of Health and Human Services [USDHHS], 2001)
- *The Planning, Program Development, and Evaluation Model* (Timmreck, 2003)
- *MAP-IT* (USDHHS, 2011)
- *SWOT* (Strengths, Weaknesses, Opportunities, Threats) *Analysis*

The PRECEDE framework was conceived in the early 1970s, whereas the PROCEED portion was developed in the early to mid-1980s. As shown in **Figure 4.10**, PRECEDE-PROCEED has eight phases. The first four phases, which make up the PRECEDE portion of the model, consist "of a series of planned assessments that generate information that will be used to guide subsequent decisions" (Green & Kreuter, 2005, p. 8). PROCEED also has four phases and "is marked by the strategic implementation of multiple actions based on what was learned from the assessments in the initial phase" (Green & Kreuter, 2005, p. 9).

At first glance, the PRECEDE-PROCEED model appears overly complicated. However, there is a logical sequence to the eight phases that outlines the health promotion planning process. The underlying approach of this model begins by identifying the desired outcome, then determines what causes it, and finally designs an intervention aimed at reaching the desired outcome. In other words, PRECEDE-PROCEED starts with the final consequences and works backward to the causes (McKenzie et al., 2013). **Table 4.5** provides an overview of the eight phases of this model.

MATCH

MATCH is an acronym for Multilevel Approach To Community Health. This planning model (see **Figure 4.11**) was developed in the late 1980s (Simons-Morton, Simons-Morton, Parcel, & Bunker, 1988). Like the PRECEDE-PROCEED model, MATCH has also been used in a variety of settings. For example, several intervention handbooks created by the Centers for Disease Control and Prevention (CDC) used MATCH (Simons-Morton et al., 1995).

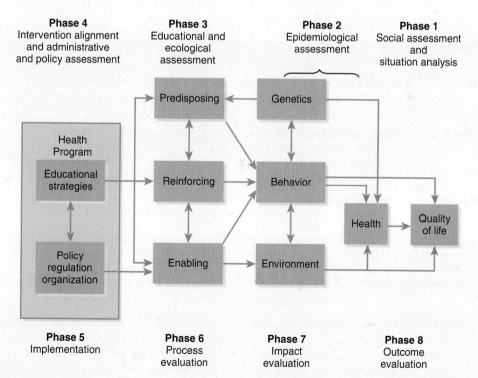

Figure 4.10 PRECEDE-PROCEED model for health program planning.

Table 4.5 The Eight Phases of the PRECEDE-PROCEED Model

Phase 1	**Social assessment** is "the assessment in both objective and subjective terms of high-priority problems or aspirations for the common good, defined for a population by economic and social indicators and by individuals in terms of their quality of life" (p. G-8), **situational analysis** is "the combination of social and epidemiological assessments of conditions, trends, and priorities with a preliminary scan of determinants, relevant policies, resources, organizational support, and regulations that might anticipate or permit action in advance of a more complete assessment of behavioral, environmental, educational, ecological, and administrative factors" (pp. G-7–8).
Phase 2	**Epidemiological assessment** is "the delineation of the extent, distribution, and causes of a health problem in a defined population" (p. G-3).
Phase 3	**Educational assessment** is "the delineation of factors that predispose, enable, and reinforce a specific behavior, or through behavior, environmental changes" (p. G-3), and **ecological assessment** is "a systematic assessment of factors in the social and physical environment that interact with behavior to produce health effects or quality-of-life outcomes" (p. G-3).
Phase 4a	**Intervention alignment** is matching appropriate strategies and interventions with projected changes and outcomes identified in earlier phases.
Phase 4b	**Administrative and policy assessment** is "an analysis of the policies, resources, and circumstances prevailing in an organizational situation to facilitate or hinder the development of the health program" (p. G-1).
Phase 5	**Implementation** is "the act of converting program objectives into actions through policy changes, regulation, and organization" (p. G-5).
Phase 6	**Process evaluation** is "the assessment of policies, materials, personnel, performance, quality of practice or services, and other inputs and implementation experiences" (p. G-6).
Phase 7	**Impact evaluation** is "the assessment of program effects on intermediate objectives including changes in predisposing, enabling, and reinforcing factors, as well as behavioral and environmental changes, and possibly health and social outcomes" (p. G-5).
Phase 8	**Outcome evaluation** is an "assessment of the effects of a program on its ultimate objectives, including changes in health and social benefits or quality of life" (p. G-6).

Reproduced from Green, L. W., & Kreuter, M. W. (2005). *Health program planning: An educational and ecological approach* (4th ed.). McGraw-Hill. Reprinted by permission of the authors. An updated version of the model will be available in the forthcoming edition, Green et al. (2022). *Health program planning, implementation, and evaluation.* Johns Hopkins University Press.

MATCH is a socio-ecological planning approach. It recognizes that intervention activities can and should be aimed at a variety of objectives and individuals. This approach is illustrated in Figure 4.11 by the various levels of influence.

The MATCH framework is recognized for emphasizing program implementation (Simons-Morton et al., 1995). This planning approach was "designed to be applied when behavioral and environmental risk and protective factors for disease or injury

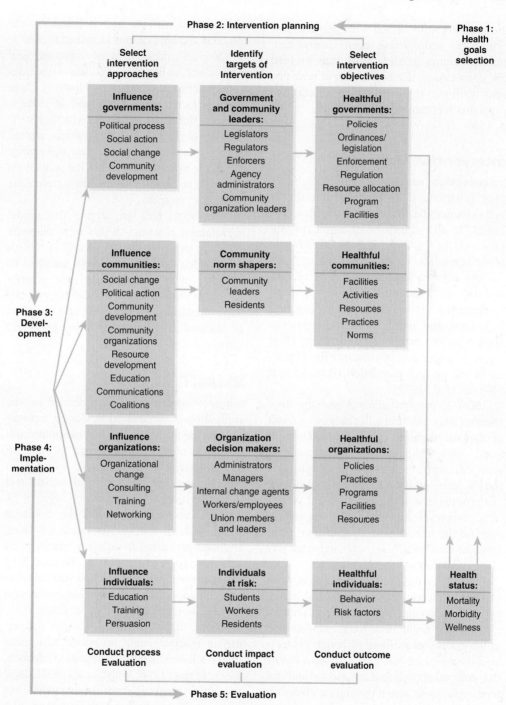

Figure 4.11 MATCH: Multilevel Approach To Community Health.

Reproduced from Simons-Morton, B. G., Greene, W. H., & Gottlieb, N. H. (1995). *Introduction to health education and promotion* (2nd ed.). Waveland Press.

are generally known and when general priorities for action have been determined, thus providing a convenient way to turn the corner from needs assessment and priority setting to the development of effective programs" (Simons-Morton et al., 1995, p. 155).

Intervention Mapping

Intervention mapping focuses on planning programs that are based on theory and evidence (Bartholomew Eldredge et al., 2016). It also draws on multiple principles used in the PRECEDE-PROCEED and MATCH models.

Intervention mapping has six steps. The first step, *needs assessment*, includes two major components: (1) scientific, epidemiological, behavioral, and social analysis of a priority population or community; and (2) an effort to get to know and understand the character of the priority population (Bartholomew Eldredge et al., 2016).

Step 2, *program outcomes and objectives*, specifies who and what will change as a result of the intervention (Bartholomew Eldredge et al., 2016). Although the identification of goals and objectives is included in all planning models, intervention mapping makes a unique contribution in how this is carried out. In this step, planners create a matrix of change objectives for the intervention. By doing so, planners can more clearly see who and what will change as a result of the intervention.

In Step 3, *program design* planners work to identify theory-based methods and practical applications that hold the greatest promise to change the health behavior(s) of individuals in the priority population. Although planners seek theory-based methods, they also ensure that practical applications are selected and that final applications match the change objectives from the matrices.

In Step 4, *program production*, planners create the intervention details and materials and protocol needed for the program's implementation. This step is based on the methods and applications identified in Step 3.

Step 5, *adoption, implementation, and maintenance*, is like Step 2 in that it includes the development of matrices. However, these matrices focus on adoption and implementation performance objectives (Bartholomew Eldredge et al., 2016). In other words, instead of concentrating on who and what will change within the priority population, the focus is on what will be done by whom among planners or program partners.

The sixth, and last, step of this model is *evaluation planning*. In this step, planners decide if determinants were well specified, if strategies were appropriately matched to methods, what proportion of the priority population was reached, and whether or not implementation was complete and executed as planned (Bartholomew Eldredge et al., 2016).

SMART

Social marketing has been defined as "the application of commercial marketing technologies to the analysis, planning, execution, and evaluation of programs designed to influence the voluntary behavior of target audiences in order to improve their personal welfare and that of their society" (Andreasen, 1995, p. 7). This process offers benefits the audience wants, reduces barriers the audience faces, and uses persuasion to influence intentions to act favorably (Albrecht, 1997). The concept of social marketing is more than 30 years old, but its application to health education/promotion is much more recent (McDermott, 2000).

Even though the use of social marketing is relatively new in health education/promotion, several different authors (Andreasen, 1995; Bryant, 1998; Walsh et al., 1993) have presented planning processes, models, or frameworks based on social marketing. The Social Marketing Assessment and Response Tool **(SMART)** is a social marketing planning framework developed by Neiger and

Thackeray (1998) and influenced primarily by Walsh and colleagues (1993). It is presented here because it provides a composite of other social marketing models and because it has been used from start to finish on multiple occasions in several social marketing interventions (Neiger & Thackeray, 2002).

SMART is composed of seven phases (see **Table 4.6**). As a social marketing model, SMART focuses on the consumers (i.e., the priority population). That focus is presented in Phases 2 through 4 of the model, the phases where the analyses of the consumers, marketing mix, and communication channels are completed. Because the results of these analyses are needed prior to developing an intervention, they are often conducted simultaneously rather than in the linear order in which they are displayed (McKenzie et al., 2013).

MAPP

MAPP is an acronym for Mobilizing for Action through Planning and Partnerships. It is a planning model created by the National Association of County and City Health Officials (NACCHO) to assist local health departments (LHDs) at the city or county level with planning. This model blends many of the strengths of the planning models already presented in this chapter. MAPP is designed to provide a structure for communities to assess health needs and align resources for strategic action (NACCHO, 2021). The process results in a community health needs assessment and community health improvement plan (CHIP).

MAPP is composed of multiple steps within three phases (see **Figure 4.12**). In the first phase of MAPP, Build the CHI Foundation, includes an analysis of stakeholders readiness and resources to engage in and support the process.

Phase 2, Tell the Community Story, involves a comprehensive, accurate, and timely community assessment of health and well-being.

Phase 3, Continuously Improve the Community, provides structured methods of continuous quality improvement and a framework for monitoring and evaluating short and long-term impact on CHIP priorities (Clayton et al., 2020).

Generalized Model (GM)

As seen in the planning models presented so far, there are various approaches and frameworks on which to develop a program. Each model seems to have its own characteristics, whether it is the terminology used (e.g., predisposing, enabling, and reinforcing or analyzing a problem or consumer analysis), the number of components (e.g., eight phases versus six steps), or the progression through the phases or steps (e.g., circular, linear, or starting with the desired end and working backward). In other words, there are many ways to get from point A to point B. However, each of the models previously presented revolves around the five primary tasks incorporated in the **Generalized Model** (McKenzie et al., 2013). These five tasks are

1. Assessing needs
2. Setting goals and objectives
3. Developing interventions
4. Implementing interventions
5. Evaluating results (see **Figure 4.13**)

"In addition, pre-planning is a quasi-step in the model but is not included formally since it involves actions that occur before planning technically begins" (McKenzie et al., 2013, p. 44). These tasks plus the quasi-step of preplanning define planning and evaluation at its core.

To better understand the planning process in health education/promotion and the various models presented, consider the following scenario. A health education specialist was hired to develop health education/promotion programs in a corporate setting.

Table 4.6 The SMART Model

Phase 1: Preliminary Planning

- Identify a health problem and name it in terms of behavior.
- Develop general goals.
- Outline preliminary plans for evaluation.
- Project program costs.

Phase 2: Consumer Analysis

- Segment and identify the priority population.
- Identify formative research methods.
- Identify consumer wants, needs, and preferences.
- Develop preliminary ideas for preferred interventions.

Phase 3: Market Analysis

- Establish and define the market mix (4Ps).
- Assess the market to identify competitors (behaviors, messages, programs, etc.), allies (support systems, resources, etc.), and partners.

Phase 4: Channel Analysis

- Identify appropriate communication messages, strategies, and channels.
- Assess options for program distribution. Determine how channels should be used.
- Assess options for program distribution.
- Identify communication roles for program partners.

Phase 5: Develop Interventions, Materials, and Pretest

- Develop program interventions and materials using information collected in consumer, market, and channel analyses.
- Interpret the marketing mix into a strategy that represents exchange and societal good.
- Pretest and refine the program.

Phase 6: Implementation

- Communicate with partners and clarify involvement.
- Activate communication and distribution strategies.
- Document procedures and compare progress to timelines.
- Refine the program.

Phase 7: Evaluation

- Assess the degree to which the priority population is receiving the program.
- Assess the immediate impact on the priority population and refine the program as necessary.
- Ensure that program delivery is consistent with established protocol.
- Analyze changes in the priority population.

Data from Chapman Walsh, D., Rudd, R. E., Moeykens, B. A., & Moloney, T. W. (1993). Social marketing for public health. *Health Affairs, 12*(2), 104–119. https://doi.org/10.1377/hlthaff.12.2.104; Neiger, B. L., & Thackeray, R. (1998). *Social marketing: Making public health sense.* Paper presented at the annual meeting of the Utah Public Health Association, Provo, UT.

The Revised MAPP Phases

Phase 1: Build the Community Health Improvement (CHI) Foundation	Phase 2: Tell the Community Story	Phase 3: Continuously Improve the Community
Decide to Conduct MAPP 2.0	Form the Assessment Design Team	Prioritize Issues for CHIP
Lead Agency Conducts Initial Power Analysis	Design the Assessments	Conduct Power Analysis on Each Issue
Establish/Revisit CHI Leadership Structures	Conduct the Community Partners Assessment	Establish Priority Issue Sub-Committees
Engage and Orient Leadership Committees	Conduct the Community Status Assessment	Create Community Partner Profiles
Define Community and Develop the CHI Mission	Conduct the Community Context Assessment	Develop Shared Goals and Long-Term Measures
Develop a Community Vision	Present Data to Community and Identify Top Issues	Develop Strategies and Conduct (Racial) Equity Impact Assessment as Appropriate
Conduct a Starting Point Assessment	Develop Issue Profiles through Root Cause Analysis	Continuous Quality Improvement Action Planning Cycles
Identify CHI Infrastructure Scope and Develop CHI Plan	Disseminate Community Assessment Findings	Ongoing Monitoring and Evaluation of CHIP

Coordinate CHI Infrastructure Workgroups
Across phases workgroups will build and evaluate critical elements of CHI infrastructure such as data capacity, broadening funding and resources, evaluation, partner engagement, and health equity and community engagement.

Figure 4.12 Mobilizing for Action through Planning and Partnerships (MAPP) model.

Reproduced from Clayton, A., Verma, P., & Weller Pegna, S. (2020). *MAPP evolution blueprint executive summary.* National Association of County & City Health Officials. https://www.naccho.org/uploads /downloadable-resources/MAPP-Evolution-Blueprint-Executive-Summary-V3-FINAL.pdf

She began her work with the quasi-step of preplanning by trying to find out as much as possible about the "community" of this corporate setting and get those in the priority population involved in the program planning process. She did this by reading all the material she could find about the company. She also spent time talking with various individuals and subgroups in the company (i.e., new employees, longtime employees, management, clerical staff, labor representatives, etc.) to find out what they wanted from a health education/promotion program. In addition, she reviewed old documents of the company (i.e., health insurance records, labor agreements, written history of the company, etc.). As part of this background work, she formed a program planning committee with representation from the various subgroups of the workforce.

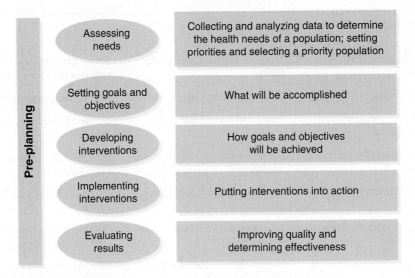

Figure 4.13 Generalized Model.

With the help of the planning committee, the health education/promotion specialist was ready to assess the needs of the priority population. She did this by reviewing the relevant literature, examining company health insurance claims, conducting a survey of employees, and holding focus groups with selected employees. As a result of the needs assessment, she was able to identify a target health problem. In this company, the problem was a higher than expected number of breast cancer cases in the priority population. This was a result in part of (1) the limited knowledge of employees about breast cancer, (2) the limited number of employees conducting breast self-examination (BSE), and (3) the low number of employees having mammograms on a regular basis.

With an understanding of the needs of the priority population, the health education specialist created specific objectives to increase the (1) employees' knowledge of breast cancer from baseline to after program participation, (2) number of women receiving mammograms by 30%, and (3) number of women reporting monthly BSE by 50%.

Using these objectives, she planned multiple intervention activities:

1. An information sheet on the importance of BSE and mammography, for distribution with employee paychecks
2. A mobile mammography van on site every other month
3. Plastic BSE reminder cards, suitable for hanging from a showerhead, for distribution to all female employees
4. An article in the company newsletter covering the company's high rate of breast cancer and the new program to help women reduce their risk
5. Posters and pamphlets from the American Cancer Society in the company's lunchroom

Next, all the listed intervention activities were carried out. Finally, the health education specialist completed an evaluation to determine if there was an increase in knowledge, mammograms, and monthly BSE. As can be seen from this scenario, health education/promotion involves careful, systematic planning to achieve successful programs.

Summary

Health education/promotion is a multidisciplinary profession that has evolved from the theory and practice of other biological, behavioral, sociological, and health science disciplines. Many of the theories and models used in health education/promotion have also evolved from these other disciplines. This chapter presented an overview of the theoretical foundations and planning models of health education/promotion. Readers were introduced to the definitions of *theory, concept, construct, variable*, and *model*. A rationale was provided to explain why it is important that health education specialists use theory in their work. Readers were then introduced to eleven of the behavior change theories that health education specialists use in their work. These theories were presented within the socio-ecological approach, which incorporates the seven levels of influence. There was also a distinction made between continuum theories and stage theories. And finally, overviews of six planning models were provided.

Review Questions

1. Define each of the following and explain how they relate to each other.
   - *Theory*
   - *Concept*
   - *Construct*
   - *Variable*
   - *Model*
2. Why is it important to use theory in the practice of health education/promotion?
3. What are behavior change theories?
4. What are the seven levels of influence within the socio-ecological approach? How do they relate to behavior change theories?
5. Identify the eleven theories presented in this chapter that focus on health behavior change. Briefly describe each of the theories and name their components.
6. What is the difference between continuum theories and stage theories?
7. Why is it important that health education specialists have a good understanding of stage models?
8. What are three advantages to using a planning model when preparing to conduct a health promotion intervention?
9. Name the six planning models presented in this chapter and list one distinguishing characteristic of each.
10. Of the six planning models presented in this chapter, which one is best known? Name the phases of this model.

Case Study

Rocio (pronoun: she/her/hers) graduated a year ago with a bachelor's degree in health education. She felt very fortunate to "beat out" 10 interviewees for the health education specialist position at the Ada County Health Department. Although the health department has a good reputation throughout the state, it turns out that Rocio is the only person on the staff hired to do health education.

Rocio's supervisor, Rick Shaw (pronoun: he/him/his), is the Environmental Health Coordinator for the health department. Rick has worked for the department for about 35 years. He holds a bachelor's degree from the same university Rocio graduated from. However, Rick received his general studies degree in health and fitness before the university formed new departments and implemented new majors including the current community/public health education major.

Throughout Rocio's tenure with the health department, she and Rick had had a good working relationship. However, when asked to plan a tobacco cessation program for a group of teenagers in the county, Rocio ran into a situation that caused her some concern. After conducting a needs assessment and writing the program goals and objectives, she could not decide which behavior change theory to use to plan her intervention so she decided to seek her supervisor's advice. When she asked Rick what theory or model he would recommend, he responded rather dramatically, "Theory-shmeary, you don't need to use that stuff; just skip the theory part and get to work planning the intervention.

Remember, this program needs to be up and running by the end of the month."

Based on this short conversation with her supervisor, Rocio was left unsure as to how to proceed. During her undergraduate preparation at the university, Rocio was told time and time again to "never plan an intervention that was not based on theory." Rocio does not want to upset her supervisor, but she also knows that her program should be grounded in theory. What are Rocio's options at this point? How should she proceed? What process would you use to address this dilemma?

Critical Thinking Questions

1. This chapter presented a number of different theories focusing on health behavior change. If you were trying to help a friend stop using nicotine, at the friend's request, what behavior change theory would you use to develop the intervention to help your friend? Defend why you selected this theory and explain how you would apply each of the constructs.

2. You have been invited by the Nelson Corporation to interview for a newly created position in the company as a health education specialist. The position has been described as one that will focus on helping employees become healthier by modifying or changing selected health behaviors. As a part of the interview, the director of human resources asks you this question: "Of all the theories related to health education/promotion you studied in your college courses, which one do you think will have the greatest application to your work here at the Nelson Corporation?" Defend your response.

3. What would you say to a person who asked you, "Tell me how the socio-ecological approach applies to changing health behavior?"

Activities

1. Interview a practicing health education specialist, asking about the theories and models the person has used in planning and implementing health education/promotion programs. Ask why those theories and models were used. Also, find out if the health education specialist has run into any problems trying to use the theories and models. Summarize the interview in a one-page paper.

2. Choosing and selecting from the components found in the planning models, create your own model. Draw a diagram of your model and, in two paragraphs, explain why you have included the components you did.

3. Choose a health behavior. Conduct a literature search to determine if the behavior you chose has been researched using one of the behavior change theories in the chapter.

Weblinks

1. **http://www.naccho.org**

   National Association of County and City Health Officials

   At this website, the MAPP model is comprehensively presented and explained (search for "MAPP" on the homepage).

2. **https://health.gov/healthypeople**

   Healthy People 2030

   Scroll down the page to learn how to use Healthy People in program planning.

3. **https://web.uri.edu/cprc/**

   Cancer Prevention Research Center (CPRC), University of Rhode Island

   Home of the Transtheoretical Model of Change—information about the model as well as measures that can be used to "stage" a person can be found at this site.

4. **http://people.umass.edu/aizen/tpb.html**

   Theory of Planned Behavior

   This is a webpage of Icek Ajzen, creator of the Theory of Planned Behavior. Information about the theory as well as example measures that can be used to measure the constructs of the theory can be found at this site.

References

Ajzen, I. (2006). *Theory of Planned Behavior Diagram*. Retrieved May 19, 2013, from http://www.people.umass.edu/aizen/index.html

Albrecht, T. L. (1997). Defining social marketing: 25 years later. *Social Marketing Quarterly, 3*(3–4), 21–23.

Andreasen, A. (1995). *Marketing sound change: Changing behavior to promote health, social development, and the environment.* San Francisco: Jossey-Bass.

Bandura, A. (1977). *Social learning theory.* Englewood Cliffs, NJ: Prentice-Hall.

Bandura, A. (1986). *Social foundations of thought and action.* Englewood Cliffs, NJ: Prentice-Hall.

Barnes, J. A. (1954). Class and committees in a Norwegian island parish. *Human Relations, 7*(1), 39–58.

Bartholomew Eldredge, L. K., Markham, C. M., Ruiter, R. A., Fernández, M. E., Kok, G., & Parcel, G. S. (2016). *Planning health promotion programs: An intervention mapping approach* (4th ed.). San Francisco: Jossey-Bass.

Bates, I. J., & Winder, A. E. (1984). *Introduction to health education.* Palo Alto, CA: Mayfield.

Bronfenbrenner, U. (1974). Developmental research, public policy, and the ecology of childhood. (1974). *Child Development, 45*(1), 1–5.

Bronfenbrenner, U. (1979). *The ecology of human development: Experiments by nature and design.* Cambridge, MA: Harvard University Press.

Bryant, C. (1998). *Social marketing: A tool for excellence.* Eighth annual conference on social marketing in public health. Clearwater Beach, FL.

Centers for Disease Control and Prevention (CDC). (2019). Community Health Assessment and Group Evaluation (CHANGE) Tool Retrieved on January 16, 2021, from https://www.cdc.gov/nccdphp/dnpao/state-local-programs/change-tool/index.html

Centers for Disease Control and Prevention (CDC), U.S. Department of Health and Human Services (USDHHS). (n.d.). *Planned approach to community health: Guide for local coordinators.* Atlanta, GA.

Chaplin, J. P., & Krawiec, T. S. (1979). *Systems and theories of psychology* (4th ed.). New York: Holt, Rinehart & Winston.

Clayton, A., Verma, P., & Weller Pegna, S. (2020). *MAPP Evolution Blueprint Executive Summary*. Washington, DC: National Association of County & City Health Officials. Retrieved January 2, 2021 from https://www.naccho.org/uploads/downloadable-resources/MAPP-Evolution-Blueprint-Executive-Summary-V3-FINAL.pdf

Crosby, R. A., Kegler, M. C., & DiClemente, R. J. (2009). Theory in health promotion practice and research. In R. J. DiClemente, R. A. Crosby, & M. C. Kegler (Eds.), *Emerging theories in health promotion practice and research* (2nd ed., pp. 4–17). San Francisco: Jossey-Bass.

Crosby, R. A., Salazar, L. F., & DiClemente, R. J. (2013a). How theory informs health promotion and public health practice. In R. J. DiClemente, L. F. Salazar, & R. A. Crosby, *Health behavior theory for public health: Principles, foundations, and application* (pp. 27–44). Burlington, MA: Jones & Bartlett Learning.

Crosby, R. A., Salazar, L. F., & DiClemente, R. J. (2013b). Social cognitive theory applied to health behavior.

In R. J. DiClemente, L. F. Salazar, & R. A. Crosby, *Health behavior theory for public health: Principles, foundations, and application* (pp. 163–185). Burlington, MA: Jones & Bartlett Learning.

DiClemente, R. J., Crosby, R. A., & Kegler, M. (2009). *Emerging theories in health promotion practice and research* (2nd ed.). San Francisco: Jossey-Bass.

DiClemente, R. J., Redding, C. A., Crosby, R. A., & Salazar, L. F. (2013). Stage models for health promotion. In R. J. DiClemente, L. F. Salazar, & R. A. Crosby, *Health behavior theory for public health: Principles, foundations, and application* (pp. 105–129). Burlington, MA: Jones & Bartlett Learning.

DiClemente, R. J., Salazar, L. F., & Crosby, R. A. (2013). *Health behavior theory for public health: Principles, foundations, and applications.* Burlington, MA: Jones & Bartlett Learning.

Edberg, M. (2020). *Essentials of health behavior: Social and behavioral theory in public health* (3rd ed.). Burlington, MA: Jones & Bartlett Learning.

Edwards, R. W., Jumper-Thurman, P., Plested, B. A., Oetting, E. R., & Swanson, L. (2000). Community readiness: Research to practice. *Journal of Community Psychology, 28*(3), 291–307.

Fishbein, M., & Ajzen, I. (1975). *Belief, attitude, intention and behavior: An introduction to theory and research.* Reading, MA: Addison-Wesley.

Fisher, J. D., & Fisher, W. A. (1992). Changing AIDS risk behavior. *Psychological Bulletin, 111*(3), 455–474.

Fisher, J. D., Fisher, W. A., & Shuper, P. A. (2009). The informational-motivation-behavioral skills model of HIV preventive behavior. In R. J. DiClemente, R. A. Crosby, & M. C. Kegler (Eds.). *Emerging theories in health promotion practice and research* (2nd ed., pp. 21–63). San Francisco: Jossey-Bass.

Gittell, R., & Vidal, A. (1998). *Community organizing: Building social capital as a development strategy.* Thousand Oaks, CA: Sage.

Glanz, K., & Rimer, B. K. (1995). *Theory at a glance: A guide for health promotion practice* (NIH publication no. 95–3896). Bethesda, MD: National Institutes of Health, National Cancer Institute.

Glanz, K., Rimer, B. K., & Viswanath, K. (Eds.). (2015a). *Health behavior: Theory, research, and practice* (5th ed.). San Francisco: Jossey-Bass.

Glanz, K., Rimer, B. K., & Viswanath, K. (2015b). Theory, research, and practice in health behavior. In K. Glanz, B. K. Rimer, & K. Viswanath (Eds.), *Health behavior: Theory, research, and practice* (5th ed., pp. 23–42). San Francisco: Jossey-Bass.

Goodson, P. (2010). *Theory in health promotion research and practice: Thinking outside the box.* Sudbury, MA: Jones & Bartlett.

Gore, T. D., & Bracker, C. C. (2005). Testing the theoretical design of a health risk message: Re-examining major tenets of the Extended Parallel Processing Model. *Health Education & Behavior, 32*(1), 27–41.

Green, L. W., Glanz, K., Hochbaum, G. M., Kok, G., Kreuter, M. W., Lewis, F. M., Lorig, K., Morisky, D., Rimer, B. K., & Rosenstock, I. M. (1994). Can we build on, or must we replace, the theories and models in health education? *Health Education Research, 9*(3), 397–404.

Green, L. W., & Kreuter, M. W. (2005). *Health program planning: An educational and ecological approach* (4th ed.). Boston, MA: McGraw-Hill.

Hayden, J. (2019). *Introduction to health behavior theory* (3rd ed.). Burlington, MA: Jones & Bartlett Learning.

Institute of Medicine (IOM). (2001). *Health and behavior: The interplay of biological, behavioral, and societal influences.* Washington, DC: National Academy of Sciences.

Kawachi, I., Kennedy, B. P., Lochner, K., & Prothrow-Stith, D. (1997). Social capital, income, equality, and mortality. *American Journal of Public Health, 87*(9), 1491–1497.

Kelder, S. H., Hoelscher, D., & Perry, C. L. (2015). How individuals, environments, and health behaviors interact. In K. Glanz, B. K. Rimer, & K. Viswanath (Eds.), *Health behavior: Theory, research, and practice* (5th ed., pp. 159–182). San Francisco: Jossey-Bass.

Kerlinger, F. N. (1986). *Foundations of behavioral research* (3rd ed.). Austin: Holt, Rinehart & Winston.

Luszczynska, A., & Sutton, S. (2005). Attitudes and expectations. In J. Kerr, R. Weikunat, & M. Moretti (Eds.), *ABC of behavior change: A guide to successful disease prevention and health promotion* (pp. 71–84). Edinburgh: Elsevier.

Mann, T. Tomiyama, A. J., Westling. E., Lew. A.-M., Samuels, B., & Chatman, J. (2007). Medicare's search for effective obesity treatments: Diets are not the answer. *American Psychologist, 62*(3), 220–233.

McDermott, R. J. (2000). Social marketing: A tool for health education. *American Journal of Health Behavior, 24*(1), 6–10.

McKenzie, J. F., Neiger, B. L., & Thackeray, R. (2013). *Planning, implementing, and evaluating health promotion programs: A primer* (6th ed.). Boston: Pearson.

McLeroy, K. R., Bibeau, D., Steckler, A., & Glanz, K. (1988). An ecological perspective for health promotion programs. *Health Education Quarterly, 15*(4), 351–377.

Minkler, M., Thompson, M., Bell, J. & Rose, K. (2001). Contributions of community involvement to organizational-level empowerment: The federal Healthy Start experience. *Health Education & Behavior, 28*(6), 783–807.

Minkler, M., & Wallerstein, N. (2005). Improving health through community organization and community building: A health education perspective.

In M. Minkler (Ed.), *Community organizing and community building for health* (2nd ed., pp. 26–50). New Brunswick, NJ: Rutgers University Press.

National Association of County and City Health Officials (NACCHO). (1991). *APEX/PH, Assessment protocol for excellence in public health*. Washington, DC: Author.

National Cancer Institute (NCI). (2002). *Making health communication programs work* (NIH Publication No. 02-5145). Washington, DC: U.S. Department of Health and Human Services (USDHHS).

Neiger, B. L., & Thackeray R. (1998). *Social marketing: Making public health sense*. Paper presented at the annual meeting of the Utah Public Health Association. Provo, UT.

Neiger, B. L., & Thackeray, R. (2002). Application of the SMART model in two successful social marketing campaigns. *American Journal of Health Education, 33*(5), 301–303.

Parvanta, C. F., & Freimuth, V. (2000). Health communication at the Centers for Disease Control and Prevention. *American Journal of Health Behavior, 24*(1), 18–25.

Patton, R. P., Corry, J. M., Gettman, L. R., & Graff, J. S. (1986). *Implementing health/fitness programs*. Champaign, IL: Human Kinetics.

Petty, R. E., Barden, J., & Wheeler, S. C. (2009). The elaboration likelihood model of persuasion: Developing health promotions for sustained behavioral change. In R. J. DiClemente, R. A. Crosby, & M. C. Kegler (Eds.), *Emerging theories in health promotion practice and research* (2nd ed., pp. 185–214). San Francisco: Jossey-Bass.

Petty, R. E., & Cacioppo, J. T. (1986). The elaboration likelihood model of persuasion. In L. Berkowitz (Ed.). *Advances in experimental social psychology* (Vol. 19, pp. 123–205). New York: Academic Press.

Prochaska, J. (2005). Stages of change, readiness, and motivation. In J. Kerr, R. Weitkunat, & M. Moretti (Eds.), *ABC of behavior change: A guide to successful disease prevention and health promotion* (pp. 111–123). Edinburgh: Elsevier.

Prochaska, J. O. (1979). *Systems of psychotherapy: A transtheoretical analysis*. Homewood, IL: Dorsey Press.

Prochaska, J. O., & DiClemente, C. C. (1983). Stages and processes of self-change of smoking: Toward an integrative model of change. *Journal of Consulting and Clinical Psychology, 51*(3), 390–395.

Prochaska, J. O., Johnson, S., & Lee, P. (1998). The transtheoretical model of behavior change. In S. A. Shumaker, E. B. Schron, J. K. Ockene, & W. L. McBee (Eds.), *The handbook of health behavior change* (2nd ed., pp. 59–84). New York: Springer Publishing Company.

Prochaska, J. O, Redding, C. A., & Evers, K. E. (2015). The transtheoretical model and stages of change.

In K. Glanz, B. K. Rimer, & K. Viswanath (Eds.), *Health behavior: Theory, research, and practice* (5th ed., pp. 125–148). San Francisco: Jossey-Bass.

Prochaska, J. O., Redding, C. A., Harlow, L. L., Rossi, J. S., & Velicer, W. F. (1994). The transtheoretical model of change and HIV prevention: A review. *Health Education Quarterly, 21*(4), 471–486.

Putman, R. D. (1995). Bowling alone: America's declining social capital. *Journal of Democracy, 6*(1), 65–78.

Redding, C. A., Rossi, J. S., Rossi, S. R., Velicer, W. F., & Prochaska, J. O. (1999). Health behavior models. In G. C. Hyner, K. W. Peterson, J. W. Travis, J. E. Dewey, J. J. Foerster, & E. M. Framer (Eds.), *SPM handbook of health assessment tools* (pp. 83–93). Pittsburgh: The Society of Prospective Medicine.

Rimer, B. K., & Glanz, K. (2005). *Theory at a glance: A guide for health promotion practice* (2nd ed.). [NIH Pub. No. 05-3896]. Washington, DC: National Cancer Institute.

Rogers, E. M. (2003). *Diffusion of innovations* (5th ed.). New York: Free Press.

Rogers, R. W. (1983). Cognitive and physiological processes in fear-based attitude change: A revised theory of protection motivation. In J. Caccioppo & R. Petty (Eds.), *Social psychophysiology: A sourcebook* (pp. 153–176). New York: Guilford.

Rogers, R. W. (1975). A protection motivation theory of fear appeals and attitude change. *Journal of Psychology, 91*(1), 93–114.

Rosenstock, I. M. (1966). Why people use health services. *Milbank Memorial Fund Quarterly, 44*, 94–124.

Rosenstock, I. M., Strecher, V. J., & Becker, M. H. (1988). Social learning theory and the health belief model. *Health Education Quarterly, 15*(2), 175–183.

Ross, H. S., & Mico, P. R. (1980). *Theory and practice in health education*. San Francisco: Mayfield.

Rotter, J. B. (1954). *Social learning and clinical psychology*. New York: Prentice-Hall.

Salazar, L. F., Crosby, R. A., & DiClemente, R. J. (2013). Health behavior in context of the "new" public health. In R. J. DiClemente, L. F. Salazar, & R. A. Crosby. *Health behavior theory for public health: Principles, foundations, and applications* (pp. 3–26). Burlington, MA: Jones & Bartlett Learning.

Sharma, M. (2017). *Theoretical foundations of health education and health promotion* (3rd ed.). Sudbury, MA: Jones & Bartlett.

Simons-Morton, B. G., Greene, W. H., & Gottlieb, N. H. (1995). *Introduction to health education and health promotion* (2nd ed.). Prospect Hts., IL: Waveland Press, Inc.

Simons-Morton, B. G., McLeroy, K. R., & Wendel, M. L. (2012). *Behavior theory in health promotion practice and research*. Burlington, MA: Jones & Bartlett Learning.

Simons-Morton, D. G., Simons-Morton, B. G., Parcel, G. S., & Bunker, J. F. (1988). Influencing personal and environmental conditions for community health: A multilevel intervention model. *Family and Community Health, 11*(2), 25–35.

Skinner, C. S., Tiro, J. & Champion, V.L. (2015). The health belief model. In K. Glanz, B. K. Rimer, & K. Viswanath (Eds.), *Health behavior and health education: Theory, research, and practice* (5th ed., pp. 75-94). San Francisco: Jossey-Bass.

Sleet, D. A., Hopkins, K. N., & Olson, S. J. (2003). From discovery to delivery: Injury prevention at CDC. *Health Promotion Practice, 4*(2), 98–102.

Spencer, L., Adams, T. B., Malone, S., Roy, L., & Yost, E. (2006). Applying the transtheoretical model to exercise: A systematic and comprehensive review of the literature. *Health Promotion Practice, 7*(4), 428–443.

Sullivan, D. (1973). Model for comprehensive, systematic program development in health education. *Health Education Report, 1*(1), (November/December), 4–5.

Timmreck, T. C. (2003). *Planning, program development, and evaluation* (2nd ed.). Boston: Jones & Bartlett.

Timmreck, T. C., Cole, G. E., James, G., & Butterworth, D. D. (2010). Health education and health promotion: A look at the jungle of supportive fields, philosophies, and theoretical foundations. In J. M. Black, S. Furney, H. M. Graf, & A. E. Nolt (Eds.), *Philosophical foundations of health education* (pp. 67–78). San Francisco: Jossey-Bass.

U.K. Office of National Statistics, Social Analysis and Reporting Division. (2001). Social capital: A review of the literature. Newport, South Wales.

Ungar, M. (2008). Putting resilience theory into action: Five principles for intervention. In L. Liebenberg & M. Ungar (Eds), *Resilience in action* (pp. 17–38). Toronto: University of Toronto Press.

U.S. Department of Health and Human Services (USDHHS). (2001). *Healthy people in health communities: A community planning guide using Healthy People 2010.* Washington, DC: Author.

U.S. Department of Health and Human Services (USDHHS). (2011). *MAP-IT: A guide to using Healthy People 2020 in your community.* Retrieved January 16, 2021, from https://www.healthypeople.gov/2020/tools-and-resources/Program-Planning

W.K. Kellogg Foundation. (2004). Retreived January 16, 2021, from https://www.wkkf.org/resource-directory/resources/2004/01/guiding-program-direction-with-logic-models

Walsh, D. C., Rudd, R. E., Moeykens, B. A., & Moloney, T. W. (1993). Social marketing for public health. *Health Affairs, 12*(2), 104–119.

Warren, M. R., Thompson, J. P., & Saegert, S. (2001). The role of social capital in combating poverty. In S. Saegert, J. P. Thompson, & M. R. Warren (Eds.), *Social capital and poor communities* (pp. 1–28). New York: Sage Foundation.

Weinstein, N. D., Rothman, A. J., & Sutton, S. R. (1998). Stage theories of health behavior: Conceptual and methodological issues. *Health Psychology, 17*(3), 290–299.

Weinstein, N. D., & Sandman, P. M. (2002). The precaution adoption process model and its application. In R. J. DiClemente, R. A. Crosby, & M. C. Kegler (Eds.), *Emerging theories in health promotion practice and research: Strategies for improving public health* (pp. 16–39). San Francisco: Jossey-Bass.

Weinstein, N. D., Sandman, P. M., & Blalock, S. J. (2008). The precaution adoption process model. In K. Glanz, B. K. Rimer, & K. Viswanath (Eds.), *Health behavior and health education: Theory, research, and practice* (4th ed., pp. 123–147). San Francisco: Jossey-Bass.

CHAPTER 5

Ethics and Health Education/Promotion

CHAPTER OBJECTIVES

After reading this chapter and answering the questions at the end, you should be able to:

- Identify and define the three major areas of philosophy.
- Define *ethics*.
- Explain the difference between ethics and morality.
- Explain why it is important to act ethically.
- Define *professional ethics*.
- Explain and briefly describe the two major categories of ethical theories.
- Identify principles that create a common ground for all ethical theories.
- Outline a guide for making ethical decisions.
- Identify ethical issues associated with the profession of health education/promotion.
- Explain how a profession can ensure that its professionals will act ethically.
- Define *code of ethics* and identify the source of the code available for health education specialists.

In recent years, there has been an increasing interest in ethical questions in all walks of life. The interest has become so great that it is difficult to avoid the topic of ethics in everyday living. Newspapers and television networks are constantly covering stories that involve ethical issues, many of which are related to health. Examples include genetic engineering, allocating and distributing of vaccinations end-of-life issues, the reduction of welfare benefits, health research, appropriate sexual behavior, and professional behavior, to name a few.

How do we determine what is ethical or unethical? By whose standards do we make such judgments? To answer these questions requires some background and perspective. In this chapter, we will provide the background and perspective to understand how ethics relates to the profession of health education/promotion. First, we will present key terms that relate to the study of ethics and examine the origin of ethics. Next, we look at reasons why people should work from an ethical base. We will then briefly look at the theories used to create ethical "yardsticks" and how these theories can be used to make ethical decisions. Within this context, a sampling of ethical issues facing health education specialists today will be presented. Finally, we conclude with a discussion on how a profession can ensure that its professionals will act ethically.

Key Terms and Origin

Ethics, the study of morality (Morrison, 2006), is one of the three major areas of philosophy. The other two are **epistemology**, the study of knowledge, and **metaphysics**, the study of the nature of reality (Thiroux, 1995). Ethics, or **moral philosophy** as it is often stated, dates back 2,000 plus years to the Greek philosopher Socrates (470–399 BCE). He, and other early philosophers, publicly posed questions and challenged people to think about how they lived. Although philosophers do not sit around publicly today to challenge people, the behavior, actions, and values of people are constantly being examined for their appropriateness.

You will note that the word *ethics* was described using the words *moral* and *morality*. The reason for this is that both words, *ethics* and *morals*, have ancient Greek and Latin roots in the words *ethos* and *mores* and both mean *character*. Thus, most associate *good character* with ethical behavior (White, 1988). Sperry (2007) has made a distinction between morality and ethics saying that morality "is the activity of making choices and of deciding, judging, justifying, and defending those actions or behaviors called moral," whereas ethics is "the science of how choices are made or should be made" (p. 38). Pigg (2010) has stated that "*ethics* defines acceptable and unacceptable behavior within the norms of a particular group" (pp. 11–12), whereas "*morality* sets standards for right and wrong in human behavior" (p. 12). Nevertheless, to avoid confusion throughout the rest of this chapter, we will use **ethical** and **moral** to mean the same thing.

White (1988) refers to the words *good, right, bad*, and *wrong* as the labels people use when making ethical judgments about human actions. Some authors have used these words to define ethics. Feeney & Freeman (1999) state, "Ethics is the study of right and wrong, duty and obligation" (p. 5). In the end, factual knowledge is not the concern of ethics but rather the virtues and values that drive human conduct (Pozgar, 2013).

Why Should People Act Ethically?

Because ethics is one of the three major areas of philosophy, a philosophical answer to the question of why people should act ethically is that to act ethically brings meaning or purpose to the life of an individual (McGrath, 1994). It provides a standard by which to live. Ethical living, in turn, provides for a better society for all. It is the right thing to do for society and self.

Personally, observation has shown "that those who are ethical tend to lead healthier, more emotionally satisfying lives" (McGrath, 1994, p. 131). Professionally, those who implement community interventions, including health education specialists, have much to gain from ethical behavior. Rabinowitz (2015) has noted that ethical practices make programs more effective, promote a sense of trust in an organization, contribute to moral credibility and leadership, and assure good standing legally and professionally. In short, ethics help guide our decision making and assist us in making better choices.

Professional Ethics

Whereas personal values and morality may guide us in our everyday living, it is important to note that they may not be sufficient to guide our professional behavior. People come to their work with different personal experiences. Because of these different experiences, they do not hold the same values nor have they learned the same moral lessons. Even those who hold the same beliefs may not apply them in the same way in a professional setting (Feeney & Freeman, 1999). Thus, in a work setting, individuals are guided by professional ethics. **Professional ethics** focuses on the "actions that are right and wrong in the workplace and are of public matter. Professional moral principles are not statements of taste or preference; they tell practitioners what they ought to do and what they ought not do" (Feeney & Freeman, 1999, p. 6). Coming to an understanding of what behaviors are appropriate in a professional role is referred to as *professional socialization* (Morrison & Furlong, 2014).

Ethical behavior is expected from professionals. "'Ethics' delineates what we consider acceptable and unacceptable conduct regarding professional practice in Health Science education. Ethical conduct is particularly important to professional health educators, since we belong to a profession with a mission to serve the individual" (Pigg, 1994, p. iii). Health education/promotion is a profession with much human interaction. Dorman (1994) adds, "As writers, reviewers, and scientists we must insist on the highest of ethical practices in publication and research. As practitioners, we must seek to actively practice ethical behavior in our service and teaching. Individually, we must aspire for a reputation which reflects a life of personal integrity. The wisdom of King Solomon probably puts it best: *'A good name is more desirable than great riches; to be esteemed is better than silver or gold'*" (p. 4). Or, as Pigg (2006) stated when he summarized the lesson on integrity he learned from observing his father throughout life, "When fame and fortune fade, only our reputations remain as important but fragile reflections of our true nature" (p. 41).

Within the larger realm of *professional ethics*, there may be some subsets of ethical behavior that are specific to certain tasks of the professional. For example, among the eight responsibilities of health education specialists is Responsibility IV "Evaluation and Research" (National Commission for Health Education Credentialing [NCHEC], 2020)

(see the discussion of the responsibilities in Chapter 6). To conduct evaluation and research, health education specialists not only need to be aware of appropriate general professional ethics but also of ethical behavior as it relates to evaluation and research processes. Such behavior falls under the area of *research ethics*. **Research ethics** "comprises principles and standards that, along with underlying values, guide appropriate conduct relevant to research decisions" (Kimmel, 2007, p. 6). An ethical principle associated with the research process is the concept of voluntary participation. That is, potential research participants should not be forced or coerced into participating in a research study, but rather should do so on a voluntary basis (see **Box 5.1** for other issues related to research process).

Ethical Theories

Philosophers do not speak with a common voice about the standards of morality. Depending on the ethical theory espoused, one philosopher may see a certain behavior as moral or ethical, whereas another may see the same behavior as immoral or unethical. For example, one philosopher may see capital punishment as a moral action to punish a person for murder, and the other sees the taking of another life, for whatever reason, as immoral. The purpose of this section is to categorize and summarize the better-known theories (see **Table 5.1**) and to suggest ways by which their content can be applied to health education/promotion practice.

Ethical theories provide frameworks whereby health education specialists and others are able to evaluate whether human actions are acceptable (Shive & Marks, 2006). The primary means by which ethical theories have been categorized has been to place them in the category of deontology, also referred to as **formalism**, or **nonconsequentialism**, or teleology, commonly called **consequentialism**, theories. **Deontological theories** (from Greek

---

Box 5.1 Examples of Ethical Issues Related to Research

The research process includes a number of steps that could have ethical ramifications. Examples of such issues are presented based on whether it is a consideration before the research begins, during the research process, or after the research is complete.

Before the research begins

- Selecting a research topic; must weigh risk (harm) to benefit (positive value)
- Recruiting participants: equitable opportunity to participate; voluntary participation; concern for vulnerable groups
- Institutional Review Board approval of research protocol

During the research process

- Obtaining participant consent and/or assent
- Using deception (active or passive) as part of the intervention
- Participant privacy: anonymity or confidentiality
- Using an untreated comparison or control group
- Data analysis: careless use of data; manipulation of data; selective use or elimination of data; over-analysis of data

After the research is complete

- Reporting results: what to report; protecting confidentiality; declaring conflict of interest; disclosing sponsorship
- Sharing results with participants; debriefing experimental, control, and comparison groups
- Publication/presentation of results: determining authorship and order of authors; avoiding duplication of published works, fragmentation into several publications, and plagiarism.

---

deontos, "of the obligatory" or *deon* meaning duty) promote the belief that certain actions are good or bad, regardless of the consequences of those actions. For example, a deontologist would argue that lying to a client or patient is wrong even if it is done to help that person. According to this theory, the mere act of lying is wrong, regardless of the benefits it may bring. Deontology theories involve making decisions based on a moral code or rules (Pozgar, 2013)—that is to say, the end

(the consequences) *does not* justify the means (the act).

Teleological theories (from Greek *teleios,* "brought to its end purpose"), on the other hand, evaluate the moral status of an act by the goodness of the consequences (Reamer, 2006). If the act produces good or happiness, it is morally okay; if it does not, it is immoral. Using the same example of lying to a patient or client, if the consequences turned out okay, the consequentialist would

Table 5.1 Summary of Ethical Theories

Category	Primary Reasoning	Examples of Such Theories
Deontology (also known as formalism or nonconsequentialism)	The end does not justify the means.	Natural law morality, deontological ethics, existentialism
Teleology (also known as consequentialism)	The end does justify the means.	Contractarian ethics, utilitarianism, pragmatism

see this act as morally okay. In short, this category of ethical theories states that the end *does* justify the means.

As can be seen from these descriptions of formalism and consequentialism, the primary point of contention is whether or not the means justify the end. Most people would say that neither category of ethical theory can answer all moral questions in their lives. In fact, Summers (2014) has stated, "humans have yet to develop an ethical theory that will satisfactorily handle all issues" (p. 62). There are times when deontology provides guidance for the ethical way to act, whereas teleology is best in other situations. What this means is that each person must carefully study the ethical theory options, combine what is compatible, and resolve what is inconsistent in those options, and attempt to work out a moral consensus for herself and society (Mellert, 1995). This is not an easy process. Many times, philosophical questions and problems are abstract or conceptual in nature. For example, is there ever a time when it is okay for a health education specialist to lie to his supervisor? Such questions are answered through philosophical thought, using reason, logic, and argument. Thus, the most important tool people can use to find these answers is the mind.

When analyzing an ethical problem, people need to depend more on thinking than feeling—using their minds and not their hearts (White, 1988). For example, if a person says, "I feel that abortion, no matter when it occurs, is morally wrong," that person is really saying there is something about abortion that makes her uneasy, unhappy, or distressed. This person is expressing a feeling, not a moral position. This person's feelings would be better stated if she were to say, "Abortion makes me feel upset." However, if a person states that abortion is immoral, then she should be prepared to provide specific reasons for holding this belief (White, 1988). For example, she may hold the belief that life begins at conception and having an abortion is ending the life of another human being. It is for these reasons that answering ethical questions is a thinking, not a feeling, process. Or, as Penland and Beyrer (1981) have stated, "If ethics is to have personal meaning it demands thoughtful examination. The answers to ethical questions are found by looking within, examining our personal belief systems and values, and using our intelligence to integrate what we have learned and what we have experienced with what we believe and value" (p. 6).

Basic Principles for Common Moral Ground

As was shown in the previous section, deontoloists and teleologists are not in agreement when it comes to the rationale to be used in making moral decisions. No single ethical theory can answer every ethical question to the satisfaction of all, yet, to live in a moral society, all must be able to work from a common moral ground. "We must search for a larger meeting ground in which the best of all these theories and systems can operate meaningfully with a minimum of conflict and opposition" (Thiroux, 1995, p. 172).

To help us with this common ground, Thiroux (1995) has identified five basic principles that can apply to human morality, regardless of the embraced theory. The principles do not provide the answers to how one should behave but rather help to provide a foundation for making ethical decisions. The first is the **value of life** principle. This is the most basic of principles. Without living human beings, there can be no ethics. Thiroux (1995) has specifically stated this principle as "human beings should revere life and accept death" (p. 180). This means that no life should be ended without strong justification. This, for example, is why topics such as abortion, suicide, euthanasia, and capital punishment raise a number of ethical questions.

The second is the principle of **goodness (rightness)**. "Good" and "right" are at the core of every ethical theory. Theorists may disagree on what is good and bad and right and wrong, but they all strive for goodness and rightness. "'Good' should not only be in abstract, but it should be seen in relation to (other) human beings. As an example, a person who is suicidal may no longer value his or her life as 'good,' but that person's mother may have a very different concept of the value of her child's life" (Tschudin, 2003, p. 56).

The principle of goodness includes two parallel principles of ethics: (1) the principle of **nonmaleficence** and (2) the principle of **beneficence**, or **benevolence**. "Briefly, nonmaleficence refers to the non-infliction of harm to others" (Balog et al., 1985, p. 91). Furthermore, nonmaleficence can "be broken into three components: not inflicting harm, preventing harm, and removing harm when it is present" (Greenberg, 2001, p. 3). Although the concepts presented in this explanation of nonmaleficence are seemingly straightforward, the application of the concepts can be difficult. For example, what is meant by harm? Are there degrees of harm like "a little harm" and "a lot of harm"? Must an action produce no harm to be acceptable from an ethical point of view? These are difficult questions to answer and make some situations difficult to respond to in an ethical way.

"Beneficence implies more than just avoiding doing harm" (Summers, 2014, p. 49). It "describes the principle of doing good, demonstrating kindness, showing compassion, and helping others" (Pozgar, 2013, p. 9). In the bioethical realm, nonmaleficence and beneficence make up the "benefit-harm ratio" in which, ideally, benefits outweigh costs and in which the "minimization of harm" rather than the "maximation of good" is more strongly emphasized (Fox & Swazey, 1997).

Thiroux's third principle is **justice (fairness)**. This principle deals with people treating other people fairly and justly in distributing goodness (benefits) and badness (burdens) (Summers, 2014; Thiroux, 1995). Justice can be examined in two ways—(1) *procedural* and (2) *distributive* (Summers, 2014). **Procedural justice** deals with whether fair procedures were in place and whether those procedures were followed, while **distributive justice** deals with the allocation of resources (Summers, 2014). Does this mean that all people will always get their fair share of goodness and badness? No, but it does mean everyone will have an equal chance at obtaining the good (Thiroux, 1995). "The bottom line is that one has indeed acted justly toward a person when that person has been given what she or he is due or owed" (Balog et al., 1985, p. 90). For example, should only those who are able to pay for them receive health education/promotion services, or should only the poor carry that burden?

The fourth principle of this common moral ground is that of **truth telling (honesty)**. At the heart of any moral relationship is communication. A necessary component of any meaningful communication is telling the truth, being honest. This may be the most difficult principle to live by. This is not to say that people will never lie or that lying might be justified, but there is a need for a strong attempt to be truthful. In the end, morality depends on what people say and do (Thiroux, 1995). Health education specialists working in a clinical setting may be faced with this principle when caught in a situation in which an ill child (and a minor by law) asks about their health problem, but the child's parent or guardian has strictly forbidden such communication.

The fifth principle is that of **individual freedom (equality principle or principle of autonomy)**. (See **Figure 5.1**.) "The word *autonomy* comes from the Greek words *autos* ("self") and *nomos* ("rule," "governance," or "law") and was originally referred to as self-governance in Greek city-states" (Greenberg, 2001, p. 3). "This principle

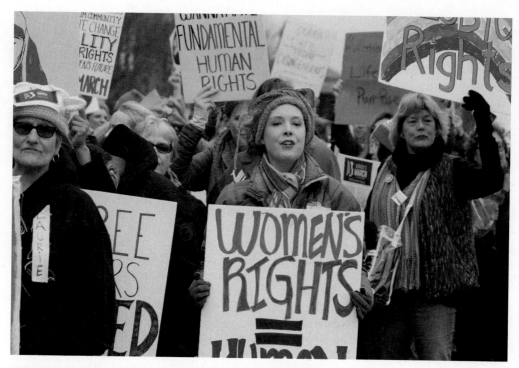

Figure 5.1 Individual freedom is an important principle of human morality.
© Anthony Ricci/Shutterstock.

means that people, being individuals with individual differences, must have the freedom to choose their own ways and means of being moral within the framework of the first four basic principles" (Thiroux, 1995, p. 187). This is to say that individual freedom is limited by the other four principles. Underlying the principle "of autonomy is the idea that we are to respect others for who they are" (Summers, 2014, p. 50). This is a principle that health education specialists deal with on a regular basis, specifically as it relates to helping others engage in enhancing health behavior. Health education specialists need to respect the rights of others to deliberate, choose, and act (Balog et al., 1985).

With the grounding of the ethical theories and the establishment of these basic principles, let us examine the process of making ethical decisions.

Making Ethical Decisions

"Ethical decision making in health education, as in other areas, involves determining right and wrong within situations where clear demarcations do not exist or are not clearly apparent to the decision maker . . . . To be considered a professional health educator, one must possess requisite skill and knowledge in making individual decisions. And, in making decisions it is imperative that one has analyzed his or her decisions in terms of standards of right and wrong, good and bad" (Balog et al., 1985, p. 88). To decide and, in turn, act in an ethical manner, people must rely on their values, principles, and ethical thinking. To assist in this process, a number of authors (e.g., Balog et al., 1985; Fisher, 2003;

Mellert, 1995; Melnick, 2015; Nelson, 2005; Reamer, 2006; Remley & Herlihy, 2007; Svara, 2007; Thompson et al., 2000) have presented guides for applying the concepts presented previously in this chapter to everyday ethical decision making. Although the number of steps and labels used to identify the steps are different from guide to guide, they are similar in that they provide a framework for making an ethical decision. Because of the limitation of space, we are presenting a single approach (see **Figure 5.2**) to ethical decision making that blends the ideas and is representative of these guides.

The ethical decision-making process should begin long before any ethical problems surface. The process begins when a person develops and sustains a personal and/or professional commitment to doing what is right. Such a commitment will go a long way toward creating a work environment that can prevent many ethical problems. This is not to say that all ethical problems will be avoided. Ethical problems can arise in situations in which two or more ethical principles appear to be in conflict, in unforeseen reactions from those with whom a health education specialist may work, or in unexpected events (Fisher, 2003). However, having a commitment to doing what is right becomes a form of "primary prevention" for many ethical problems.

Aligned with a commitment to doing what is right is familiarity with what the health education/promotion profession expects of practicing professionals. Stated differently, what are the expected norms for those who practice health education/promotion? Such expectations can be found in the profession's code of ethics and responsibilities of health education specialists (CNHEO, 2020; NCHEC, 2020). With a commitment to doing what is right and knowing what is expected of practicing health education specialists, they are enhancing their *moral sensitivity*. Rest et al. (1999) explained **moral sensitivity** as being aware that an ethical problem exists and

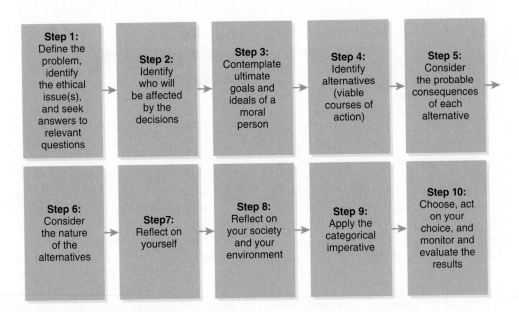

Figure 5.2 Steps in ethical decision making.

Data from Balog, J. E., Shirreffs, J. H., Gutierrez, R. D., & Balog, L. F. (1985). Ethics and the field of health education. *The Eta Sigma Gamma Monograph Series, 4*(1), 65–110; Mellert, R. B. (1995). *Seven ethical theories.* Kendall Hunt; Nelson, W. A. (2005). An organizational ethics decision-making process. *Healthcare Executive, 20*(4), 8–14; Reamer, F. G. (2006). *Social work values and ethics* (3rd ed.). Columbia University Press; Remley, T. P., & Herlihy, B. (2007). *Ethical, legal, and professional issues in counseling* (2nd ed.). Merrill, Prentice Hall; and Svara, J. (2007). *The ethics primer for public administrators in government and nonprofit organizations.* Jones & Bartlett Learning.

having an understanding of what impact different courses of action may have on the people involved.

The first step to take when confronted with an ethical decision is to define the problem/concern, identify the ethical issue(s), clarify the facts, and seek answers to relevant questions (Mellert, 1995; Melnick, 2015; Nelson, 2005; Reamer, 2006; Remley & Herlihy, 2007; Svara, 2007). This first step is one of clarification and gathering relevant information. Several questions need to be answered. What is the problem/concern that makes you believe there is an ethical decision to be made? Is there a legal question that needs to be answered? What do you know? What do you need to find out? Does a decision have to be made? If so, by when, and in what context? Are these decisions within the realm of your authority, or does someone else with other responsibilities/authority/resources determine them?

Second, identify the individuals, groups, and organizations that are likely to be affected by this ethical decision (Nelson, 2005; Reamer, 2006) and what stakes they have in the outcome (Svara, 2007). When making an ethical decision, it is important to understand all who will be impacted because one solution may create additional ethical problems for others.

Third, consider the ultimate goals and ideals you are striving for and ask, "What are the most noble aspirations that pertain to this concrete situation?" (Mellert, 1995, p. 156). How should you as an ethical person want to act in this situation? Consider the ethical theory you embrace and the principles for common ethical ground. How do these goals and ideals apply to this decision? Ultimate goals and ideals do not always apply to every decision and sometimes may not be appropriate, but, to the extent that they do apply, let them help with the decision.

Fourth, identify all of the possible alternatives to solving the problem (viable courses of action), the people involved in each, and the potential benefits and risks of each (Reamer, 2006). It is important to brainstorm the various alternatives to help organize subsequent analyses (Reamer, 2006). Consider ethical and health theories, a code of ethics (Melnick, 2015), and consult with colleagues and, if necessary, experts. Be aware that there may not be a "best alternative"; you may have to deal with an ethical dilemma. An **ethical dilemma** is a situation that forces a decision that involves breaking some ethical norm or contradicting some ethical value. It involves making a decision between two or more possible actions in which any one of the actions can be justified as being the right decision, but whatever action is taken, there always remains some doubt as to whether the correct course of action was chosen. The effect of an action may put others at risk, harm others, or violate the rights of others. (Pozgar, 2013, pp. 534–535)

Fifth, "consider the probable consequences of each alternative" (Mellert, 1995, p. 157). Look at both the short- and long-term consequences of each alternative. How will these consequences affect you, others, and the environment? In other words, weigh the strengths and weaknesses of the alternatives based on the consequences (Balog et al., 1985). Maybe the consequences are different, or maybe they are not and thus, may not be important in the final decision.

Sixth, "consider the nature of the alternatives" (Mellert, 1995, p. 157). Consider the deontologist approach to the decision-making process in selecting an alternative. Does the alternative lead to an act or a behavior that is wrong? Would you be violating anyone's basic rights? Does it go against basic human ideals and intrinsic moral values? If you answer *yes* to any of these questions, you do not necessarily need to eliminate the alternative from further consideration but should give greater consideration to alternatives that do not violate this portion of your reflection.

Seventh, "reflect on yourself" (Mellert, 1995, p. 157). What impact will a proposed course of action have on you as a moral person? Will it enhance or detract from your moral stature? If it detracts, maybe other alternatives should be considered. If you cannot accept a course of action due to your internal values and your own moral beliefs, then consider that there must be something morally questionable about the considered action (Mellert, 1995). Although you may be striving to be objective as you work toward a decision, be aware that your emotions will also play a part. Your emotions will influence your judgment and may help guide you in your decision making (Remley & Herlihy, 2007).

Eighth, "reflect on your society and your environment" (Mellert, 1995, p. 158). Will your action mesh with that of society and the environment? Moral acts are unselfish acts in that they do not prefer one's own interests at the expense of the interests of others (Mellert, 1995). Will society in general see your action as morally correct? (See **Figure 5.3**.)

Ninth, "apply the categorical imperative" (Mellert, 1995, p. 158). Would you want your

course of action to be a role model for others? If others were faced with the same decision, is this how you would want them to act?

Tenth, choose the best alternative, provide a reasoned justification for the choice (Svara, 2007), "act courageously and decisively" (Mellert, 1995, p. 158), monitor and evaluate the results, and if necessary, make adjustments (Svara, 2007). "Choosing among conflicting options is difficult, but at least one can feel confident that the choice did not ignore an important alternative" (Svara, 2007, p. 109). Having said this, you still may not feel comfortable after the choice has been made.

Context of Ethical Decision Making

In considering the components in this decision-making process, it is important to note that moral decision making does not

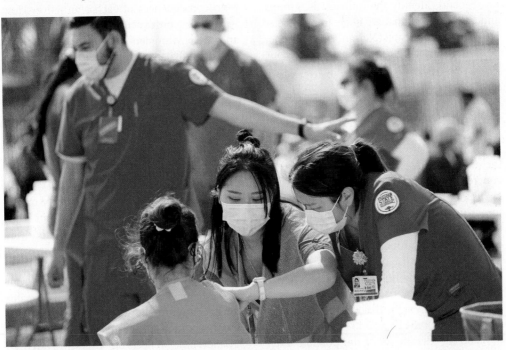

Figure 5.3 The COVID pandemic highlighted a number of vaccination-related ethical challenges centered around access to vaccinations which can be influenced by socioeconomic and racial ethnic minority status causing to question whether or not all lives are of equal value.

Courtesy of Cary Edmondson/California State University, Fresno.

occur in a vacuum (Mellert, 1995). If it did, every decision would be resolved with the "right" alternative for all. Each decision is surrounded by the context in which it must be made. Mellert feels that, when working through the process, a person must consider and be aware of the context. When making ethical decisions, people must have a sense of the following:

1. **Place.** Be aware of the appropriateness of an action in a particular environment. One action may be appropriate in one setting but not in another.
2. **Time.** Be aware of the history leading up to the decision and other similar decisions. Learn from past decisions.
3. **Identity.** Who am I? How does this moral decision relate to me?
4. **Social relationships.** Be aware that making moral decisions will impact social relationships. There is a good chance that not everyone will agree with your decision and action.
5. **The ideal.** When making a moral decision, aim for the noblest ideals of humanity.
6. **The concrete.** Never lose sight of the fact that choices arise from concrete events.
7. **Seriousness.** When making a moral decision, do so with an attitude that is appropriate to the situation.

Applying the Ethical Decision-Making Process

Now let us see if we can apply this decision-making process to the profession of health education/promotion. A health education specialist, let's call her Anne (pronouns: she/her/hers), is employed by an organization and is in charge of the organization's employee health promotion program. Based on the results of the health risk assessments (HRA) taken by employees, Anne is aware that one employee, "high up in the organization" (e.g., school principal or department manager), is a consistent abuser of alcohol. The person's supervisor is aware of the situation but has ignored it. The employee in question is well liked within the organization and is a good employee. To the best of Anne's knowledge, alcohol has not impacted this person's work performance, but she feels it has the potential to do so. Anne is not sure if the alcohol has impacted the employee's personal life. What should Anne do with this information? Let's look at how we might analyze this situation using the 10-step process presented on the previous pages.

Step 1. Define the problem, identify the ethical issue, and gather relevant information.

The problem is that the employee is abusing a substance, and the health education specialist knows it, as does the employee's supervisor. Is it an ethical problem? Anne knows that an alcohol-impaired person can harm themselves and others, either intentionally or unintentionally, and thus has an obligation to protect their health (see Article I, Section 4, of Appendix A). Anne also knows she has an obligation to protect the privacy of the employees (see Article I, Section 6, of Appendix A). To Anne, this appears to be an ethical situation because of the two competing issues. Anne has decided to get more information before acting. She decides to look at the employee handbook to see if anything like this appears there. She also decides to ask her own supervisor for guidance and check with the Human Resources (HR) Department for information. And, finally, she looks to see when the employee is scheduled for their HRA feedback appointment.

Step 2. Identify who will be affected.

Anne is aware that, depending on what actions are taken, the parties impacted by those actions are the employee, the employee's supervisor, the organization and its reputation, family members of the employee, and even Anne herself and her supervisor.

Step 3. Contemplate the ultimate goals and ideals.

Anne wants to do what is ethically right. From a theoretical point of view, Anne embraces the deontological viewpoint of dealing with ethical situations. In other words, she believes that the ends do not justify the means. She is trying to make sense of how that applies to this situation.

Step 4. Identify the alternatives (viable courses of action).

Anne sees the following as viable courses of action: (1) Approach the employee's supervisor and ask them to handle it; (2) Talk to the employee about it at their scheduled HRA feedback appointment; (3) Turn the information over to the HR Department to let someone there deal with the problem; (4) Turn the information over to their supervisor so that it can be dealt with at the managers' level; (5) Do nothing until something happens because of the employee's alcohol use; or (6) Do nothing at all.

Step 5. Consider the consequences of the alternatives.

Here are the consequences Anne sees with each of the alternatives she identified in Step 4: Alternative 1—The supervisor may do nothing or may now be forced to act because someone else is aware of the situation. This may lead to the employee's dismissal, or the employee may get the help they need, or the supervisor may decide not to act on the information. Alternative 2—This alternative would protect the employee's privacy, bring the problem to the attention of the employee, and let the employee act without others knowing about it. Anne also knows that the employee may not take the feedback session well and "blow up" at Anne. Alternative 3—This alternative places the situation in the hands of those trained to deal with them effectively. Depending on the organization's policy, it may also lead to the employee's dismissal, or the employee may get the help they need. Alternative 4—Similar to Alternatives 2 and 4, it places the problem in someone else's hands and would probably have much the same consequences as those two alternatives. Alternative 5—Nothing may ever come of the employee's alcohol abuse, or some serious harm may come to the employee or someone around them. Or Alternative 6—Doing nothing at all, which would change nothing. The employee possibly will continue as a good employee with no problem for themselves or others, or harm could come to the employee, their coworkers, or members of the employee's family.

Step 6. Consider the nature of the alternatives.

Anne does not feel that by acting she would be violating any human ideals or intrinsic moral rules or values. She does feel; however, that she cannot do "nothing." She does not like the alternatives, but she feels an ethical obligation to act. Anne may be facing an ethical dilemma.

Step 7. Reflect on yourself.

Anne knows that if she does nothing, she will not be able to live with herself because she sees herself as a moral person. But she is concerned about being seen as the "goody-goody" employee or even a "tattle tale" or an employee who cannot be trusted with confidential information.

Step 8. Reflect on society and the environment.

Anne had a hard time reasoning through this step of the process. Because a large percentage of U.S. adults consume alcohol, she feels that society in general may see the employee's situation as "none of her business." But she still sees a need to act.

Step 9. Apply the categorical imperative.

Anne feels she needs to act because it is her duty. She wonders what kind of health education specialist she would be if she was not concerned about the health of a coworker and the possible harm that coworker could bring to self or others. She feels that she needs to be a role model for others.

Step 10. Choose an alternative, provide a rationale, act, and monitor the results.

Anne decided to act by talking to the employee about the alcohol abuse at her scheduled HRA feedback appointment. She chose this approach not only because it does not violate the employee's privacy but because it also tries to protect both the employee's health and that of those around them. If this approach does not induce the employee to change, Anne feels that she may need to take further action.

As you can see, moral decisions are not easy to make. They are not to be taken lightly, and responsible action is important. Remember, this decision will not occur in a vacuum; the "ideal" decision may not be the best decision. What do you think about Anne's actions?

Ethical Issues and Health Education/ Promotion

As previously noted, ethical concerns interface with all aspects of our lives. That includes our professional lives too. "Ethical issues permeate almost every decision and action undertaken in health education" (Goldsmith, 2006, p. 33). Although some of the ethical issues faced by health education specialists are specific to the profession, such as the ethical issues surrounding getting clients to begin a health-enhancing behavior, using interventions to protect and promote at the population level, and dealing with the potential pervasiveness of most things in life impacting peoples' health (Dawson & Verweij, 2007), the majority of concerns affecting most professions are similar (Hiller, 1987). Here are some situations that are specific to preventive care and public health programs.

Bayles, (1989) has organized the substantive obligations of professions and professionals, regardless of the profession, from which most professional ethical situations arise. The following is a list of these obligations, with several questions that relate the obligations to the practice of health education/promotion. [Note: These obligations closely align with the *Code of Ethics for the Health Education Profession* (Coalition of National Health Education Organizations [CNHEO], 2020).]

1. **Obligations and availability of services.** The primary issue related to this obligation is the equality of opportunity for making professional services available to all citizens. Examples of ethical issues associated with this obligation include the right to legal counsel, access to health care, and refusal to accept clients for lack of ability to pay. (Who should receive health education/promotion? What about clients who are hard to reach? In what settings should it be offered? Should clients have to pay for health education/ promotion, or should health education/ promotion be denied if a person cannot pay? Should health education specialists ever terminate an intervention before it is complete? Is there ever a time when a health education specialist should use an intervention in which the possible outcomes are questionable?)

2. **Obligations between professionals and clients.** Once the services of a professional have been secured, a number of ethical issues can arise from the professional–client relationship. (See **Figure 5.4**) "The fiduciary model presents the best ethical ideal for the professional–client relationship" (Bayles, 1989, p. 100). In such a model, the professional is honest, candid, competent, loyal, fair, and discreet. At the same time, the client keeps commitments to the professional, is truthful to the professional, and does not request unethical acts from the professional.

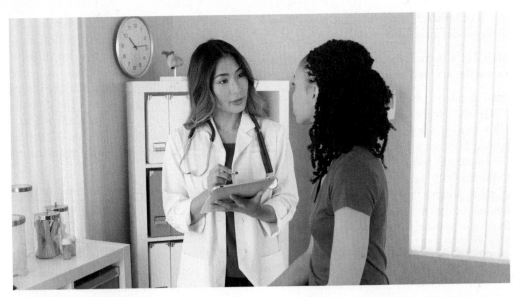

Figure 5.4 The professional–client relationship is an obligation that is often encountered by health education specialists.

(Is there ever a time when health education specialists should not be candid or honest with their clients? How should health education specialists respond when their clients ask them about their personal behavior? Is there ever a time when health education specialists should not obtain informed consent before proceeding with an intervention?) (See **Box 5.2**).

Box 5.2 Informed Consent: An Ethical Obligation

The term **informed consent** is often associated with medical procedures or research projects, but it is also important in health education/promotion. The concept behind informed consent is that people—whether patients, research participants, or participants in a health education/promotion program—should be given sufficient information from which to make informed choices about whether they want a certain medical procedure, or to participate in a research project or health education/promotion program. From an ethical standpoint, it is based on the common ground principle of individual freedom. That is, freedom to choose after being well informed on the consequences of participation.

Although receiving a medical procedure or participating in a clinical trial often carries more risks than participating in a health education/promotion program, individuals should not be allowed to participate in any health education/promotion program without giving their informed consent (McKenzie et al., 2013). In practice, the informed consent process should include (1) the health education specialist discussing the details of the program (i.e., purpose of the program, description of the intervention, risks and benefits associated with participation, alternative programs that will accomplish the same thing, and the freedom to discontinue participation at any time) with the prospective participant; (2) the participant having an opportunity to ask questions about the program; (3) the participant understanding what they have been told; and (4) the participant signing a written informed consent document (Cottrell & McKenzie, 2011).

3. **Obligations to third parties.** This obligation revolves around what others need to know about the professional–client relationship. Often, professionals are confronted with the issue of whether to share client information with family members of the client, people in a supervisory capacity (e.g., teachers, employers), legal authorities (e.g., police, lawyers), or peers (e.g., professional colleagues). What duty does a health education specialist have to communicate information with parents of a student when the student has shared information in confidence? Is there ever a time when a health education specialist can share confidential information? How about with the insurance company of a client? With the client's employer?) (See **Box 5.3**).

4. **Obligations between professionals and employers.** Employed professionals have obligations to employers that are similar to the obligation they have to their clients (see #2). "However, the obligation to obey employers is stronger than an obligation to clients. It includes acting as, and only as, authorized" (Bayles, 1989, p. 158). On the other hand, "employers' obligations to professional employees are universal, role related, and contractual" (Bayles, 1989, p. 159). Ethical issues related to this obligation often involve due process, confidentiality, and professional

---

Box 5.3 Privacy, HIPAA, and GINA

One of the most basic concepts associated with providing a service (e.g., health education) to other people is that of privacy. **Privacy** has been defined as "the claim of individuals, groups, or institutions to determine for themselves when, how, and to what extent information about them is communicated to others" (Westin, 1968, p. 7). Thus, when people have agreed to participate in a health education/promotion program, it becomes the duty of the health education specialist to protect the information provided by participants.

The importance of privacy for health education specialists, and all others associated with health care, was further emphasized with the enactment of the Health Insurance Portability and Accountability Act of 1996 (officially known as Public Law 104-191 and referred to as HIPAA) and the Genetic Information Nondiscrimination Act of 2008 (officially known as Public Law 110-233 and referred to as GINA). The HIPAA and GINA regulations apply to protected health information (PHI), whether transmitted orally, in writing, or electronically, that is generated by an employer, a health plan, a health clearinghouse, or a healthcare provider, or in connection with financial or administrative activities related to health care (Fisher, 2003). Failure to implement the standards can lead to civil and criminal penalties (U.S. Department of Health and Human Services [USDHHS], n.d.). The two techniques that are used to protect the privacy of program participants are anonymity and confidentiality. **Anonymity** exists when no one, including those conducting the program, can relate a participant's identity to any information pertaining to the program. In applying this concept, health education specialists would need to ensure that collected information had no identifying marks attached to it such as the participant's name, social security number, or any other less common information. In practice, because of the nature (the need to know about the participants) of most health education/promotion programs, anonymity is not often used. Its most common application in health education/promotion is in conducting research projects.

Conversely, the concept of confidentiality is common in health education/promotion programs. **Confidentiality** exists when only those responsible for conducting a program can link information about a participant with the individual and do not reveal such information to others. Thus, health education specialists need to take every precaution to protect participants' information. Often, this means keeping the information "under lock and key" while the program is being conducted, then destroying (e.g., shredding) the information when it is no longer needed.

support. (Should health education specialists always implement "company" policy when they know it is wrong or could bring harm to a client? What if a health education specialist has a conflict of interest between his personal life and what his employer says he must do? Is there ever a time when health education specialists should publicly speak against their employers?)

5. **Obligations to the profession.** "These obligations rest on the responsibilities of a profession as a whole to further social values" (Bayles, 1989, p. 179). Issues associated with this obligation include conducting research, reforming the profession, and maintaining respect for the profession. (Is there ever a reason why health education specialists should not behave in a professional manner? What duty does a health education specialist have to report the inappropriate behavior of a colleague? What obligations do health education specialists have to keep up-to-date on the content of their fields?)

Having identified problems that may cut across all professions, let us examine those that are more specific to health education/promotion. First, Penland & Beyrer (1981) state that ethical issues are defined by two criteria. "First they must be 'issues'; that is, there must be controversy related to the problem or topic. There must be 'two sides,' supported by people with two different viewpoints" (p. 6). Issues, by definition, are controversial. For example, the need for youth to know sexual information is not an issue; however, from whom and when such information should be provided may be an issue.

"The second criterion for an ethical issue in health education is that it must involve a question of right and wrong" (Penland & Beyrer, 1981, p. 6). "Can health education/promotion programs in the worksite change health behavior?" may be a controversial

issue, but it does not deal with rightness and wrongness. Thus, it is not an ethical issue, but "does an employer have the right to make all employees attend the health education/promotion program?" is an ethical issue.

Now that we know what constitutes an ethical issue, let us look at some of the ethical issues health education specialists are likely to face. The literature is abundant with examples of ethical issues in health education/promotion. Issues cited include abstinence-only and abstinence-plus sexuality education (Wiley, 2002), community organization and community participation (Bromly et al., 2015; Minkler et al., 2012), ethics instruction (Modell & Citrin, 2002), global health (Stapleton et al., 2014), health education research (Bastida et al., 2010; Buchanan et al., 2002; Minkler et al., 2002; Minkler et al., 2008; Paul & Brooks, 2015), health disparities (Shaw-Ridley & Ridley, 2010), health literacy (Marks, 2009), health promotion evaluation (Thurston et al., 2003), health risk appraisals (The Society of Prospective Medicine Board of Directors [SPM], 1999), health screenings (Melnick, 2015), practice of health education/practice (Kahan, 2012; Shive & Marks, 2006), research/scientific inquiry/publishing (Margolis, 2000; McKenzie et al., 2009; Pigg, 1994, 2006; Price & Dake, 2002; Price et al., 2001), service by health education specialists (Price et al., 2001; Young & Valois, 2010), social marketing (Rothschild, 2000; Siegel & Lotenberg, 2007), the teaching of health (Telljohann et al., 2001), topical areas (Eve et al., 2008; Knight et al., 2014), and the teaching of ethics (Goldsmith, 2006). McLeroy et al., (1993) have identified other areas of ethical concern, which reflect the inclusion of health education as a component of health promotion. The major categories of issues raised by McLeroy and colleagues (1993) include

1. "Assigning individual responsibility to the victim for becoming ill due to personal failures" (p. 314)—for example, becoming ill because one does not

exercise or continues to use tobacco products.

2. "Attempting to change individuals and their subsequent behaviors rather than the social environment that supports and maintains unhealthy lifestyles" (p. 314)—for example, telling employees to manage their stress when it is environmental stressors causing the stress.

3. Using "system interventions to promote health behaviors" (p. 315)—for example, public policy strategies or coercive strategies to modify unhealthy actions.

4. Overemphasizing behavior change as a program outcome instead of focusing more on changes in the social and physical environment.

5. Overemphasizing the importance of health, forgetting that health is a means to an end, not an end in itself.

6. Educating the public on the concept of risk and how to properly use risk factor information.

7. Underemphasizing professional behavior, regardless of the health education/promotion setting—for example, keeping up-to-date, serving as a role model, and providing ethics education for the next generation of health education specialists.

As you can see, there are a number of ethical issues that can arise in the process of carrying out the work of a health education specialist. Rabinowitz (2015) has provided several issues that need to be considered when planning, implementing, and evaluating community interventions. They are presented in **Box 5.4**.

Ensuring Ethical Behavior

The majority of this chapter has been used to examine ethical theory, identify and deal with ethical issues, and discuss why it is important to act ethically. What we have yet to discuss is the answer to the question "how the profession can ensure that professionals will behave ethically?" The answer is it cannot. Professionals who act unethically usually do so (1) for personal financial gain and reputation and (2) for the benefit of clients or employers without considering the effects on others (Bayles, 1989). However, a profession can put procedures into place to work toward ethical behavior by all.

Certain professional procedures or practices are limited to those who are in professional preparation programs and those who have already been admitted to the profession. Traditional ways of doing this have been through (1) selective admissions into academic programs, (2) retention standards to remain in academic programs, (3) graduation from academic programs, (4) completion of internships, (5) the process of becoming credentialed (i.e., certified or licensed to practice), and (6) continual updating to retain the credential. While proceeding through these steps, individuals may have to provide evidence of good moral character.

Upon entering the field, professionals are expected to behave according to a system of norms. As noted previously in this chapter, this system of norms (or professional moral consensus, as some refer to it) is often placed in writing and referred to as a code of ethics. More specifically, a **code of ethics** is a "document that maps the dimensions of the profession's collective social responsibility and acknowledges the obligations individual practitioners share in meeting the profession's responsibilities" (Feeney & Freeman, 1999, p. 6). Such a document is not only useful for the professional but also for those who use the services of the professional. An ethical code's principal function is to "organize in a systematic way basic ethical standards, rules, and principles of professional conduct" (Pritchard, 2006, p. 85). In other words, "codes serve to *constrain*

Box 5.4 Ethical Issues that Need to Be Considered with Community
Interventions

---

1. **Confidentiality.** Probably the most familiar of ethical issues—perhaps because it is the one most often violated—is the expectation that communications and information from participants in the course of a community intervention or program (including conversations, written or taped records, notes, test results, etc.) will be kept confidential.
2. **Consent.** There are really three faces of consent: program participants giving program staff consent to share their records or information with others for purposes of service provision; participants giving informed consent to submit to particular medical or other services, treatment, research, or program conditions; and community members consenting to the location or operation of an intervention in their neighborhood.
3. **Disclosure.** Like consent, disclosure in this context has more than one meaning: disclosure to participants of the conditions of the program they are in; disclosure of participant information to other individuals, agencies, etc.; and disclosure—by the program and by the affected individuals—of any conflict of interest that the program represents to any staff or board members.
4. **Competence.** By offering services of any kind, an organization is essentially making a contract with participants to do the job it says it will do. Implied in that contract is that those actually doing the work, and the organization as a whole, are competent to accomplish their goals under reasonable circumstances.
5. **Conflict of interest.** A conflict of interest is a situation in which someone's personal (financial, political, professional, social, sexual, family, etc.) interests could influence their judgment or actions in a financial or other decision, in carrying out their job, or in their relationships with participants. In community interventions, conflicts of interest may change—to the community's disadvantage—how a program is run or how its money is spent.
6. **Grossly unethical behavior.** This is behavior far beyond the bounds of the normally accepted ethical standards of society. In some cases, grossly unethical behavior may stem from taking advantage of a conflict of interest situation. In others, it may be a simple case of dishonesty or lack of moral scruples. Both individuals and organizations can be guilty of some instances of it, and in both cases, it is often a result of someone managing to justify the unjustifiable. Community programs need to be clear about their own ethical standards, and to hold individuals to them and to any other standards their professions demand. In most cases, staff members guilty of grossly unethical behavior should be dismissed as quickly as possible and prosecuted where it is appropriate.
7. **General ethical responsibilities.** Ethical behavior for a community intervention is more than simply following particular professional codes and keeping your nose clean. It means actively striving to do what is right for participants and for the community, and treating everyone—participants, staff members, funders, the community at large—in an ethical way.

---

and set limits by identifying behaviors that should be avoided. They *guide* or instruct by identifying obligations and desirable qualities" (Svara, 2007, p. 75). And, "they can *inspire* and set forth the broad goals that the adherents are supposed to promote" (Svara, 2007, p. 76). They also provide the consumers of health education/promotion services with an understanding of what they should expect from the provider.

Svara (2007) has noted that most codes of ethics have four different types of statements in them. **Box 5.5** lists these four different types of statements and references to where they may be found in the *Code of Ethics for the Health Education Profession* (CNHEO, 2020).

In addition to a code of ethics, a profession should also have a means by which to deal with (discipline) professionals who violate the code of ethics. "A wide range of enforcement mechanisms are possible" (Taub et al., 1987, p. 82). Such mechanisms may range from self-monitoring (also referred to as self-regulating) to a more formal process in which a committee of peers reviews ethics cases. Self-regulation is most effective when the person responsible for the potential violation of the code has enough professional and peer pressure to believe appropriate mediation is the best outcome for all. Formal ethical violations, most often evaluated by a committee of that professional organization, can recommend various avenues of resolution. First or minor violations of ethical behavior often carry disciplinary measures of "warnings." Repeated or major violations can lead to more serious penalties like limitations on the ability to practice and "even outright expulsion from the profession (that is, decertification or rescinding the member's license to practice)" (Gold & Greenberg, 1992, p. 145). In determining the sanctions, review committees may base their decision on a variety of factors including but not limited to (1) the type of violation (e.g., violation of privacy vs. sexual misconduct), (2) number of prior violations by the professional, (3) the willfulness of the violation, and (4) the level of responsibility of the professional (Svara, 2007).

> **Box 5.5** Types of Ethical Statements and Examples Found in the *Code of Ethics for the Health Education Profession*
>
> ---
>
> **"Don't" statements**
>
> Ex. There are no "Don't" statements in the *Code of Ethics for the Health Education Profession* (CNHEO, 2020), but they are assumed. All statements are made in the positive of what health education specialists will do, not what they shouldn't do. For example, instead of saying that health education specialists should never violate one's right to privacy, Article I. 4. states, "Health Education Specialists are ethically bound to respect privacy, confidentiality, and dignity of individuals and organizations" (CNHEO, 2020, p. 1).
>
> **Obligations and Responsibilities**
>
> Ex. Article II, Section 4:E.—"Health Education Specialists disclose potential benefits and harms of proposed services, strategies, and actions that affect individuals, organizations, and communities" (CNHEO, 2020, p. 3).
>
> **Virtues, Personal Qualities, and/or Values**
>
> Ex. Article I: 2.—"Health Education Specialists respect and support the rights of individuals and communities to make informed decisions about their health, as long as such decisions pose no risk to the health of others" (CNHEO, 2020, p. 1).
>
> **Aspirations**
>
> Ex. Article II, Section 6:A.—"Health Education Specialists foster an inclusive educational environment free from all forms of discrimination, coercion, and harassment" (CNHEO, 2020, p. 4).

Reproduced from Coalition of National Health Education Organizations. (2020). *Code of ethics for the health education profession.* http://www.cnheo.org/code-of-ethics.html

Ensuring Ethical Behavior in the Health Education/ Promotion Profession

Previously, we identified a number of steps that a profession can take to try to ensure ethical behavior from its professionals. Let's look at how the health education/promotion profession has dealt with this, starting with admission into a health education professional preparation program at a college or university.

Currently, the admission procedure into the profession of health education/promotion is not clear. Some colleges and universities preparing health education specialists have selective admission standards, but most have open admissions, meaning that students can enter the health education/promotion program if admitted to the institution. Once in the program, all academic institutions have varied retention standards, minimum grade point averages, and graduation requirements. With regard to the amount of education required in the profession, a bachelor's degree is required to sit for the certified health education specialist (CHES®) examination (see Chapter 6); however, there is no consensus in the profession that a bachelor's degree should be the standard. Many feel a master's degree is more appropriate. Regardless of whether a bachelor's or master's degree is required to take the credentialing examination, the earned credentials (CHES® or MCHES®) are not universally accepted, either in or out of the profession, as necessary to practice health education/promotion.

A professional code of ethics has existed for decades within the field. The first was created in 1976 by the Society for Public Health Education (SOPHE) while another was later written by the American Association for Health Education in 1994. In 1995, the National Commission for Health Education Credentialing, Inc. (NCHEC) (see Chapter 6 for more on NCHEC) and the Coalition of National Health Education Organizations (CNHEO) (see Chapter 8 for more on CNHEO) cosponsored a conference, "The Health Education Profession in the Twenty-First Century: Setting the Stage," at which it was recommended that efforts be expanded to develop a profession-wide code of ethics. Soon after

that conference, the CNHEO began work on such a code. After several years of work, in 1999, the *Code of Ethics for the Health Education Profession* was created and approved by all members of CNHEO, thus replacing the earlier codes developed by SOPHE and AAHE. That code was most recently updated in 2020 (see Appendix A for a copy of the code and more information on its development). However, like the codes before it, this code does not include a formal procedure for enforcement. So currently, the profession has informal enforcement via "the subtle influences colleagues exert on one another" (Iammarino et al., 1989, p. 104). "One of the true weaknesses of our present code of ethics is no accountability to its standards" (Goldsmith, 2006, p. 36).

Most recently, as a result of the Health Education Specialist Practice Analysis II 2020 (HESPA II 2020) project, an eighth area of responsibility was added to the competencies of the health education profession (see the discussion of the responsibilities in Chapter 6), Ethics and Professionalism. Specific competencies and subcompetencies related to ethical practice, the role of each professional to be an authoritative resource, professional development to enhance/maintain proficiency, and the need to promote the health education profession to others have been added to the responsibilities of a health education specialist. This addition will ensure that those health education specialists who seek certification or who are certified will work toward upholding these responsibilities. As stated earlier, since certification is not universally accepted, this new ethics competency will require time and research to understand professional impact (NCHEC, 2020).

Although moving in the right direction, the health education/promotion profession has much opportunity to refine its ethical foundations.

Summary

Ethical questions impact all aspects of life. Individuals on both a personal and professional level are constantly being confronted with ethical situations. To deal with these situations, people must have a basic understanding of how to make an ethical decision. To prepare readers for this task, this chapter presented key terms, such as philosophy, ethics, and morals; the philosophical, practical, and professional viewpoints of why people and professionals should work from an ethical base; the two major categories of theories (deontology and teleology) used to create ethical "yardsticks" for making ethical decisions; a set of principles and a guide for ethical decision making; a sampling of the ethical issues facing health education specialists today; and a discussion about how a profession can ensure that its professionals will act ethically.

Review Questions

1. What are the three major areas of philosophy? What does each of them mean?
2. In your own words, how do you define *ethics*?
3. What do the definitions of *ethics* and *morals* share? How are they different?
4. Why is it important to act ethically and who determines what qualifies as ethical?
5. What is meant by the term *professional ethics*? What is *research ethics*? In general terms, why are professional ethics important to you? How might that change over the course of your career?
6. Summarize the difference between the two major categories of ethical theories (deontology and teleology)?
7. Outline Thiroux's five principles that create a common ground for all ethical theories?
8. What should be included in a process for making ethical decisions? Are there things that should not be included in ethical decision making?
9. What is meant by the term *moral sensitivity*? Do you feel this should have a legitimate place in the health field?
10. Name five ethical issues currently facing the profession of health education/promotion. Can an issue be seen as ethical by one person while seen as unethical by another? Give an example of a health-related issue that might create this dynamic.
11. What does the profession currently do to ensure its professionals act ethically? What, if anything, might the profession change/improve to encourage more of their own to act ethically?
12. Define *code of ethics*. Should ethics play a role in all health-related decisions? Can you describe a situation in which ethics would not play a role?

Case Study

Pat (pronouns: they/them/theirs) accepted a position as a patient educator with the Hamilton Township Hospital after graduating with their bachelor's degree last spring. They are one of five health education specialists employed by the patient education department. About three months after Pat was hired, they observed Robert (pronouns: he/him/his), the most experienced patient educator in the department, engage in what they believed was unethical behavior. Pat observed Robert accepting a really nice windbreaker (worth about $80) from a pharmaceutical company representative.

In return, the pharmaceutical rep asked Robert to recommend the pharmaceutical company's glucometer during the diabetes education sessions he ran. Robert said that "that would be no problem." Do you agree with Pat—do you think this is unethical behavior? On what ethical principles do you base your response? Is there something in the *Code of Ethics for the Health Education Profession* (Appendix A) that supports your position? Say you agree with Pat; what would be your course of action? Do you think Robert's supervisor should be involved? Why or why not? Do you think Robert should be sanctioned by the profession? If so, how could it be enforced?

Critical Thinking Questions

1. Ethical dilemmas are rarely crystal clear and there is often more than one point of view to any given situation. How would you handle a coworker behaving in an unethical manner? Would your response change if you knew it was an isolated event? That it would continue? That it might result in a coworker being fired? That you might be viewed negatively for "whistle blowing"?

2. Do you think it is ethical to use disincentives to change people's health behavior? For example, charging smokers more for health insurance, or fining a person for not wearing a facial covering or texting while driving. Provide a rationale for your response.

3. If you were asked by one of your professors to help design a professional ethics course for health education/promotion majors or minors at your college/university, what would you suggest be included in the course? Why?

4. Several professions (e.g., medicine and law) have procedures for dealing with members' unethical behavior. In fact, if the offense is extreme enough a lawyer can be disbarred, and a physician could lose their license to practice medicine. Do you think the profession of health education/promotion should create a similar process to review unethical behavior and if necessary, take away the certification of certified health education specialists (CHES® or MCHES®)? Defend your response.

5. Do you think that all health education/promotion majors/minors should be required to take an ethics course while in college? Why or why not? If you responded yes to the question, do you think that a general ethics course open to all university students would be sufficient, or do you think the course should be specific to the profession? Why?

Activities

Directions for activities 1–4. You will find four scenarios that include an ethical issue. Using the 10-step decision-making process put forth in this chapter, write a response to one of the scenarios. In your response, include a response for each of the 10 components. Your responses to the 10 components should state your course of action.

1. You have been hired to work for the city health department to complete a project that was begun by your predecessor and funded with money from a local foundation. The grant requires the health department to develop X number of programs on the topic of hepatitis and then to present these programs to X number of people representing specific priority groups in the community. After being hired, you discover that the administrator of the

grant, your supervisor, has not adhered to the grant guidelines. Only half of programs have been developed as the grant required. Furthermore, the number of presentations is less than required, and presentations have been given to people not in the identified priority groups. In addition, your supervisor has taken some of the travel funds allocated to pay for your travel to and from presentations and has diverted them into his personal travel fund to attend a national conference in Las Vegas. It is now time for you to develop your year-end report, which will be sent directly to the local foundation office. Your supervisor has provided you with a copy of the original grant proposal and says to make sure your figures agree with those in the proposal. In other words, he expects you to "fudge" the data. What will you do?

2. As the health and fitness director of a large corporate wellness program, you have been asked to provide data to your supervisor that supports the effectiveness of your program. The trend in the company has been to cut programs that do not "carry their weight." The "bottom line" is important. In your review of the data related to your program, it is obvious that the data are not strong. However, in fairness to you, the program has been in operation for only two years, and it is too early to see the type of results management is looking for. You are the only one who has access to the data, and no one will know if the data you submit are accurate. How will you handle this situation?

3. You are a high school health teacher. The school board has just adopted a policy that prohibits the teaching or discussing of information related to contraceptives or abortion in the district. The only approach that can be mentioned in the classroom is abstinence. You have read research that indicates that the abstinence approach is not as effective as some may think. After class one day, one of your students approaches you and informs you that she is pregnant. She requests your help and asks for the name and location of an abortion clinic. She also asks that you not tell anyone else about this. What will you do?

4. You are the health education specialist for a large city hospital. Your supervisor has asked you to develop a program on "safer sex" practices for the LGBTQ population in the community. Because of your strong religious convictions, your personal values and beliefs are opposed to the LGBTQ lifestyle and the "safer sex" approach. In addition, you feel uncomfortable dealing with homosexuals in general and especially with anyone who is HIV-positive. How will you handle this situation?

5. Read thoroughly the *Code of Ethics for the Health Education Profession* presented in Appendix A, then provide written answers to the following questions.
   - What is your overall opinion of the code? Does it include everything you thought it would? Were there any surprises?
   - Do you think it should include any "Don't" statements? (Refer back to Box 5.5.) If yes, which ones? If no, why not?
   - Is there anything in the code you feel should not be there? If so, what and why?
   - If you could add something else to the code, what would it be?
   - Do you think the profession should incorporate a means of enforcement in the code? Why or why not?

6. Select one of the ethical theories presented in Table 5.1 to study further. Find and read from other sources explaining the theory. Then develop a presentation on the theory's application

to the practice of health education/
promotion.

7. Make an appointment to meet with one
of your professors or with a practicing
health education specialist. Inform him
or her that you would like to spend
about 15 to 20 minutes discussing
professional ethics. At the meeting ask
if they have ever observed a professional
situation that involved an ethical issue.

If so, ask him or her to describe the
situation without revealing the parties
who were involved. Then ask how
the situation was resolved. After your
meeting, summarize the discussion in
writing and compare the steps taken in
the situation to the components of the
10-step process presented in this chapter.
Do you think the situation was handled
properly? Why or why not?

Weblinks

1. **http://www.cnheo.org**

   Coalition of National Health Education
   Organizations (CNHEO)

   This is the home page for the CNHEO.
   The coalition has as its primary mission
   the mobilization of the resources of the
   health education/promotion profession
   to expand and improve health education/
   promotion, regardless of the setting. At this
   site you can print out a copy of the *Code of
   Ethics for the Health Education Profession*.

2. **http://www.ethics.org/**

   Ethics & Compliance Initiative

   The Ethics & Compliance Initiative
   (ECI) is composed of three nonprofit
   organizations that collaborate to provide
   ethics and compliance research and best
   practices.

3. **http://www.hhs.gov**

   U.S. Department of Health and Human
   Services (USDHHS)

   Search the USDHHS homepage for
   "Health Information Privacy"; this will

bring you to a page where you can get
more information about the National
Standards to Protect the Privacy of
Personal Health Information.

4. **https://www.appe-ethics.org/**

   Association for Practical and Professional
   Ethics (APPE)

   The APPE is a professional organization
   that works to advance scholarship,
   education, and practice in practical
   and professional ethics. It offers
   both individual and institution
   memberships.

5. **https://www.who.int/health-topics
   /ethics-and-health**

   The World Health Organization (WHO)

   The WHO examines ethical questions
   related to health, health care and
   public health; examines ethical issues
   that arise; and challenges healthcare
   professionals to raise and address
   questions related to access and
   allocation of health care.

References

Balog, J. E., Shirreffs, J. H., Gutierrez, R. D., & Balog,
L. F. (1985). Ethics and the field of health education.
The Eta Sigma Gamma Monograph Series, 4(1),
65–110.

Bastida, E. M., Tseng, T-S., McKeever, C., & Jack, Jr., J.
(2010). Ethics and community-based participatory

research: Perspectives from the field. *Health Promotion
Practice, 11*(1), 16–20.

Bayles, M. D. (1989). *Professional ethics* (2nd ed.).
Wadsworth.

Bromley, E., Mikesell, L., Jones, F., & Khodyakov, D.
(2015). From subject to participant: Ethics

and the evolving role of community in health research. *American Journal of Public Health, 105*(5), 900–908.

Buchanan, D., Khoshnood, K., Stopka, T., Shaw, S., Santelices, C., & Singer, M. (2002). Ethical dilemmas created by the criminalization of status behaviors: Case examples from ethnographic field research with injection drug users. *Health Education & Behavior, 29*(1), 30–42.

Coalition of National Health Education Organizations (CNHEO). (2020). *Code of ethics for the health education profession.* Retrieved December 20, 2020, from http://www.cnheo.org/code-of-ethics.html

Cottrell, R. R., & McKenzie, J. F. (2011). *Health promotion and education research methods: Using the five-chapter thesis/dissertation model* (2nd ed.). Jones & Bartlett.

Dawson, A., & Verweij, M. (Eds.). (2007). *Ethics, prevention, and public health.* Oxford University Press.

Dorman, S. M. (1994). The imperative for ethical conduct in scientific inquiry. In R. M. Pigg (Ed.), Ethical issues of scientific inquiry in health science education. *The Eta Sigma Gamma Monograph Series, 12*(2), 1–5.

Eve, D. J., Marty, P. J., McDermott, R. J., Klasko, S. K., & Sanberg, P. R. (2008). Stem cell research and health education. *American Journal of Health Education, 39*(3), 167–179.

Feeney, S., & Freeman, N. K. (1999). *Ethics and the early childhood educator.* National Association for the Education of Young Children.

Fisher, C. B. (2003). *Decoding the ethics code: A practical guide for psychologists.* Sage Publications.

Fox, R. C., & Swazey, J. P. (1997). Medical morality is not bioethics: Medical ethics in China and the United States. In N. S. Jecker, A. R. Jonsen, & R. A. Pearlman (Eds.), *Bioethics: An introduction to history, methods and practice* (pp. 237–251). Jones and Bartlett.

Gold, R. S., & Greenberg, J. S. (1992). *The health education ethics book.* Wm. C. Brown Publishers.

Goldsmith, M. (2006). Ethics in health education: Issues, concerns, and future directions. *The Health Education Monograph Series: Foundations of Health Education, 23*(1), 33–37.

Greenberg, J. S. (2001). *The code of ethics for the health education profession: A case study book.* Jones & Bartlett Publishers.

Hiller, M. D. (1987). Ethics and health education: Issues in theory and practice. In P. M. Lazes, L. Kaplan, & G. A. Gordon (Eds.), *The handbook of health education* (pp. 87–108). Aspen.

Lammarino, N. K., O'Rourke, T. W., Pigg, R. M., & Weinberg, A. D. (1989). Ethical issues in research and publication. *Journal of School Health, 59*(3), 101–104.

Kahan, B. (2012). Using a comprehensive best practices approach to strengthen ethical health-related practice. *Health Promotion Practice, 13*(4), 431–437.

Kimmel, A. J. (2007). *Ethical issues in behavioral research: Basic and applied perspectives* (2nd ed.). Blackwell Publishing.

Knight, R., Schoveller, J., Greyson, D., Kerr, T., Gilbert, M., & Shannon, K. (2014). Advancing population and public health ethics regarding HIV testing: A scoping review. *Critical Public Health, 24*(3), 238–295.

Margolis, L. (2000). Ethical principles for analyzing dilemmas in sex research. *Health Education & Behavior, 27*(1), 24–27.

Marks, R. (2009). Ethics and patient education: Health literacy and cultural dilemmas. *Health Promotion Practice, 10*(3), 328–332.

McGrath, E. Z. (1994). *The art of ethics: A psychology of ethical beliefs.* Loyola University Press.

McKenzie, J. F., Neiger, B. L., & Thackeray, R. (2013). *Planning, implementing, and evaluating health promotion programs: A primer* (6th ed.). Pearson.

McKenzie, J. F., Seabert, D. M., Hayden, J., & Cottrell, R. R. (2009). Textbook writing: A form of professional development. *Health Promotion Practice, 10*(1), 10–14.

McLeroy, K. R., Bibeau, D. L., & McConnell, T. C. (1993). Ethical issues in health education and health promotion: Challenges for the profession. *Journal of Health Education, 24*(5), 313–318.

Mellert, R. B. (1995). *Seven ethical theories.* Kendall Hunt.

Melnick, A. L. (2015). Case finding: Screening, testing, and contact tracing. In R. Gaare Bernheim, J. F. Childress, R. J. Bonnie, & A. L. Melnick (Eds.), Essentials of public health ethics (pp. 119–143). Jones & Bartlett Learning.

Minkler, M., Fadem, P., Perry, M., Blum, K., Moore, L., & Rogers, J. (2002). Ethical dilemmas in participatory action research: A case study from the disability community. *Health Education & Behavior, 29*(1), 14–29.

Minkler, M., Pies, C., & Hyde, C. A. (2012). Ethical issues in community organizing and building. In M. Minkler (Ed.), *Community organizing and community building for health* (3rd ed., pp. 110–129). Rutgers University Press.

Minkler, M., Vásquez, V. B., Tajik, M., & Petersen, D. (2008). Promoting environmental justice through community-based participatory research: The role of community and partnership capacity. *Health Education & Behavior, 35*(1), 119–137.

Modell, S. M., & Citrin, T. (2002). Ethics instruction in an issues-oriented course on public health genetics. *Health Education & Behavior, 29*(1), 43–60.

Morrison, E. E. (2006). *Ethics in health administration: A practical approach for decision makers.* Jones & Bartlett.

Morrison, E. E., & Furlong, B. (2014). *Health care ethics: Critical issues for the 21st Century* (3rd ed.). Jones & Bartlett Learning.

National Commission for Health Education Credentialing, Inc. (2020). *Health education responsibilities.* Retrieved December 20, 2020, from https://www.nchec.org/health-education-responsibilities

Nelson, W. A. (2005). An organizational ethics decision-making process. *Healthcare Executive, 20*(4), 8–14.

Paul, C., & Brooks, B. (2015). The rationalization of ethical research: Revisionist accounts of the Tuskegee Syphilis Study and the New Zealand "unfortunate experiment." *American Journal of Public Health, 105*(10), e12–e19.

Penland, L. R., & Beyrer, M. K. (1981). Ethics and health education: Issues and implications. *Health Education, 12*(4), 6–7.

Pigg, R. M. (Ed.). (1994). Ethical issues of scientific inquiry in health science education. *The Eta Sigma Gamma Monograph Series, 12*(2), 1–150.

Pigg, R. M. (2006). Conflict and consensus on ethics in publishing. *The Health Education Monograph Series: Foundations of Health Education, 23*(1), 38–41.

Pigg, R. M., Jr. (2010). Three essential questions in defining a personal philosophy. In J. M. Black, S. Furney, H. M. Graf, & A. E. Nolte (Eds.), *Philosophical foundations of health education* (pp. 11–15). Jossey-Bass.

Pozgar, G. D. (2013). *Legal and ethical issues for health professionals* (3rd ed.). Jones & Bartlett Learning.

Price, J. H., & Dake, J. A. (2002). Ethical guidelines for manuscript reviewers and journal editors. *American Journal of Health Education, 33*(4), 194–196.

Price, J. H., Dake, J. A., & Islam, R. (2001). Selected ethical issues in research and publication: Perceptions of health education faculty. *Health Education & Behavior, 28*(1), 51–64.

Price, J. H., Dake, J. A., & Telljohann, S. K. (2001). Ethical issues regarding service: Perceptions of health education faculty. *American Journal of Health Education, 32*(4), 208–215.

Pritchard, M. S. (2006). *Professional integrity: Thinking ethically.* University Press of Kansas.

Rabinowitz, P. (2015). *The community health toolbox: Ethical issues in community interventions.* Retrieved April 4, 2016, from http://ctb.ku.edu/en/table-of-contents/analyze/choose-and-adapt-community-interventions/ethical-issues/main

Reamer, F. G. (2006). *Social work values and ethics* (3rd ed.). Columbia University Press.

Remley, T. P., & Herlihy, B. (2007). *Ethical, legal, and professional issues in counseling* (2nd ed.). Merrill, Prentice Hall.

Rest, J., Narvaes, D., Bebeau, M. J., & Thoma, S. J. (1999). *Postconventional moral thinking: A neo-kohlbergian approach.* L. Erlbaum Associates.

Rothschild, M. L. (2000). Ethical considerations in support of marketing of public health issues. *American Journal of Health Behavior, 24*(1), 26–35.

Shaw-Ridley, M., & Ridley, C. R. (2010). The health disparities industry: Is it an ethical conundrum? *Health Promotion Practice, 11*(4), 454–464.

Shive, S. E., & Marks, R. (2006). The influence of ethical theories in the practice of health education. *Health Promotion Practice, 7*(3), 287–288.

Siegel, M., & Lotenberg, L. D. (2007). *Marketing public health: Strategies to promote social change* (2nd ed.). Jones & Bartlett.

Sperry, L. (2007). *Dictionary of ethical and legal terms and issues: The essential guide for mental health professionals.* Routledge.

Stapleton, G., Schröder-Bäck, P., Laaser, U., Meerschoek, A., & Popa, D. (2014). Global health ethics: An introduction to prominent theories and relevant topics. *Global Health Action, 7*(s2), 1–7.

Summers, J. (2014). Principles of healthcare ethics. In E. E. Morrison & B. Furlong, *Health care ethics: Critical issues for the 21st Century* (3rd ed., pp. 47–63). Jones & Bartlett Learning.

Svara, J. (2007). *The ethics primer for public administrators in government and nonprofit organizations.* Jones & Bartlett.

Taub, A., Kreuter, M., Parcel, G., & Vitello, E. (1987). Report of the AAHE/SOPHE Joint Committee on Ethics. *Health Education Quarterly, 14*(1), 79–90.

Telljohann, S. K., Price, J. H., & Dake, J. A. (2001). Selected ethical issues in the teaching: Perceptions of health education faculty. *American Journal of Health Education, 32*(2), 66–74.

The Society of Prospective Medicine Board of Directors (SPM). (1999). Ethics guidelines for the development and use of health assessments. In G. C. Hyner, K. W. Peterson, J. W. Travis, J. E. Dewey, J. J. Foerster, & E. M. Framer (Eds.), *SPM handbook of health assessment tools* (pp. xxii–xxvi). The Society of Prospective Medicine.

Thiroux, J. P. (1995). *Ethics: Theory and practice* (5th ed.). Prentice Hall.

Thompson, I., Melia, K., & Boyd, K. (2000). *Nursing ethics* (4th ed.). Churchill Livingstone.

Thurston, W. E., Vollman, A. R., & Burgess, M. M. (2003). Ethical review of health promotion program evaluation proposals. *Health Promotion Practice, 4*(1), 45–50.

Tschudin, V. (2003). *Ethics in nursing: The caring relationship* (3rd ed.). Butterworth Heinemann.

U.S. Department of Health and Human Services. (n.d.). *Health information privacy.* Retrieved April 9, 2016, from http://www.hhs.gov/ocr/privacy

Westin, A. F. (1968). *Privacy and freedom.* Atheneum.

White, T. I. (1988). *Right and wrong: A brief guide to understanding ethics.* Prentice Hall.

Wiley, D. C. (2002). The ethics of abstinence-only and abstinence-plus sexuality education. *Journal of School Health, 72*(4), 164–167.

Young, M., & Valois, R. F. (2010). Magic, morals, and health: Plus 40 years. *American Journal of Health Education, 41*(1), 18–19.

CHAPTER 6

The Health Education Specialist: Roles, Responsibilities, Certifications, and Advanced Study

CHAPTER OBJECTIVES

After reading this chapter and answering the questions at the end, you should be able to:

- Define *credentialing*.
- Discuss the history of role delineation and certification.
- Explain the differences among *certification, licensure,* and *accreditation*.
- List and describe the eight major responsibilities of a health education specialist.
- Discuss the need for advanced study in health education/promotion.
- Outline factors to consider in applying for master's degree programs.

Although education about health has been around since the beginning of human intelligence, health education/promotion as a profession is, relatively speaking, an infant. When any infant begins to mature, it takes on its own identity. This chapter chronicles major historical events that have helped shape the identity of health education/promotion since the 1970s. The current identity of health education/promotion is also presented in terms of roles, responsibilities, certification, and accreditation.

The importance of advanced study and continuing education in the health education/promotion profession is also discussed.

Quality Assurance and Credentialing

As a profession matures and grows, it becomes increasingly important that professional preparation become standardized and that individual practitioners perform the same set of skills at a high level of competency. Quality assurance and credentialing often go hand-in-hand and are utilized to help ensure a profession's excellence. It is important to be familiar with these terms as they apply to health education/promotion. In the business world, the term **quality assurance** means "the planned and systematic activities necessary to provide adequate confidence that the product or service will meet given requirements" (Quality Assurance Solutions, 2020). **Credentialing** is one means by which professions such as health education/promotion demonstrate quality assurance. In other words, credentialing would be the "planned and systematic activities" used to increase confidence that the product or service—in this case, health education specialists—is meeting the requirements of the profession. Credentialing is a process whereby an individual, such as a health education specialist, or a professional preparation program demonstrates that established standards are met. When people or programs meet specific standards established by a credentialing body, they are recognized for having done so. We say, "They earned their credentials," which indicates that they are meeting their profession's requirements. Credentialing can take the form of accreditation, licensure, or certification.

Accreditation is "The process by which an agency or organization evaluates and recognizes an institution as meeting certain predetermined standards" (McKenzie et al., 2018, p. 319) Thus, the health education/promotion program at any particular institution may be accredited by one of several outside agencies discussed later in this chapter. For example, the health education/promotion program at Alpha University could be accredited by Beta Accrediting Group. Such a process takes place after the program at Alpha University creates a self-study document that shows how it meets the Beta Accrediting Group's standards. Accrediting procedures may also include an on-campus visit by representatives from Beta. Throughout the process, factors such

as student–teacher ratio, curriculum, faculty qualifications, budget, evaluation procedures, and diversity are examined closely.

Licensure is "the process by which an agency or government [usually a state] grants permission to individuals to practice a given profession by certifying that those licensed have attained specific standards of competence" (Cleary, 1995, p. 39). Licensure applies to most medical professionals, such as doctors, nurses, dentists, and physical therapists. The only health education specialists who are licensed in the United States at the present time are school health education specialists in some states.

Certification "is a process by which a profession grants recognition to an individual who, upon completion of a competency-based curriculum, can demonstrate a predetermined standard of performance" (Cleary, 1995, p. 39). Note that certification is granted to an individual, not a program, and it is given by the profession or an independent certifying agency, not by a governmental body. Certification is available for all health education specialists, regardless of specialty area. One who is certified is recognized as a **Certified Health Education Specialist (CHES)** and may use the initials **CHES** after one's name and academic degree. In the fall of 2010, an advanced certification became available. Those who obtain this advanced certification are **Master Certified Health Education Specialists (MCHES)** and may use the initials **MCHES** after their names. See **Figure 6.1** for an overview of quality assurance mechanisms available for health education programs in the United States.

History of Role Delineation and Certification

Certification in health education got its formal start around 1978. At that time, individual certification for health education specialists

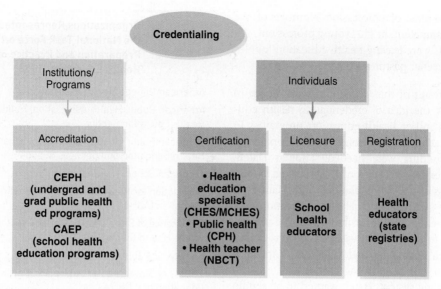

Figure 6.1 Overview of health education credentialing in the United States.

Note: CHES, Certified Health Education Specialist; CAPE, Council for the Accreditation of Educator Preparation; CEPH, Council on Education for Public Health; CPH, Certified in Public Health; MCHES, Master Certified Health Education Specialist; NBCT, National Board Certified Teacher; NCATE, National Council for the Accreditation of Teacher Education; SABPAC, SOPHE/AAHE Baccalaureate Approval Committee; SOPHE, Society for Public Health Education; TEAC, Teacher Education Accreditation Council.

Modified from Cottrell, R. R., Auld, M. E., Birch, D. A., Taub, A., King, L. R., & Allegrante, J. P. (2012). Progress and directions in professional credentialing for health education in the United States. *Health Education and Behavior, 39*(6), 681–694. https://doi.org/10.1177%2F1090198112466096

was not available, except for school health education specialists, who had to be licensed or certified in the state where they taught.

Program accreditation was available only for school health and master's level public health professional preparation programs. Many public health programs outside of schools of public health, and all community health education programs, were not accredited nor was accreditation available for these programs. This gave rise to a situation in which there were great discrepancies in professional preparation. One program might look entirely different from another program, and one health educator might have very different skills than another. To say that an individual was a health educator had little meaning. In describing the situation, Helen Cleary (see **Figure 6.2**), who was president of the Society for Public Health Education (SOPHE) in 1974, wrote the following:

What I found in my travels [as SOPHE president] was a profession

in disarray. Many, many health educators could neither define themselves nor their role. It was clear that the preparation of most was so varied that there was no common core. There was no professional identity,

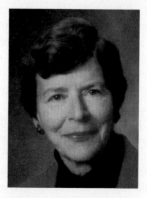

Figure 6.2 Helen P. Cleary—the person most responsible for establishing certification for health education specialists.

Courtesy of The National Commission for Health Education Credentialing.

no sense of a profession. Numbers of competent, bright, young professionals were leaving health education for greener pastures. (Cleary, 1995, p. 2)

As a result of this situation, Cleary began to pursue the idea of credentialing health educators and/or health education programs. To undertake such a project, outside expertise and funding were needed. Thomas Hatch, director of the Division of Associated Health Professions in the Bureau of Health Manpower of the Department of Health, Education, and Welfare, expressed an interest in the project. Prior to funding the project; however, they needed assurances that members of the profession would work together to create a credentialing system. Hatch wanted to be certain that those who practiced health education in different settings would have enough in common to develop one set of standards.

In response to Hatch's concern, a conference, known as the Bethesda Conference on Commonalities and Differences, was held in February of 1978 in Bethesda, Maryland. The conference's planning committee was composed of representatives from the eight organizations composing the Coalition of Health Education Organizations. This planning committee formulated two questions to be answered at the conference: (1) What are the commonalities and differences in the function of health educators practicing in different settings? and (2) What are the commonalities and differences in the preparation of health educators? (Cleary, 1995, p. 3).

After much discussion, conference attendees concluded that health education was one profession and that a credentialing system was necessary. "It was the consensus of the participants that standards were essential if they were to provide quality service to the public and if they were to survive as a viable profession" (Cleary, 1986, p. 130). Further, the conference planning committee members were asked to continue as a task force to develop the credentialing system. Thus, the

Table 6.1 Organizations Represented on the National Task Force on the Preparation and Practice of Health Educators, 1978

American College Health Association

American Public Health Association, Public Health Education Section

American Public Health Association, School Health Education and Services Section

American School Health Association

Association for the Advancement of Health Education (AAHE)

Conference of State and Territorial Directors of Public Health Education

Society for Public Health Education, Inc.

Society of State Directors of Health, Physical Education and Recreation

National Task Force on the Preparation and Practice of Health Educators was born (see **Table 6.1**).

In January of 1979, funding became available to embark on the project, and **role delineation** for health educators got underway. Alan Henderson was hired as the project director. Under his leadership, a working committee of the task force began the difficult job of defining the health education specialist's role. In describing this process, Cleary (1995) notes, "For the first time in the profession's history, specialists in school health education and in community health education faced each other across the table and learned that each was dealing with similar concepts, but using different terminology and, as well, applying them in different settings" (p. 5).

Once the initial phase of role delineation was completed, the next step was to verify and refine the role of a health educator. Funding for this became available in March 1980. Health education specialists working in all areas of health education were surveyed to verify the role of a health educator. Survey results were positive; there were no significant differences among practitioners in different settings.

In addition to the survey, a conference for college and university health education faculty members was held in Birmingham, Alabama, in February of 1981. The conference provided the opportunity for academics to review the initial role delineation work and discuss its potential impact on the field. The planning committee chairman was Warren E. Schaller from Ball State University, and 238 academics from 125 institutions attended.

Many conference participants were happy with the work and direction of the task force, but others were not. Differences of opinion surrounding the health educator as a content expert vs. a process expert emerged and probably reflected the different types of professional preparation programs the faculty represented. Although these differences were real, they were not divisive enough to alter the work of the task force.

The third step in the role delineation process involved creating a curriculum framework based on the verified role of a health educator. Initially, the task force decided to develop a curriculum guide, which is a fairly specific set of rules used to develop a curriculum. Little room is left for interpretation because the curriculum must meet the standards established in the guide. Betty Mathews from the University of Washington and Herb L. Jones from Ball State University were recruited to do the actual writing.

After a draft copy of the curriculum guide was developed, it had to be pretested. Eleven regional workshops were held around the country to obtain feedback on the guide. Again, differences surfaced regarding whether health educators were specialists in content or process. Furthermore, some felt entry-level preparation should be at the bachelor's degree level, whereas others believed it should be at the master's degree level. Feedback was also obtained from professional associations and practitioners in the field.

To deal with some of the criticisms and to make the curriculum guide less rigid, it was ultimately transformed into a curriculum framework. A framework merely provides a frame of reference around which a curriculum can be developed. As Cleary (1995) notes, "It does not tell a faculty what to teach or how to teach it. It simply tells them what the students should know when they have completed the program of studies" (p. 9). Marion Pollock was the individual responsible for transforming the curriculum guide into a curriculum framework.

At this juncture, it was important to check with those in the profession to determine if they wanted to continue with the development of a credentialing system and, if so, what kind of system they wanted. The Second Bethesda Conference was held in February of 1986, with 99 attendees. Participants were divided into five groups and asked to answer several predetermined questions. When reports from the groups were analyzed, four of the five were in favor of a certification system for individuals and some form of credentialing for professional preparation programs. They recommended that the task force continue to develop the credentialing system.

Over the next two years, the task force continued to work toward the development of a certification system for individual health education specialists. The Professional Examination Service (PES), which developed certification and licensure exams for many other professions, was contracted to assist with this process. Not only was its experience in test development vital to the process, but it was also willing to provide start-up funds to get the process off the ground.

By June of 1988, the National Task Force on the Preparation and Practice of Health Education had functioned for 10 years. With the certification of individual health education specialists about to become a reality, it was time to establish a more permanent structure to manage the certification process. As a result, the **National Commission for Health Education Credentialing, Inc. (NCHEC)** was formed to replace the National Task Force. Today, NCHEC still oversees and administers the health education certification process. NCHEC's mission "is to enhance the professional practice of Health Education by promoting and sustaining a credentialed body of Health Education Specialists. To meet this mission, NCHEC certifies health education specialists, promotes professional development, and strengthens professional preparation and practice" (NCHEC, n.d.-d).

Individual Certification

When a new certification program is initiated, charter certification is usually available for a limited time. Charter certification allows qualified individuals to get certified on the basis of their academic training, work experience, and references without taking an exam. After the charter period expires, anyone seeking certification must meet all criteria for certification and pass the examination. The CHES charter certification period began in October of 1988 and ended in 1990. After charter certification, when the first exam was held in 1990, 644 candidates passed it to become Certified Health Education Specialists.

The CHES voluntary professional certification program established for the first time a national standard for health education practice. All health education/promotion students are strongly urged to obtain national certification upon graduation (see Practitioner's Perspective). Certification includes the following benefits (NCHEC, n.d.-c):

- Establishes a national standard of practice for all health education specialists.
- Attests to the individual health education specialist's knowledge and skills.
- Assists employers in identifying qualified health education practitioners.
- Develops a sense of pride and accomplishment among certified health education specialists.
- Promotes continued professional development for health education specialists.

Currently, eligibility to sit for the CHES exam is based exclusively on academic qualifications. You must "possess a bachelor's, master's,

---

Practitioner's Perspective

Mitchell Kron

CURRENT POSITION/ TITLE: Disease Investigator

EMPLOYER: Central District Health

DEGREE/INSTITUTION: B.S. Public Health with an emphasis in Health Education & Promotion, 2018, Boise State University

My job responsibilities: On a broader level, Disease Investigators reach out to individuals who test positive for infectious diseases to conduct an investigation. The goals of the investigation include learning how the individual contracted the disease, finding out who the person may have exposed to the disease while they were contagious, and providing disease prevention education. My Disease Investigator position, specifically, involves conducting COVID-19 case investigations for my local health department. The familiar term for our responsibilities is Contact Tracing. After we elicit contacts from the individual who tests positive, we reach out to the people exposed to the virus to see if they are experiencing any symptoms. We educate about quarantine guidelines, answer any questions, and direct them to any needed resources.

How I obtained my job: Central District Health (CDH) has always been on my list of places where I could see myself starting a career. When I saw the job posting for the open position on social media, I filled out the application and sent my resume and cover letter. During my interview, the hiring staff was excited to see that I had obtained my CHES credential. My Program Managers know the value of having Certified Health Education Specialists on staff because we have training, knowledge, and skillsets that translate well into many department positions, including Disease Investigator. CDH offered me a position almost immediately after my interview, and I started making calls just a few days later.

What I like most about my job: Helping slow the spread of COVID-19 in my community has been very gratifying. We receive many thank you's from community members nearly every day. Doctors, nurses, first responders, teachers, and even children thank us for our efforts in fighting the pandemic. It feels good to know you are helping save lives.

What I like least about my job: The most difficult part of my job is speaking with people who have lost loved ones to COVID-19. Sometimes it makes you feel like what we are doing is not helping. However, when we talk with people who have lost loved ones or are currently ill, they appreciate the education and support we provide. It is also tricky to have conversations with people who want to politicize the virus by saying COVID-19 is a hoax, no big deal, or they don't trust the government. We have to remember that public health is nonpartisan, and we are doing our best to keep our communities and loved ones safe and healthy. Communicating that message to people is essential, even if they do not want to believe what you say. Sometimes you will change someone's mind, but sometimes the people who need help the most will continue to refuse it.

Why I decided to obtain my Certified Health Education Specialist (CHES) credential: As soon as I found out about the credential, I knew it was something I wanted to acquire. I take pride in my profession and in being a health advocate. Having a nationally accredited certification will give you an edge in the hiring process, as it did for me. Some Health Educator positions may require a CHES certification before even considering applicants.

How I prepared for the CHES: Planning study groups with my peers who were also taking the exam was a big help. We scheduled about three hours per week for several weeks leading up to the exam. We would quiz each other on the competencies and responsibilities of a CHES, make flashcards for key terms, and help each other understand topics from study guides. I also completed a lot of practice tests, which were helpful.

How the CHES credential has helped me: The CHES credential helped me get the position I currently have, and it will very likely help me get another position in the department. Passing the exam and getting the credential also gave me the confidence to know that I have what it takes to succeed in the field.

How my work relates to the responsibilities and competencies of a CHES: My daily tasks fall under several areas of responsibility and competencies. We collect primary data about COVID-19 symptoms during investigations, which helps determine how to educate the public about watching for symptoms (1.3.5). We implement health education by educating contagious people to avoid spreading the virus to the community and household members (3.3). We deliver health education as designed by the CDC and Central District Health, making the messaging consistent (3.3.6, 7.2.8). There are many mixed messages surrounding COVID-19, so we help individuals understand which information is valid (6.1.2). When we communicate with the public, we must remember we represent the local health department so providing guidance, and building relationships is essential (6.3.3). Finally, the most significant part of the job is communication. We are advocating for the health of a diverse community. We must be able to identify the health literacy of the audience and tailor the messaging to fit. For example, sometimes you speak with someone with a strong health background—that conversation would be significantly different from someone with a lower level of health knowledge (7.1.2, 7.1.3).

Reproduced from National Commission for Health Education Credentialing. (2015). *Areas of responsibilities, competencies, and sub-competencies for health education specialists – 2015.* https://assets.speakcdn.com/assets/2251/2015_hespa_competencies_and_sub-competencies.pdf or doctoral degree from an accredited institution of higher education; *AND* (1) an official transcript (including course titles) that clearly shows a major in health education, e.g., Health Education, Community Health Education, Public Health Education, School Health Education, etc. Degree/major must explicitly be in a discipline of Health Education/Promotion; *OR* (2) an official transcript that reflects at least 25 semester hours or 37 quarter hours of course work (with a grade 'C' or better) with specific preparation addressing the Eight Areas of Responsibility and Competency for Health Educators" (NCHEC, n.d.-a).

Graduate Health Education Standards

The roles and responsibilities document, *A Competency-Based Framework for Professional Development of Certified Health Education Specialists* (NCHEC, 1996), defined the skills needed for the entry-level health education/promotion professional. This document provided guidance for professional preparation programs at the bachelor's degree level but not at the graduate degree level. Although many health education specialists with advanced master's and doctoral degrees had obtained certification, it attested only to the fact that they had entry-level skills. The need existed for an advanced level of certification.

In June of 1992, the Joint Committee for Graduate Standards was established. After much work, discussion, and review, the Joint Committee for Graduate Standards developed a draft document that contained additional responsibilities, competencies, and subcompetencies specific to graduate-level preparation (Joint Committee for Graduate Standards, 1996).

In February of 1996, 134 health education specialists from more than 100 colleges and universities gathered at the National Congress for Institutions Preparing Graduate Health Educators. At this meeting in Dallas,

Texas, the draft document of graduate-level competencies was presented to attendees. After revisions were made, the final version was presented to the AAHE and SOPHE boards of directors, who granted approval in March of 1997. These graduate-level competencies served to guide the health education curriculum of professional preparation programs but were not used for individual certification purposes. In the fall of 2010, advanced certification became available through NCHEC. Those who obtain this advanced certification are designated Master Certified Health Education Specialists (MCHES). A graduate degree is not required to obtain the MCHES designation; rather, MCHES indicates that an individual is practicing advanced-level competencies.

Competencies Update Project

Since the initial Role Delineation Project began in the 1980s, health education/promotion had evolved and matured. Changes in the profession created a need to reverify the competencies and subcompetencies of a health education specialist. The **Competencies Update Project (CUP)** began in 1998 and was completed in 2004 (Gilmore et al., 2005). This was the first of four updates that have been completed since the competencies were first developed. The majority of the CUP work was conducted by a three-person steering committee comprising Gary Gilmore, chair; Alyson Taub; and Larry Olsen (see **Figure 6.3**). The profession owes a deep debt of gratitude to these individuals for the time and effort they invested in this project.

NCCA Accreditation and Five-Year Updates

The National Commission for Certifying Agencies (NCCA) accredits professional credentials offered by certifying agencies.

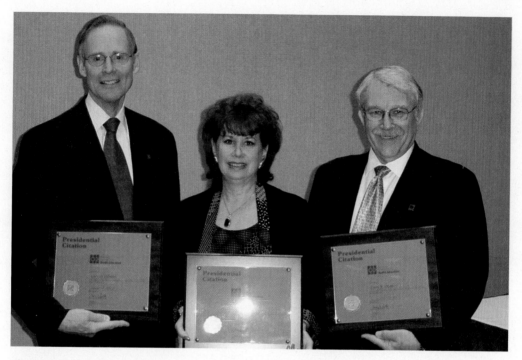

Figure 6.3 CUP Steering Committee. From left, Gary Gilmore, chair; Alyson Taub; and Larry Olsen.
Courtesy of The National Commission for Health Education Credentialing.

Essentially, the NCCA accredits the credentials provided by accrediting bodies. The NCHEC and the health education profession thought it important that the CHES and MCHES credentials be accredited by the NCCA. To obtain accreditation from NCCA, an accrediting agency must follow recognized best practices. Both the CHES and MCHES credentials have been accredited by the NCCA (NCHEC, 2015).

One of the best practices required by the NCCA is updating the job analysis and thus the competencies for the agency's field every five years. To meet the five-year update requirement, NCHEC, along with AAHE and SOPHE, commissioned the 2010 job analysis study (NCHEC & SOPHE, 2020) This study was needed to update the health education competencies, last revised in 2005 by the CUP project. Results of the study were released in 2010, called the Health Education Job Analysis 2010 model (*HEJA 2010* model).

Again, to keep the five-year update requirement, in the Spring of 2013, NCHEC and its partners SOPHE and ProExam began work for the Health Education Specialist Practice Analysis 2015 (HESPA). The 18-month project was completed and results were published in 2015 (National Commission for Health Education Credentialing and Society for Public Health Education, 2015).

The areas of responsibility remained essentially the same over the first three revisions as they were in the initial entry-level framework with only minor wording changes. This changed with the fourth revision, which became known as the Health Education Practice Analysis II 2020 (HESPA II 2020 model). Begun in 2017 and completed in 2020, this latest revision identified eight areas of responsibility (NCHEC, 2020). **Table 6.2** shows a comparison of the HESPA 2015 model's seven responsibilities with the eight responsibilities in the HESPA II 2020 model.

Table 6.2 Comparison of HESPA 2015's Seven Areas of Responsibility with HESPA II 2020's Eight Areas of Responsibility

HESPA 2015 Model	HESPA II 2020 Model
I. Assess needs, resources, and capacity for health education/promotion	I. Assessment of Needs and Capacity
II. Plan health education/promotion	II. Planning
III. Implement health education/promotion	III. Implementation
IV. Conduct evaluation and research related to health education/promotion	IV. Evaluation and Research
V. Administer and manage health education/promotion	V. Advocacy
VI. Serve as a health education/promotion resource person	VI. Communication
VII. Communicate, promote, and advocate for health, health education/promotion, and the profession	VII. Leadership and Management
	VIII. Ethics and Professionalism

By examining this comparison table, it can be seen that the first four responsibilities essentially cover the same areas as in the previous models. While the other areas appear somewhat different, the competencies and subcompetencies associated with these areas are still included, but rearranged. The competencies listed in HESPA 2015 under responsibility V to administer and manage have now been incorporated into Responsibility VII in the new model with the addition of a leadership focus. The competencies listed under Responsibility VI in the HESPA 2015 model have been divided between Responsibilities VI and VII in the new model. The competencies associated with communication in Responsibility VII of the HESPA 2015 model have been moved to a new Responsibility VI in HESPA II 2020, which puts added emphasis on the importance of communication. The competencies in responsibility VII of HESPA 2015 related to advocating for health, health education/health promotion, and the profession

have been divided between HESPA II 2020 responsibility V, Advocacy; and responsibility VII, Ethics and Professionalism. Overall, by adding the eighth area of responsibility, the HESPA II 2020 model has placed greater emphasis on advocacy and communication than have previous models. The Task Analysis Panel that reviewed and revised the responsibilities, competencies and subcompetencies felt strongly that advocacy and communication play a greater role in the work of health education specialists now than they did previously and thus the additional emphasis on these two areas was warranted.

The important point here is that the health education/promotion profession has and continues to carefully and systematically review and validate the responsibilities, competencies and subcompetencies of a health education specialist. The CHES exam is based on these standards and the health education/promotion curricula of professional preparation programs should be grounded on them as well.

International Efforts in Quality Assurance

Outside of the United States, efforts to ensure quality in health education/promotion have also occurred. According to Allegrante, Barry, Auld, et al. (2009), Canada, Australia, New Zealand, member states of the European Union and Council of Europe, Spain, Japan, Israel, the People's Republic of China, India, and Taiwan have all endeavored to improve health education or health promotion practice.

In an effort to promote international exchange and understanding related to the core competencies of health education/promotion and various credentialing mechanisms, a working group of 26 health education/promotion scholars and leaders from around the world met at the National University of Ireland in the summer of 2008. This meeting, now known as the Galway Consensus Conference, was a first effort to identify and codify agreement around quality assurance and credentialing on an international basis.

At this conference, the Domains of Core Competencies were developed (Allegrante et al., 2009). The domains are broader than competencies, but using these broad domains, competencies and credentialing systems can be developed by nations around the world. The Domains of Core Competencies align nicely with the NCHEC Responsibilities of a Health Education Specialist (NCHEC, 2020). Several of the Domains are exactly the same as the NCHEC responsibilities including assessing, planning, implementing, evaluating, leadership, and advocacy. Two Domains, catalyzing change, and partnerships, are not identified as one of the eight major NCHEC Responsibilities but would still be considered important skills that would actually be delineated at the competency or subcompetency level by NCHEC.

Since the Galway Consensus Conference, a new round of efforts to enhance professional preparation standards and credentialing

has emerged in North America, throughout Europe, and in other regions and countries of the world such as Australia, Canada, Latin America, and New Zealand (Allegrante et al., 2012). In Europe, professional standards for health promotion have been developed and reviewed (Speller et al., 2012).

The International Union for Health Promotion and Education (IUHPE) has established an accreditation system (IUHPE, 2016). The goal of the IUHPE European Health Promotion Accreditation System is, "to promote quality assurance, competence and mobility in Health Promotion practice, education and training globally" (IUHPE, 2020). This accreditation is to provide recognition to individual practitioners as well as education and training courses.

Accreditation Task Forces

"Accreditation is a process by which a recognized professional body evaluates an entire program against predetermined criteria or standards" (Cleary, 1995). In most cases, colleges and universities that train students to enter a given profession are accredited by a recognized professional body that operates independently of the school. If a program does not meet the standards of the recognized professional body, it can be refused accreditation or lose its accreditation status. A nonaccredited program might have difficulty recruiting new students, recruiting quality faculty, placing program graduates in jobs, obtaining grant funds and may be restricted in its participation in the profession. Accreditation helps ensure that all students entering the profession have similar training and preparation. Accreditation has been a major focus for the health education/promotion profession since 2000. In January 2000, the SOPHE and AAHE cosponsored a meeting in Dulles, Virginia, to explore the issue of accreditation. Twenty-four professionals who were broadly representative of health education/promotion professional preparation programs or other stakeholders were invited to attend. Meeting participants reached consensus that a "coordinated accreditation system" was needed.

As a result of this meeting, the SOPHE/ AAHE National Task Force on Accreditation in Health Education was established, and Dr. John Allegrante and Dr. Collins Airhihenbuwa agreed to serve as co-chairs (Allegrante et al., 2004). The Task Force was charged to (1) "gather background information and refine plans for a comprehensive, coordinated quality assurance system that meets commonly accepted standards of accreditation, and (2) develop processes for ensuring profession-wide involvement in the discussion and design of such a system to foster its adoption and utilization" (SOPHE, 2000, p. 5).

After a comprehensive study of the issue, the task force completed its work in the spring of 2004 and submitted its final report to the AAHE and SOPHE boards of directors (Allegrante et al., 2004). In this report, four principles were given to guide the profession:

1. Health education is a single profession, with common roles and responsibilities.
2. Professional preparation in health education provides the health education specialist with knowledge and skills that form a foundation of common and setting-specific competencies.
3. Accreditation is the primary quality assurance mechanism in higher education.
4. The health education profession is responsible for assuring quality in professional preparation and practice (Allegrante et al., 2004, p. 676).

On the basis of these four principles, the task force developed eight important recommendations that were included within the study's final report. Since the release of the report, many of the recommendations have been implemented. Below is a summary of the eight recommendations, each followed by a comment on the progress that has been made on that recommendation:

1. Accreditation should replace approval as the accepted quality assurance mechanism for health education professional preparation. (This is accomplished. CEPH is now accrediting standalone undergraduate programs. The last SABPAC program approvals expired in 2019 [E. Auld, personal communication, December 1, 2020]. CEPH accreditation is the only quality assurance option open to standalone undergraduate health education programs.)
2. The National Council for the Accreditation of Teacher Education (NCATE) should be the accrediting body for school health education programs, and the Council on Education for Public Health (CEPH) should be the accrediting body for community/public health education programs. (NCATE has evolved into a new organization—CAEP—but it will be the credentialing body for school health education, and CEPH has accepted the responsibility to serve as the accrediting body for undergraduate community/ public health education programs. This recommendation has been accomplished.)
3. Future accreditation should be based on the best practices of existing accreditation systems. (This is accomplished with CEPH and CAEP.)
4. Students prepared in health education at the graduate level should meet *all* health education competencies with graduate-level proficiency. (This recommendation has been met. To achieve the MCHES designation, all competencies must be met in addition to additional advanced-level competencies.)
5. Separate designations should be developed to identify undergraduate level practitioners from graduate level practitioners. (The NCHEC certification process designates those with entry-level skills [CHES]

and those with advanced skills [MCHES]. This recommendation has been met.)

6. Undergraduate and graduate certification of individual health education specialists should be provided by NCHEC. In order to be eligible for CHES and MCHES certification, students must be graduates from schools/programs that are accredited. (This recommendation is in progress. NCHEC is the entity responsible for certifying entry-level and advanced-level health education specialists. NCHEC has agreed in principle to only certify students from accredited programs and will move to implement this recommendation when accreditation is widely available and enough time has expired to allow programs to transition to the new accreditation process.)

7. The results of the Task Force should be shared with those professional associations that include public/community health education specialists as members. (Numerous articles have been written in professional journals and presentations made at professional meetings regarding the task force recommendations.

8. Implementation of the Task Force results will require a profession-wide effort and resources from stakeholders for an extended period of time. (This has occurred as many of the recommendations noted above have been accomplished.)

Both the AAHE and SOPHE boards accepted the final Task Force report and then instituted a second committee to transition from the National Task Force recommendations to an implementation phase of the process. Dr. David Birch and Dr. Kathleen Roe co-chaired this committee called the National Transition Task Force on Accreditation in Health Education.

The work of this task force culminated in a three-day meeting of health education/promotion professional preparation programs in Dallas, February 23–25, 2006 (Taub et al.,

2009). At this "Third National Congress on Institutions Preparing Health Educators," accreditation issues were presented, discussed, and debated. Some attendees felt accreditation should move forward as quickly as possible. Others were reluctant to move in the direction of accreditation and wanted more discussion and debate. Several small programs expressed concern that they would not be able to meet accreditation requirements. Some present were concerned that the CEPH was being considered as the accreditation body and that using CEPH would push all health education/promotion programs to become public health programs. Others felt that if the roles and responsibilities utilized by NCHEC were used as the basis for accreditation, CEPH would be a suitable accrediting body. At the end of the conference, most participants supported the initiation of a coordinated accreditation system (Taub et al., 2009). To follow up the work of the National Transition Task Force and the Third National Congress, a third task force was initiated late in 2006. This task force, co-chaired by Dr. David Birch and Dr. Randy Cottrell, was named the National Implementation Task Force for Accreditation in Health Education. Its charge was to continue preparing the health education/promotion profession for accreditation (Cottrell et al., 2009, 2012).

Health Education Program Accreditation

In health education/promotion, accreditation is available through two accrediting bodies. Health education/promotion programs that are affiliated with a college of education and prepared school health education teachers may receive "national recognition" through the Council for Accreditation of Educator Preparation (CAEP). CAEP's mission is to "advance excellent educator preparation through evidence-based accreditation that assures quality and supports continuous improvement to strengthen P-12 student learning" (CAEP, 2020b). As the mission implies, CAEP is dedicated to quality assurance for education in the broad sense. It accredits entire schools of education. Individual program reviews, such as for health education, math education, etc., are a part of the CAEP accreditation process, and successfully reviewed programs that receive "National Recognition." School health teacher preparation programs seeking national recognition through CAEP submit a portfolio to CAEP for review based on discipline-specific standards. Specialized Professional Associations (SPAs) recognized by CAEP develop the standards for their respective disciplines and conduct the recognition reviews; thus, professionals with discipline-specific content expertise make recognition decisions for programs such as health education, science, language arts, and math teacher preparation within teacher preparation institutions of higher education. The SPA for health education is the Society for Public Health Education (CAEP, 2020a).

The Council on Education for Public Health (CEPH) accredits public health schools and programs at the graduate and undergraduate levels (CEPH, 2020a). This would include public health programs that have a health education concentration or focus. In the past, only graduate public health programs and undergraduate public health programs in the same unit as a Master of Public Health (MPH) degree program could be accredited. This left many undergraduate health education programs with no accrediting body. Beginning in January of 2014, standalone undergraduate programs (those not affiliated with a graduate program) could also be accredited through CEPH. In June of 2016, CEPH announced the first four accredited standalone undergraduate public health programs. They included East Carolina University, Rutgers University, The University of Nebraska at Omaha, and The University of North Carolina at Wilmington. As of December 2020, 18 standalone baccalaureate programs have been accredited and 14 additional programs are in the application process (CEPH, 2020c).

The accreditation of standalone undergraduate public health programs marks a major milestone for the health education profession. Professional preparation, especially at the undergraduate level, has not been uniform in the profession (Cleary, 1986). Some programs focus more on content, such as drugs, sexuality, stress, and physical fitness, whereas other programs emphasize process courses, such as planning, implementing, and evaluating. Some programs stress individual behavior change, and others stress population-based approaches to change. In 1987, the National Task Force on the Preparation and Practice of Health Educators attempted to develop a registry of health education programs. This effort, however, had to be abandoned. There was too much variety in faculty, administrative arrangements, courses, and philosophies of the various professional preparation programs to agree on criteria for inclusion in the registry (Cleary, 1995). This clearly indicated a lack of consistency and quality control in the profession. Hopefully, with the initiation of standalone baccalaureate program accreditation, this situation will be improved and the quality of undergraduate health education professional preparation will be enhanced.

Even with the lack of quality control in the profession, the number of undergraduate public health professional preparation programs has grown significantly over the past 25 years. Many of these programs evolved from community health education programs while others were newly developed. Approximately 50,000 undergraduate students graduated in public health between 1992 and 2012, and half of these graduations occurred after 2008 (Leider et al., 2015).

Responsibilities and Competencies of Health Education Specialists

The skills needed to practice health education/promotion are clearly delineated as responsibilities, competencies, and subcompetencies. **Responsibilities** are "the major categories of performance expectations of a proficient health education specialist" (NCHEC & SOPHE, 2020, p. 99). They provide a general idea of what health education specialists do but do not provide the detail necessary to practice health education/promotion.

Under each responsibility, there are three to six **competencies**. A competency is defined as a "skill or ability necessary for successful performance as a health education specialist" (NCHEC & SOPHE, 2020, p. 99). Each competency is further broken down into multiple **subcompetencies**. A subcompetency is a "cluster of simpler but essential related skills or abilities within a competency" (NCHEC & SOPHE, 2020, p. 100). All students graduating from a health education professional preparation program as well as all practicing health education specialists should be able to demonstrate proficiency in all of the health education specialist competencies and subcompetencies.

The most recent set of responsibilities, competencies, and subcompetencies of health education specialists, based on HESPA II 2020, is available in the publication, *A Competency Based Framework for Health Education Specialists 2020* (NCHEC & SOPHE, 2020) and can be found in Appendix B of this text. The number of responsibilities increased from seven to eight between the HESPA 2015 and the HESPA II 2020 models. The number of competencies in the HESPA II 2020 model is 35 compared with 36 in HESPA 2015. The total number of subcompetencies in the HESPA II 2020 model is now 193 compared with 258 in HESPA 2015. Of the 193 HESPA II 2020 sub-competencies, 114 were validated at the entry level, 59 at the advanced I level, and 20 at the advanced II level (see **Table 6.3**). The reduction in total number of subcompetencies was intentional to reduce overlap, clarify intent, and make it

Table 6.3 HESPA 2015 Model Hierarchical Approach

Level of Practice	Subcompetencies
Entry-Level (less than five years of experience; baccalaureate or master's degree)	114 entry-level subcompetencies
Advanced 1 (five or more years of experience; baccalaureate or master's degree)	114 entry-level subcompetencies **PLUS** 59 Advanced 1 sub-competencies
Advanced 2 (doctorate and five or more years of experience)	114 entry-level subcompetencies **PLUS** 59 Advanced 1 subcompetencies **PLUS** 20 Advanced 2 subcompetencies

Data from National Commission for Health Education Credentialing, & Society for Public Health Education. (2020). *A competency-based framework for health education specialists – 2020.* Author. Reprinted by permission of the National Commission for Health Education Credentialing, Inc. (NCHEC) and Society for Public Health Education (SOPHE).

easier for professional preparation programs to monitor student progress in obtaining the skills necessary to address each subcompetency (NCHEC & SOPHE, 2020).

The *HESPA II 2020* framework should be used by health education specialists and students on a regular basis. This is not a document that should be placed on a shelf to gather dust (see Appendix B). The NCHEC suggests that the competencies be used by students as a personal inventory to assess progress toward becoming a health education specialist, as a resource when preparing for the CHES.MCHES exam, as a means to assess strengths/weaknesses and direct continuing education efforts, and for professional preparation programs as a guide for curricular development (NCHEC & SOPHE, 2020).

Because the eight major responsibilities identified in the *HESPA II 2020 model* are the core of what a health education specialist does, it is important to have a basic understanding of them when entering the profession. The following sections briefly describe each responsibility.

Responsibility I: Assessment of Needs and Capacity

The first major area of responsibility listed for health education specialists involves assessing needs, assets, and the capacity for health education/promotion. This responsibility provides the foundation for program planning (Bensley & Brookins-Fisher, 2009). In fact, "Conducting a needs assessment may be the most critical step in the planning process..." (McKenzie et al., 2017, p. 68). A **needs assessment** is a process that helps program planners determine what health problems might exist in any given group of people, what assets are available in the community to address the health problems, and the overall capacity of the community to address the health issues. Other terms used to describe this process include *community*

analysis, community diagnosis, and *community assessment* (McKenzie et al., 2017).

In a needs assessment, "**Capacity** refers to both individual and collective resources that can be brought to bear for health enhancement" (Gilmore, 2012, p. 9). More specifically, assessing capacity identifies the assets—skills, resources, agencies, groups, and individuals—that can be brought together in a community to solve problems and empower a community. According to the World Health Organization (n.d.) **community empowerment** "refers to the process of enabling communities to increase control over their lives." It is, however, more than just allowing or encouraging people to be involved and participate in their communities. Community empowerment necessitates a renegotiation of power. It requires those in power to share their power with community members; thus, giving up some of their power. "Power is a central concept in community empowerment and health promotion invariably operates within the arena of a power struggle" (World Health Organization, n.d.). For that reason, it is critical to include community members on any planning team and to give them a real voice in the decision-making process.

All health education specialists, regardless of the setting in which they are employed, must have the skills to assess the needs and capacity of those groups or individuals to whom their programs are directed. For example, a school health education specialist needs to base curriculum on the needs of the students, a health education specialist in the corporate setting needs to plan programs based on the needs of the company's employees, and public health education specialists should base their health education/promotion efforts on the needs of the community they serve (NCHEC & SOPHE, 2020).

Health education/promotion programs should not be based on the whim of the health education specialist or any small group of decision makers. Resources are too valuable to waste on programs that do not address the needs of the population being served. As McKenzie et al. (2017) note, "...failure to perform a needs assessment may lead to a program focus that prevents or delays adequate attention directed to a more important health problem" (p. 68). Conversely, "We know our health education programs are on target when we base them on accurate needs assessment data and a careful interpretation of their meaning" (Doyle & Ward, 2001, p. 124). Ultimately, a well-conceived and well-conducted needs assessment determines if a health education/promotion program is justified. It also defines the nature and scope of a program (Gilmore, 2012).

To conduct a needs assessment, health education specialists should know how to locate and obtain valid sources of information related to their specific population(s) or to populations with similar characteristics. For example, this may entail a literature review or accessing information from local, county, or state health departments. In addition to examining preexisting information, called **secondary data**, it may be necessary for health education specialists to gather data of their own, known as **primary data**. They may have to conduct mail, electronic, and/or telephone surveys; hold focus group meetings (see **Figure 6.4**); and/or use a nominal group process. After all of this information is collected, the health education specialist must be able to analyze the data and determine priority areas for health education/promotion programming.

The following example demonstrates the importance of a needs assessment. A health education internship student was placed with the Shriners Hospital for Burned Children in Cincinnati, Ohio. The hospital identified a problem with children being burned around campfires during the summer months and asked the student intern to develop a fire

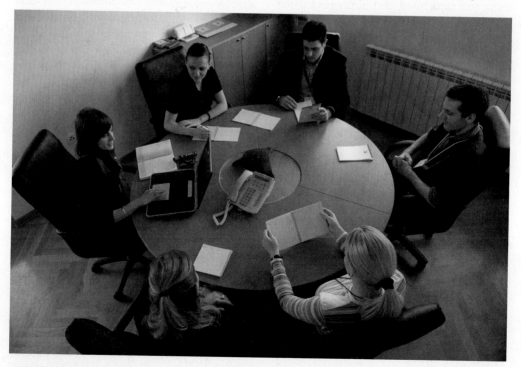

Figure 6.4 A group of health education specialists meeting to discuss information gathered during the assessment phase that will be used to guide the planning phase.

© Lucky winner/Alamy Stock Photo.

safety program for young campers. Fortunately, the site supervisor also required the student to conduct a needs assessment before planning the program. After conducting focus groups, interviewing camp counselors, and reviewing the literature, it was concluded that campers were the wrong group to target with the program. Instead, a program for the camp leaders and counselors was needed. If the needs assessment had not been done, valuable time and resources would have been spent developing a program for the wrong priority population.

Responsibility II: Planning

Planning involves more than just determining a location and time for a health education/promotion program. Planning begins by reviewing the health needs, problems, concerns, and capacity of the priority population obtained through the needs assessment. Early in the planning process, it is important to recruit interested stakeholders, such as community leaders, representatives from community organizations, resource providers, and representatives of the community population, to support and help develop the program. Without the help of these stakeholders, it may be impossible to develop effective programs. To be effective in the planning process, the health education specialist should have strong written and oral communication skills, leadership ability, and the expertise to help diverse groups of people to reach consensus on issues of interest. Furthermore, as part of the planning process, it may be necessary for the health education specialist to identify and obtain resources to support the program. This often involves the development of grants and/or contracts with outside organizations or funding agencies.

As part of the planning process, health education specialists must be competent to develop goals and objectives specific to the proposed health education/promotion program. These goals and objectives are the foundation on which the program is established. Writing specific and measurable objectives is critical. No health education/promotion program should be initiated without objectives or considered complete until an evaluation of the objectives is conducted. Writing good objectives is a skill you can only obtain through guided practice and experience. After program goals and objectives are written, the next step is to develop appropriate interventions that will meet these goals and objectives.

Many different types of interventions are available to health educators. These interventions can involve educational strategies like brochures, presentations, simulations, health fairs, case studies, role playing, etc. They could also involve changing the social physical environment like removing candy from a vending machine. Sometimes interventions involve community mobilization bringing together like-minded individuals and groups to work on a common problem or issue. Various communication strategies like radio, TV, direct mail, email, and social media can also be utilized as health education strategies. In addition, some strategies involve changing rules, regulations, policies or laws to enhance health, such as instituting nonsmoking policies in a workplace or mandating the use of seatbelts in automobiles.

Consider the following example of a planning process. A health education specialist, who is working in the university health service wellness center, analyzes the results of a recently conducted needs assessment. Next, the health education specialist recruits a variety of individuals to form a committee that will help develop a plan for the university. This committee includes representatives of the Greek system, student life organizations, resident life (dorms), athletics, health education/promotion program, provost's office, campus security, and local chamber of commerce. Together, they review the needs assessment data and agree that alcohol-related incidents are a health problem on campus that needs to be addressed.

First, the planning group uses existing baseline data on alcohol-related incidents to establish written objectives for the overall program. Next, they plan a variety of strategies to increase awareness of alcohol-related problems, modify alcohol-drinking behaviors, and reduce the number of reported alcohol incidents on campus. They organize a campus-wide alcohol awareness day, and they devise strategies with local bar owners to reduce excessive drinking. They also establish an agreement with campus security and the provost to refer any student involved in an alcohol-related incident to a mandatory alcohol education program that they will develop. In addition, they create posters and flyers promoting responsible drinking, train a bevy of peer student leaders to speak to dorm and Greek groups, and plan a variety of nonalcoholic alternative events for the campus community. For each and every strategy, they write specific objectives, establish implementation timelines, assign tasks to committee members, and establish a budget. If the planned strategies are successful, the program objectives will be met.

An important aspect of planning includes observing the **Rule of Sufficiency**. This rule states that any strategies chosen must be sufficiently robust, or effective enough, to ensure the stated objectives have a reasonable chance of being met. For example, in the preceding scenario, do you think the primary objective (e.g., reduce the number of alcohol-related incidents on campus by 20%) has a reasonable chance of being reached if all the listed program strategies are implemented? On the other hand, if the only intervention strategy used was to hand out a pamphlet on alcohol abuse to students, the intervention will not be robust enough to achieve the stated objective. In that case, the Rule of Sufficiency would not be met. Either the intervention strategies need to be enhanced, or the program should not be implemented. Time and resources are wasted

if interventions are not sufficient to create the desired change. Furthermore, if interventions fail to meet their objectives, then both the reputation of the health education specialist and the health education/promotion profession suffer.

Responsibility III: Implementation

After a needs assessment is conducted and analyzed, objectives are written, and intervention strategies are developed, it is time to implement the program. This involves "coordinating the logistics to implement the plan, train volunteers and staff, delivering the program, monitoring the progress, and evaluating the effectiveness and sustainability of the program" (NCHEC & SOPHE, 2020, p. 41). For many health education specialists, implementation is the most enjoyable of the responsibilities because it involves actually delivering the program to participants.

To successfully implement a program, the health education specialist must have a thorough understanding of the people in the priority population. What is their current level of understanding regarding the issue at hand? What will it take to get the people to participate? Do they need financial assistance or childcare? What time of the day should the program be offered? What location(s) would be most convenient? Although some of these questions can be answered from the initial needs assessment, it may also be necessary to obtain additional information about the priority population before proceeding with implementation. As always, it is critical to have representation from the priority population on the planning committee as their input is vital to the success of a health education initiative.

When conducting various health promotion and education programs, it is important for the health education specialist to be comfortable using a wide range of educational methods, strategies, or techniques. In school health, for example, it is not enough to simply lecture students about "proper" health behaviors. A successful health education specialist uses many teaching strategies such as brainstorming, debate, daily logs, position papers, guest speakers, problem-solving, decision making, demonstrations, role playing, drama, music, and current events. In community health, most programs require going beyond developing and distributing a simple pamphlet on a given health topic. Again, a wide variety of strategies should be used, including television, radio, newspapers, billboards, celebrity spokespersons, behavioral contracting, wellness coaching, community events, contests, incentives, support groups, and many more. As a general rule, health education specialists should always use multiple intervention activities when planning and implementing programs.

Health education specialists should also include population-based approaches to create health-improvement changes. Instead of focusing on individuals, population-based approaches focus on policies, rules, regulations, and laws to modify behaviors of a priority group or population. For example, instead of working one-on-one with individuals to enhance exercise levels, it might be more effective to work toward funding new walking and biking trails, having bike racks available at bus stations, initiating a city-wide walk/bike-to-work day, advocating for improved pedestrian safety laws, and so forth.

After a program is in place and operating, the responsibility of the health education specialist is not over. The health education specialist should continue to monitor the program to make certain that everything is going as planned. If problems are noted, it may be necessary, even while the program is in progress, to revise the objectives or the intervention activities.

When implementing program strategies or interventions, health education specialists may need to apply a variety of subcompetencies such as presentation skills, group facilitation skills, pretest/posttest administration, data collection, and technology utilization, all of which must be demographically and culturally sensitive. During the intervention phase, a health education specialist typically has the most contact with the public. The Code of Ethics for health education specialists (see Appendix A) should be strictly followed, and one should always dress and act in an appropriate professional manner.

Responsibility IV: Evaluation and Research

Accurate evaluations must be conducted to measure the success of health education/promotion programs. These evaluations help reveal whether implemented programs are meeting their specified objectives. Programs not properly evaluated may be wasting valuable time, money, and other resources. Furthermore, an unevaluated program cannot "prove its worth." So, it may risk being reduced or even eliminated when resources are short and downsizing occurs.

To conduct an effective evaluation, the health education specialist must first establish realistic, measurable objectives. As previously mentioned, this is an important part of the planning process. After objectives are in place, the health education specialist must develop a plan that will accurately assess if the program objectives have been met. Depending on the setting, this process may involve developing and administering tests, conducting surveys, observing behavior, tracking epidemiologic data, or other methods of data collection. Evaluation plans can be simple or extremely sophisticated, depending on the program being evaluated, the expectations of the program planners, and the requirements of funding agents.

After data are collected, they must be analyzed and interpreted. Reports are then developed and distributed to the appropriate parties. Ultimately, the evaluation results should be used to modify and improve current or future program efforts. In some cases, evaluation results may indicate that a program needs to be discontinued and funding redirected to other, more productive efforts. Health education specialists must have the fortitude to make these difficult decisions when needed.

In addition to evaluation, research is a vital activity for any profession, including health education/promotion. A profession moves forward and improves in large part as a result of the quality of its research and the new information it generates. **Health education research** can be defined as "a systematic investigation involving the analysis of collected information or data that ultimately is used to enhance health education knowledge or practice, and answers one or more questions about a health-related theory, behavior or phenomenon" (Cottrell & McKenzie, 2011, p. 2). Although more complex research skills are required at advanced levels, entry-level health education specialists should be able to read, synthesize, and use research results to improve their practice.

Responsibility V: Advocacy

Health education specialists are expected to advocate for, support, encourage, back, promote and/or sponsor initiatives that promote the health of priority populations. This means they will need to be integrally involved in the development, passage, and implementation of legislation, laws, rules, policies, and procedures designed to enhance health. Advocacy was validated as a standalone Area of Responsibility in HESPA II 2020 for the first time (NCHEC & SOPHE, 2020). This reflects the increased importance of and emphasis on advocacy efforts by health education specialists.

There are four competencies and 18 subcompetencies specifically related to advocacy (NCHEC & SOPHE, 2020). Utilization of coalitions and sustaining their efforts are important for successful advocacy initiatives. Being

able to identify existing coalitions as well as initiating, coordinating, and evaluating new coalition efforts are included in the advocacy competencies and subcompetencies.

In addition to advocating for health, it is also important for health education specialists to advocate for their own health education programs. Programs that are well evaluated and effective need to be promoted to employers, peers, the profession, and the community. While this may seem like "blowing one's own horn," it is vital that others know the value of health education initiatives. This is especially important in times of limited resources when budget cuts are being considered.

Finally, it is important for health education specialists to advocate for their profession. This can be done by joining and participating in professional associations such as the Society for Public Health Education (SOPHE), the American Public Health Association (APHA), and/or the American School Health Association (ASHA), to name a few. These organizations are strong advocates for the health education profession and need the support and involvement of all health education specialists. Furthermore, advocating for certification of health education specialists and the accreditation of professional preparation programs is critical for advancing and standardizing the health education profession. When health education specialists hold positions with hiring authority, they should advertise for and hire degreed and certified health education specialists. It is important that health education specialists talk to legislators, policymakers, personnel directors, allied health workers, coworkers, family, and friends about the value of health education/promotion.

Responsibility VI: Communication

Health education specialists must interact with various groups of people, including other health professionals, consumers, students, employers, employees, and fellow health education specialists. They must be skilled in written communication, oral communication, and mass media use including social media. Health education specialists need to feel comfortable working with individuals, small groups, and large groups, as the situation warrants. In essence, communication is the primary tool of the health education specialist. As previously noted, it is one of the "10 Essential Public Health Services" (Krisberg, 2020). Without communication skills, it is impossible to health educate.

It is often necessary for health education specialists to serve as communication filters between medical doctors/researchers and students or clients. Health education specialists must be able to "translate" difficult scientific concepts so that constituents can understand the information necessary to improve and protect their health. For example, a physician may tell a patient to start an exercise program, reduce fat in the diet, or manage stress better. Although many patients have a general idea of what these recommendations mean, they may not have the knowledge or skills to implement them. Most physicians cannot take the time to teach patients how to incorporate these changes into their lifestyles. Health education specialists can communicate detailed information on exercising safely, teach the client to recognize high-fat foods by reading food labels, and instruct the patient in progressive neuromotor relaxation. This may involve conducting one-on-one instruction, developing a videotape for patients to watch, creating brochures for distribution to patients, teaching classes, or coordinating support groups.

Health education specialists are often called on to communicate important health messages to the public and to serve as resource persons for those needing health information. It is not unusual for a student to seek out the health teacher for assistance when having a health-related problem. In the corporate setting, health education specialists get questions on a wide range of topics, including nutritional supplements, cancer signs and symptoms, the best type of shoe to wear for jogging, and many more.

Because it is impossible for health education specialists to know all of the information that could be needed in a given position, they must have the skill to access resources they need. It may be necessary to visit the library; use computerized health retrieval systems; access health databases; find information on specific diseases; obtain local, regional, state, and national epidemiological data; and so on. It is critical that the health education specialist be able to differentiate valid information from questionable, misleading, false, or fraudulent information. As part of this resourcing process, it may also be necessary for health education specialists to select or develop their own effective educational resources for distribution to their priority populations.

Consider, for example, Melissa (she/her/hers), the entry-level, health education specialist who was hired by a large metropolitan hospital. Her duties included developing health education/promotion programs for the community and resource materials for hospital patients. Her first assignment was to develop an initiative to address the problem of incontinence in older adults. This subject had not been covered in her professional preparation program. However, because of the skills she had previously learned, she was able to locate a variety of resources on the topic, evaluate their validity, select relevant information, and then communicate this information to older adults in the hospital who exhibited incontinence problems. She did this through the development of a brochure and a short five-minute video that could be broadcast on demand via the hospital closed circuit TV system. She was also able to place the information on a website that physicians could direct their patients to during office visits.

Being able to simply retrieve information is not enough. Health-education specialists must be able to establish effective consultative relationships with people who seek assistance, whether they are students, clients, employees, or other health education specialists. Health education specialists must instill confidence and communicate effectively in a nonthreatening manner. In some situations, health education specialists may decide to market their skills to individuals or groups as resource consultants. They may even decide to focus their career entirely as a resource person.

Responsibility VII: Leadership and Management

A great deal of leadership and management is needed to bring a health education/promotion program to fruition. Even though some management and administrative tasks may be performed by entry-level health education specialists, management and administrative responsibilities are generally handled by professionals at more advanced levels of practice. For example, experienced health education specialists often become program managers or staff supervisors. Good management and supervisory skills require training in a variety of administrative, organizational, psychological, financial, and business disciplines. They must also develop good human relations skills and strive to be inclusive and culturally sensitive.

An effective leader/manager works with others in the organization to establish a vision, mission, and strategic plan. A strategic plan must be utilized to be of value to the organization. A leader/manager must, therefore, keep the strategic plan at the forefront of the organization's activities and establish an evaluation plan to determine if strategic goals and objectives are met.

Health education specialist leaders must facilitate cooperation among personnel, both within programs and between programs. Some public-school systems, for example, have initiated coordinated school health programs. This involves coordinating the activities and services of school nurses, counselors, psychologists, food-service personnel, physical educators, health education specialists, teachers, administrators, support staff, parents, and public-health agencies. The ultimate goal is to develop both curricular and extracurricular programs to improve the health status of students, faculty, staff, and the community as a whole. Furthermore, health education specialists in school settings may serve as curriculum coordinators or project directors and can occasionally be responsible for managing grants and program budgets.

Similar examples can be seen in the community setting. For example, a health department decides to apply for grant funds to reduce the incidence of tobacco use in its community. The health education specialist may form a coalition by bringing together individuals or groups with a vested interest in reducing tobacco use. Coalition members might include representatives from the American Cancer Society, American Lung Association, American Heart Association, local medical society, local dental association, public health department, public school system, and YMCA/YWCA. Coordination and integration of the services offered by these various groups would be critical to the successful development of a grant proposal and ultimately to the success of the funded program. It may even be necessary for the health education specialist to conduct or coordinate in-service training programs to ensure that all coalition members have similar knowledge of tobacco prevention programs. Obviously, leadership and management skills are needed throughout this entire process.

Beyond leadership and management in the work setting, these skills are also needed by community organizations and professional associations. It is important that good leaders step forward to chair committees and accept leadership positions as officers and board members. There are many nonprofit health organizations, foundations, and state and national professional associations that only thrive when they have good leaders and managers.

Responsibility VIII: Ethics and Professionalism

"Ethics refers to the moral principles generally accepted as the proper way to conduct oneself while working as a health education specialist" (NCHEC & SOPHE, 2020, p. 64). There is an official Code of Ethics for the Health Education Profession (see Appendix A) that health education specialists should be following in all of their professional endeavors (CNHEO, 2020). Following ethical practices should be standard practice. Occasionally; however, health education specialists may be confronted with ethical dilemmas that may not have black-and-white answers. It is always good practice for a health education specialist to review the Code of Ethics to make certain that the code is being followed.

"Professionalism relates to the accepted conduct, aims or qualities that characterize someone working in the health education profession. Examples of professionalism include practicing in accord with accepted standards, participating in continuing education, belonging to professional associations, serving on committees, attending conferences and providing leadership to the profession" (NCHEC & SOPHE, 2020, p. 64). Professionalism also includes obtaining and promoting CHES certification to colleagues, employers and the public.

Certainly, ethics and professionalism have been included in all of the previous iterations of the NCHEC Responsibilities and Competencies documents. They were, however, imbedded within each of the seven responsibilities. For the first time, HESPA II 2020 pulled the ethics and professionalism competencies and subcompetencies from the other responsibilities and placed them under a separate eighth responsibility. By doing so, ethics and professionalism now stand out and are more visible than in previous framework documents. This places an even greater responsibility on professional preparation programs to make sure their students exhibit professionalism and practice ethical behaviors. Ultimately, however, each individual health education specialist is responsible for their own professional and ethical behaviors. Remember, it takes hard work and time to establish one's professional reputation, but one unprofessional or unethical incident can ruin that reputation forever.

Summary of Responsibilities and Competencies

The responsibilities, competencies, and subcompetencies required for health education specialists do not function independently; they are highly interrelated. All of the responsibilities demand excellent communication skills. Conducting an accurate needs assessment requires research skills to identify and gather appropriate resources. Planning should be based on a valid and reliable needs assessment. When implementing programs, be prepared to serve as a resource person. Evaluation relies on goals and objectives established during the planning process. Coordinating people and managing programs are necessary in planning, implementing, and evaluating programs. Leadership is needed to effectively conduct health education programs and in service to the profession and various community agencies. In all work of health education specialists, professionalism and ethics are an expectation.

It is not enough to be proficient in one, two, or even seven of the responsibility areas. All eight responsibilities are critical for effective health education/promotion to take place. It is beyond the scope of this text to teach the reader how to perform these tasks. Rather, it is the intent of this text to familiarize readers with the responsibilities, competencies, and skills they will be taught in later classes and ultimately practice in their employment settings.

Multitasking

It is often necessary for health education specialists to use several competency-related skills simultaneously. This requires **multitasking**, the skill of coordinating and completing multiple projects at the same time. In college, health education/promotion students are often given a project at the beginning of a term. There is a specific amount of time to complete the project, and when the term ends, the project is completed. In the work world, things do not function this way. Health education specialists work on multiple projects at the same time, and each project is usually in a different stage of completion.

Organization is the key to successful multitasking. For example, one health education/promotion internship student used a visual concept to help her stay organized while working on multiple projects. Using a bulletin board, unfinished projects and tasks were represented by floating balloon images. Once completed, these "balloons" were placed at the bottom of the bulletin board in the hand of a stick figure that represented the health education specialist. Other effective tools for multitasking include spreadsheets, timelines, and "to do" lists. With use of a smartphone, such lists can be readily at one's fingertips for referencing and updating.

Technology

As in most professions, health education specialists must be familiar with and comfortable using computers and other forms of technology. Because computer software and hardware are constantly changing, it is important to keep up to date on the latest technological aids. Entry-level health education specialists are expected to have required technology skills by the time they enter their internships and certainly by the time they accept their first position.

In addition to basic computer skills, **social media** skills are becoming a vital component of health education. Social media involves use of the media and other technologies to allow for social interaction. Learning to use such social media as Facebook, Twitter, YouTube, LinkedIn, Myspace, Instagram, Blogger, Skype, Zoom, and many more is no longer an option. It is a must in many health education settings and positions. Social media can be used for program promotion, social publishing, marketing, personal networks, e-commerce, information sharing, discussion forums, and many other existing and yet-to-be conceived uses. **Social Networking** is a specific type of social media that has many uses. Social networking involves connecting individuals (or organizations) that are tied (connected) by one or more specific factors, such as friendship, kinship, common interest, financial exchange, occupational or professional interests, or beliefs. More specifically, social networking services can be used by health education specialists to connect people with similar health interests, such as losing weight, exercising, stopping smoking, or reducing stress. They can also be used to link people who have a common cause, such as passing nonsmoking legislation or advocating for gun control. In addition, they are helpful for sending information or updates about programs sponsored by a given health agency such as the American Lung Association. Social networking has been used to send emails to pregnant women in developing countries to remind them of appointments and to provide educational messages. The possible uses for social networking in health education are limited only by one's imagination and creativity.

Role Modeling

Being a healthy role model is not listed anywhere in the roles and responsibilities of a health education specialist, but it has been discussed and debated within the profession (Bruess, 2003; Davis, 1999) and is worth consideration in an entry-level health education course. Some people feel that health education specialists should not be expected to be healthy role models. This expectation may discriminate against professionals who suffer from disease conditions that cause obesity or preclude a regular exercise regimen. Furthermore, they contend that being a healthy role model puts too much pressure on health education specialists, especially because there is no accepted definition for what "healthy" means. On the other hand, many in the profession believe that being a healthy role model is important to effectively carry out the responsibilities of the profession. Some even argue that ethically, health education specialists must be role models.

The authors of this text tend to believe that role modeling is an important aspect of being a health education specialist. The purpose of presenting this issue is to stimulate health education/promotion students to enter the debate. Do you feel that health education specialists should be role models? What does it mean to be a role model? Do you think health education specialists who are not role models will be less effective in their work or that those who are role models will be more effective? Are you a role model now for fellow students? Should you be? Do you want to be a role model in the future?

Advanced Study in Health Education

After receiving a bachelor's degree in health education/promotion, students should not stop the educational process. At the very least, health education specialists should continue to learn on their own. One way of doing so is to participate in one or more professional associations (see Chapter 8). Such memberships allow the opportunity to read professional publications and attend state, regional, and national meetings of the associations.

If you are a CHES, an average of 15 continuing education contact hours are *required* each year (75 across five years) to maintain certification. These may be obtained by reading professional journals and submitting responses to questions on selected articles, by attending various professional meetings and workshops, by taking additional coursework, or by participating in other professional development activities.

At some point, health education specialists with a bachelor's degree should consider getting a master's degree. In some areas of the country and in some health education/promotion settings, such as medical care and worksite health education/promotion, the master's degree is often considered the entry-level degree. In other words, to be considered for employment in these settings, the health education specialist must hold an appropriate master's degree (see Practitioner's Perspective).

Practitioner's Perspective

Chakoma Tahuri Haidari

CURRENT POSITION/TITLE: Health Policy Analyst

EMPLOYER: Central District Health

DEGREE/INSTITUTIONS: B.S., Health Science, Boise State University

UNDERGRADUATE MAJOR: Health Science (Emphasis: Public Health)

GRADUATE MAJOR: Public Health (Emphasis: Systems Analysis and Innovation)

Background: I am originally from Afghanistan but was born and raised in Tashkent, Uzbekistan. My family and I came to the United States as refugees and I am the first generation to be pursuing a higher education degree in my family. When I came to the United States, I realized that I have a lot of opportunities and that I could choose whatever I wanted to pursue. I always wanted to be a doctor so that I could help people. At that time, I did not really know what public health was or that it even existed. When I got the opportunity to learn about public health, I realized that my passion truly is within disease prevention and health promotion. I immediately switched my major from Biology to Health Sciences with the emphasis in Public Health. I feel lucky that I got the opportunity to pursue my goals and continue my education. Not many people get the opportunity to make their dreams come true, especially for someone like me, a girl who came here as a refugee.

I currently work full time at Central District Health as a Health Policy Analyst. In my current role, I get to work on tobacco prevention, tobacco cessation, and comprehensive cancer. Through my job, I have been exposed to policy development and health promotion programs. Health disparities are growing in our communities. My passion is to work toward eliminating these disparities by addressing social determinants of health and promoting health equity. I hope to improve public health outcomes through systems change and policy. As a public health professional, I am the voice for those that don't have the opportunity to advocate for their health. I feel a responsibility to be the representative of my community and advocate for equal opportunities. We need to meet people where they are by looking at their environment and understanding what drives their health outcomes.

Overall impression of graduate school: I always wanted to get my Masters. However, I was not sure if I would get the opportunity or if the timing was right. I took a three-year break and finally decided that it was now or never. I was certainly nervous but also dedicated. Honestly, the application process was not as intimidating as I thought it would be. I asked a lot of questions to make sure that I understood what I was about to get myself into. I remember being very stressed the first semester and questioning whether I could be successful in graduate school. However, meeting the professors and my classmates, I realized that we all shared similar thoughts and feelings. As I successfully completed my first semester, I was excited and ready for the next. Graduate school has made me a stronger public health professional. We discuss topics and issues that are often left out. There are a lot of opportunities to improve skills such as public speaking, communication, writing, research, and many others.

What I like most about graduate school: I have been very pleased by the Master of Public Health program at Boise State University. The faculty are amazing and care about the success of the students. Most importantly, I really like the program itself. Even though I had been working in public health for a couple of years, I am still learning new concepts and ideas that are giving me a different perspective. I also like that we have cohorts; you really get to know your classmates and feel that you can rely on each other for feedback and support. The professors and the advisor have always allowed me to focus my projects around what I am passionate about. I always recommend the program to undergraduate students as I personally was in their shoes wondering if graduate school was for me and if the program was right. I am really glad I made the decision to apply to the program.

What I liked least about graduate school: Being in graduate school is not easy and it comes with challenges like anything else. I like to have a balance in life. Since I was the first generation and so new to graduate school, I get stressed very easily. I also work full time while attending school full time. Trying to balance my work, school, and personal life has definitely been a learning process. However, you learn how to manage your time and be present in all aspects of your life. For me, it is keeping a planner and prioritizing everything. I also had to make decisions that were right for me considering that I have a family and other responsibilities.

Recommendations for health education students considering graduate study: I always recommend that students ask questions to make sure they have a good understanding of the program and its expectations. One thing that helped me a lot as an undergraduate student was internships. I actually

(continues)

interned at Central District Health before I was hired. The internship really helped me get some experience and also understand how public health works in the real world or at least in my community. Gaining internship knowledge and experience helped me better understand public health theories and concepts that I would learn in graduate school. I also highly recommend getting a mentor. Mentors are so important and can help you grow. I can ask my mentor questions that I normally would not feel comfortable asking others. They share valuable information that can guide you throughout the graduate program and in your career.

In school settings, the master's degree brings additional financial rewards and, in some states, progress toward more permanent teaching certificates or licenses. It is usually advised, however, not to complete a master's degree in teaching prior to obtaining your first teaching position. Hiring a new teacher with a master's degree, vs. hiring a new teacher with a bachelor's degree, is more expensive for a school district. This factor may put a person with a master's degree and no teaching experience at a disadvantage in the hiring process.

In community or public health settings, the master's degree may bring additional financial rewards, as well as promotions within the agency. It may also open the door to higher-level positions with other public health agencies or public health departments.

Master's Degree Options

There are multiple types of master's degrees. Typical choices include a Master's of Education (MEd), Master's of Science (MS), Master's of Arts (MA), Master's of Public Health (MPH), and Master's of Science in Public Health (MSPH) (Bensley & Pope, 1994). Some colleges and universities may offer only one degree option, while others may offer more than one.

The MEd degree is typically found in institutions in which the health education/ promotion program is located in a College of Education or Teacher's College. Although many students in these programs focus on school health, this does not mean that everyone who obtains this degree must pursue a career in public schools. Some colleges and universities offer MEd degrees, which emphasize areas such as community health and corporate health promotion.

The MS and MA degrees are usually found in universities in which the health education/ promotion program is located in colleges other than education. Because there is no accepted accreditation for these programs, schools have much flexibility to develop programs that meet the needs of the local job market. These degrees offer a variety of emphasis areas, including public health, community health education/ promotion, and corporate health promotion.

When considering differences between the MS, MA, and MEd degrees, remember that the MS may be the more scientific or research-oriented degree, whereas the MA and MEd may be more practitioner oriented. This distinction, however, is not always true. Prospective students need to carefully examine the stated mission and degree requirements for any graduate-level health education/ promotion program.

As their names imply, the MPH and MSPH are degree choices for those wishing to work in the broad fields of public health. At one time, working in the field of public health meant one would work in a city, county, or state public health department. The definition of public health, however, has been greatly expanded and now includes many other settings including voluntary agencies, public schools, worksites, hospitals, and so forth. The MSPH degree is typically more research oriented than the MPH degree; otherwise, the degrees are similar. The MPH can be generic or awarded in a variety of specialty areas such as health education, global health, nursing, dietetics, or epidemiology. The MPH with an emphasis in health education/promotion is the degree of most interest to health education specialists. It is similar and often identical to an MS or MA degree in community health education.

Most MPH degree-granting colleges and universities are accredited by the CEPH. Thus, the requirements to obtain an MPH are more standardized than the requirements to obtain the MS, MA, or MEd degrees, which typically are not accredited by any professional body. Resulting in part from accreditation, the MPH degree may enjoy a higher status and more credibility than other health education/promotion degree designations. To obtain MPH accreditation, the curriculum must meet the CEPH standards. To demonstrate that CEPH standards are met, the program develops and writes an extensive and detailed self-study and also hosts a two- to three-day campus visit by a CEPH site visit team.

The MPH in health education/promotion has the reputation of being a more prestigious degree than the MS, MA, or MEd. As of December 2020, there were 67 accredited schools of public health (up from 48 in 2013) and 133 accredited masters-level graduate public health programs (up from 88 in 2013) (CEPH, 2020b). As can be seen, the field of public health is growing. Not all of these public health programs, however, provide a concentration in health education/promotion. From one college to another, there are variations in degree and concentration options. Students will need to look at each CEPH-approved program's website to determine which offer a specialization in health education. Before applying to a graduate program, carefully examine program requirements and master's degree options within the context of your future career goals.

Selecting a Graduate School

Determining which college or university to attend is a decision that goes hand-in-hand with deciding which degree to pursue. In terms of practicality, factors such as cost, financial aid, location, and size must be considered (Cottrell & Hayden, 2007; US News and World Report, 2012). Prospective graduate students should search the websites of various universities of interest to see which programs they offer. A current list of CEPH-accredited schools and programs in public health can be found online at the CEPH's website, <http://www.ceph.org>. The Health Education and Promotion Program Directory <https://www.healtheddirectory.org/program-search> lists only health education/promotion programs and can be filtered by state, program level, and type of program (NCHEC, n.d.-b).

College or university reputation is an important factor to consider when selecting a health education/promotion graduate program. There is a definite hierarchy among colleges and universities in the United States. Graduating from one of the more prestigious institutions may lend instant credibility to the graduate degree and enhance job opportunities.

Next, consider the reputation of the health education/promotion program at a given institution. To learn about various programs, bachelor's-level health education specialists can talk to other professionals in the field whom they admire and trust. A visit or call to current or former college professors may also be a good source of information. Contacting recent graduates from a graduate program of interest is also a good way to learn about a particular program and may help in the decision-making process (Cottrell & Hayden, 2007).

After narrowing your list to several programs, carefully review each program's admission requirements and application forms. These can typically be found online as nearly all universities now have electronic applications and electronic references. If you need more information about program curricula or application procedures, contact the program's administrator via email, phone or to schedule an in person visit to the campus.

Admission Requirements

As an undergraduate health education/promotion student, it is not too early to be concerned about admission requirements to graduate school. Although admission requirements vary greatly from one university to another, the undergraduate grade point average (GPA) has traditionally been an important factor. In general, a student should strive to achieve an overall undergraduate GPA of at least a 3.0 on a 4.0 scale to be considered by most graduate programs. Some institutions do not specify a minimum GPA (Bensley & Pope, 1994). Instead, they tend to use more individual and subjective criteria in their admission process. In either case, it is important for new health education/promotion students to attempt from the first term of their freshman year to achieve the best grades possible. Too often, low grades in the first year or two of college prevent otherwise good students from being accepted into the master's degree program of their choice.

In addition to GPA requirements, most graduate programs require a completed application form, a letter of application, and several letters of reference. To be considered for admission, some programs also require students to submit scores from a standardized performance test such as the Graduate Record Exam or Miller Analogy Test. These scores may be a major component in the decision-making process, or they may simply be used in conjunction with other applicant information to provide a more well-rounded view of the prospective student.

Financing Graduate Study

Funding a graduate degree may not be as burdensome as funding undergraduate education. Many colleges and universities award assistantships or fellowships to graduate students on a competitive basis. Typically, these graduate awards pay all or part of the graduate tuition and provide students with a monthly stipend to cover living expenses during their graduate studies. In return, students agree to work for the health education/promotion program.

If the award is a **graduate teaching assistantship** (or fellowship), the student teaches a specified number of undergraduate courses each term. These are usually introductory health education/promotion courses that meet general university requirements, or they are the first courses for health education/promotion majors. Sometimes, graduate teaching assistants assist full-time faculty to teach their courses. In this case, students may help prepare lessons, teach occasional classes, and grade student tests/papers. If the award is a **graduate research assistantship** (or fellowship), the student usually works closely with one or more faculty members on a particular research project. Students might be assigned to do literature reviews, assist with data collection, enter data into the computer, or a host of other research-related activities (Cottrell & Hayden, 2007).

Graduate assistantships and fellowships not only provide an excellent alternative for funding graduate education but also provide valuable health education/promotion work experience for the student. Furthermore, a graduate assistantship may provide an advantage in the job market or for admission into a doctoral-level program after the master's degree program is completed.

Summary

Since the late 1970s, many people have dedicated much time and hard work to defining and developing the roles and responsibilities of a health education specialist. The initial stages of this work were known as the Role Delineation Project. Eventually, a set of responsibilities, competencies, and subcompetencies were agreed upon for health education specialists, regardless of whether they ultimately wished to work in schools, communities, clinics, or corporate settings. These responsibilities, competencies, and subcompetencies encouraged college and university professional preparation programs to develop their curricula based on a standardized set of skills for all health education/promotion students. These standards were also the basis for establishing individual certification within the profession.

In 1997, three additional responsibilities with accompanying competencies and subcompetencies were identified for graduate preparation in health education/promotion. With the completion of the CUP in 2005, the initial seven responsibilities and the three graduate responsibilities were united into seven revised responsibility areas that were common to all health education specialists regardless of setting, degree, or experience. With the release of HESPA II 2020, the number of responsibilities was increased from seven to eight. All health education/promotion professional preparation programs should now be training students based on the HESPA II 2020 standards.

Accreditation of standalone undergraduate public health education programs is now available through the CEPH. Master's-level public health education programs are still accredited via the CEPH. With accreditation now available for all health education programs, it is expected that professional preparation continuity and quality will continue to be enhanced.

Continued study in health education/promotion is necessary to stay current with health information and new techniques for conducting health education/promotion programs. All health education specialists should seek certification, read professional journals, join one or more professional associations, and take an active role in their functioning. CHESs and MCHESs must obtain continuing education credits to maintain their certification. Most bachelor's-level health education specialists should consider a master's degree at some point in their career. Decisions concerning graduate study should not be taken lightly. Undergraduate health education/promotion students need to be aware of the admission requirements for graduate school and work toward meeting those requirements. Graduate assistantships or fellowships provide an excellent alternative to fund graduate education.

Review Questions

1. Define *credentialing* and explain the differences among certification, licensure, and accreditation.
2. Outline the major events of the Role Delineation Project. What is the significance of the CUP, HEJA 2010, HESPA 2015, and HESPA II 2020? As a health education specialist, why should you be proud of these efforts?
3. Review the "Responsibilities and Competencies for Entry-Level Health Educators" (Appendix B)." Do you think they are more focused on health content or the process skills needed to be a health education specialist? Defend your position and explain why you believe the health education/promotion profession has moved in this direction.

4. Identify two ways health education specialists can stay up to date in the field.
5. Explain the importance of accreditation for standalone undergraduate public health education programs.
6. What are the differences among the following academic degrees: MA, MEd, MS, MPH, and MSPH?
7. What technology skills are important for current and future health education specialists?
8. Briefly describe the process for applying to graduate school and discuss the potential benefits of serving as a graduate assistant.

Case Study

Reba (she/her/hers) is a junior-level undergraduate student majoring in public health with a concentration in community health education. She has been asked by one of her faculty members to attend a recruiting event for high school seniors. The purpose of the event is to allow high school seniors the opportunity to interact with college students who are in a major that the high school seniors are considering. After a brief presentation, Reba is answering questions from the seniors. One of the high school students asks, "You mention that your public health studies program is accredited by CEPH. Why is that important to me in considering which college program to attend?" The next question she gets is, "You mentioned that students graduating from your program are eligible to take an exam to be a Certified Health Education Specialist. If you have the degree, why do you need additional certification? What are the advantages of obtaining this certification?" How would you respond to these questions?

Critical Thinking Questions

1. If Helen Cleary and her contemporaries had not begun the Role Delineation Project, and if there were no certification (CHES, MCHES) available to health education specialists, how do you think the profession would be different today? Think in terms of professional preparation, professional recognition, employment opportunities, and so on.
2. An accreditation system is now available for all graduate and undergraduate public health education/promotion professional preparation programs. How do you think enhanced opportunities for accreditation will impact the profession? What do you see as the potential positive outcomes and the potential negative outcomes of accreditation? Do you feel that only students graduating from accredited programs should be allowed to sit for the CHES exam?
3. Review the National Health Education Competencies that resulted from the HESPA II 2020 model (see Appendix B). Do you feel they accurately represent professional practice? Why or why not? What changes do you think should be made in terms of eliminating competencies, adding competencies, or moving subcompetencies from one level to the other?

Activities

1. Read each competency and entry-level subcompetency of a health education specialist (see Appendix B). Score each competency and subcompetency using the following scale:
   a. I currently have the skill to meet this competency/subcompetency.
   b. I am uncertain if I have the skill to meet this competency/subcompetency.
   c. I do not have the skill to meet this competency/subcompetency.

   After rating each competency and subcompetency, make a list of things you can do to enhance your skills. Keep this table and periodically reevaluate your skills throughout your program of study.

2. Identify one or more universities you may wish to attend for graduate school. Go online and read about the program, its curriculum, degrees offered, financial aid and graduate assistant opportunities, and application procedures.

3. Make an appointment with a professor at your school to talk about graduate school. Ask about schools the professor attended and the degrees earned. Finally, ask for advice on what degree to earn and what school to attend.

Weblinks

1. **http://www.nchec.org/**

   National Commission for Health Education Credentialing (NCHEC)

   Use this website to learn more about becoming a CHES. The site provides helpful information about health education certification including application procedures. It even has a section spotlighting what roles certified health education specialists are playing in the COVID-19 pandemic.

2. **http://www.ceph.org/**

   Council on Education for Public Health

   The council is responsible for accrediting programs in public health. A complete list of accredited schools and programs of public health can be found at this site. This site can help identify accredited public health education graduate programs to which one may want to apply.

3. **https://www.healtheddirectory.org/program-search**

   Health Education and Promotion Program Directory

   A directory of only health education/promotion programs. It is searchable by state, program level, and type of program

4. **https://www.sophe.org/**

   Society for Public Health Education (SOPHE)

   Excellent professional organization to which you may want to become a member. SOPHE is a professional association that sponsors journals, state and national conferences, a career hub, and numerous other resources and activities. Participation in SOPHE is an excellent way to help one stay current in the profession. SOPHE represents health education specialists in all settings and offers student memberships at reduced rates.

5. **https://www.ashaweb.org/**

   American School Health Association (ASHA)

   ASHA sponsors professional journals, conferences, resources for those health education specialists focusing on teaching health education in schools. Health Education students with a school health focus should join ASHA. ASHA offers student memberships at reduced rates.

6. **https://www.apha.org/**

   American Public Health Association (APHA)

   APHA is a professional association that sponsors professional journals, conferences, and resources for those

health education specialists focusing on the public health arena. APHA offers student memberships at reduced rates.

7. **http://www.usnews.com/education /best-graduate-schools/articles/2012 /04/06/7-critical-steps-to-find-the -right-grad-school**

   Excellent article on how to find the right graduate school for you to attend.

References

Allegrante, J. P., Airhihenbuwa, C. O., Auld, M. E., Birch, D. A., Roe, K. M., & Smith, B. J. (2004). Toward a unified system of accreditation for professional preparation in health education: Final report of the National Task force on Accreditation in Health Education. *Health Education & Behavior, 35*(6), 347–358.

Allegrante, J. P., Barry, M. M., Airhihenbuwa, C. O., Auld, M. E., Collins, J. L., Lamarre, M. C., Magnusson, G., McQueen, D. V., Mittelmark, M. B. (2009). Domains of core competency, standards, and quality assurance for building global capacity in health promotion: The Galway Consensus Conference Statement. *Health Education & Behavior, 36*(3), 476–482.

Allegrante, J. P., Barry, M. M., Auld, M. E., & Lamarre, M. C. (2012). Galway revisited: Tracking global progress in core competencies and quality assurance for health education and health promotion. *Health Education & Behavior, 39*(6), 643–647.

Allegrante, J. P., Barry, M. M., Auld, M. E., Lamarre, M. C., & Taub, A. (2009). Toward international collaboration on credentialing in health promotion and health education: The Galway Consensus Conference. *Health Education & Behavior, 36*(3), 427–438.

Bensley, L. B., Jr., & Pope, A. J. (1994). A study of graduate bulletins to determine general information and graduation requirements for master's degree programs in health education. *Journal of Health Education, 25*(3), 165–171.

Bensley, R. J., & Brookins-Fisher, J. (2009). *Community health education methods: A practical guide* (2nd ed.). Jones and Bartlett Publishers.

Bruess, C. E. (2003). The importance of health educators as role models. *American Journal of Health Education, 34*(4), 237–239.

Cleary, H. P. (1986). Issues in the credentialing of health education specialists: A review of the state of the art. In William B. Ward (Ed.), *Advances in health education and promotion,* (pp. 129–154). Jai Press.

Cleary, H. P. (1995). *The credentialing of health educators: An historical account 1970–1990.* The National Commission for Health Education Credentialing.

Coalition for National Health Education Organizations (CNHEO) (2020). Code of Ethics for the Health Education Profession [Document]. http://cnheo.org /ethics.html

Cottrell, R. R., Auld, M. E., Birch, D. A., Taub, A., King, L. R., & Allegrante, J. P. (2012). Progress and directions in professional credentialing for health education in the United States. *Health Education & Behavior, 39*(6), 681–694.

Cottrell, R. R., & Hayden, J. (2007). The why, when, what, where, and how of graduate school. *Health Promotion Practice, 8*(1), 16–21.

Cottrell, R. R., Lysoby, L., Rasar King, L., Airhihenbuwa, C. O., Roe, K. M., & Allegrante, J. P. (2009). Current developments in accreditation and certification for health promotion and education: A perspective on systems of quality assurance in the United States. *Health Education & Behavior, 36*(3), 451–463.

Cottrell, R. R., & McKenzie, J. F. (2011). *Health promotion and education research methods.* Jones and Bartlett Publishers.

Council for Accreditation of Educator Preparation. (2020a). *SPA Standards and Report Forms.* Retrieved December 2, 2020, from http://caepnet.org /accreditation/caep-accreditation/spa-standards-and -report-forms

Council for Accreditation of Educator Preparation. (2020b). *Vision, Mission, & Goals.* http://caepnet.org /about/vision-mission-goals

Council on Education for Public Health. (2020a). *Accreditation Criteria and Procedures.* Retrieved December 2020, from https://ceph.org/about /org-info/criteria-procedures-documents/criteria -procedures/

Council on Education for Public Health. (2020b). *List of Accredited Schools and Programs.* Retrieved December 15,

2020, from https://ceph.org/about/org-info/who-we-accredit/accredited/#programs

Council on Education for Public Health. (2020c). *Who We Accredit.* Retrieved December 2, 2020, from https://ceph.org/about/org-info/criteria-procedures-documents/criteria-procedures

Davis, T. M. (1999). Health educators as positive health role models. *Journal of Health Education, 30*(1), 60–61.

Doyle, E., & Ward, S. (2001). *The process of community health education and promotion.* Mayfield Publishing.

Gilmore, G. D. (2012). *Needs and capacity assessment strategies for health education and health promotion.* Jones and Bartlett Publishers.

Gilmore, G. D., Olsen, L. K., Taub, A., & Connell, D. (2005). Overview of the National Health Educator Competencies Update Project, 1998–2004. *American Journal of Health Education, 36*(6), 363–372.

International Union for Health Promotion and Education. (2020). *The IUHPE Health Promotion Accreditation System.* Retrieved December 1, 2020, from https://www.iuhpe.org/index.php/en/the-accreditation-system

Joint Committee for Graduate Standards. (1996). *National Congress for Institutions Preparing Graduate Health Educators.* Program Booklet, 1.

Krisberg, K. (2020). Equity at center of revised 10 essential public health services. *The Nation's Health, 50*(9), 1–10. https://www.thenationshealth.org/content/50/9/1.5

Leider, J. P., Castrucci, B. C., Plepys, C. M., Blakely, C., Burke, E., & Sprague, J. B. (2015). Characterizing the growth of the undergraduate public health major: U.S., 1992–2012. *Public Health Reports. 130,* 104–113.

McKenzie, J. F., Neiger, B. L., & Thackeray, R. (2017). *Planning, implementing & evaluating health promotion programs* (7th ed.). Pearson Education.

McKenzie, J. F., Pinger, R. P., & Seabert, D. M. (2018). *An Introduction to Community & Public Health Planning* (9th ed.) Jones & Bartlett Learning.

National Commission for Health Education Credentialing. (n.d.-a). *CHES® exam eligibility.* Retrieved December 16, 2020, from https://www.nchec.org/ches-exam-eligibility

National Commission for Health Education Credentialing. (n.d.-b). *Health education and promotion program directory.* Retrieved December 19, 2020, from https://www.healtheddirectory.org/program-search

National Commission for Health Education Credentialing. (n.d.-c). *Health education credentialing.* Retrieved December 1, 2020, from http://www.nchec.org/credentialing/credential

National Commission for Health Education Credentialing. (n.d.-d). *Mission and purpose.* Retrieved December 21, 2020, from http://www.nchec.org/aboutnchec/mission

National Commission for Health Education Credentialing. (1996). *A competency-based framework for professional development of certified health education specialists.* National Commission for Health Education Credentialing.

National Commission for Health Education Credentialing. (2015). *NCHEC receives distinguished recognition.* http://www.nchec.org/news/posts/nchec-receives-distinguished-recognition

National Commission for Health Education Credentialing. (2020). *Areas of Responsibility, Competencies and Sub-Competencies for Health Education Specialist Practice Analysis II 2020.* Retrieved December 1, 2020, from https://assets.speakcdn.com/assets/2251/hespa_competencies_and_sub-competencies_052020.pdf

National Commission for Health Education Credentialing & Society for Public Health Education. (2015). *A competency-based framework for health education specialists—2015.* Author. Reprinted by permission of the National Commission for Health Education Credentialing, Inc. (NCHEC) and Society for Public Health Education (SOPHE).

National Commission for Health Education Credentialing & Society for Public Health Education. (2020). *A competency-based framework for health education specialists—2020.* Author. Reprinted by permission of the National Commission for Health Education Credentialing, Inc. (NCHEC) and Society for Public Health Education (SOPHE).

Quality Assurance Solutions. (2020). *Quality Assurance Definition.* Retrieved December 1, 2020, from https://www.quality-assurance-solutions.com/Quality-Assurance-Definition.html

Society for Public Health Education. (2000). Future directions for quality assurance of professional preparation in health education. *News & Views, 27* (3).

Society for Public Health Education & American Association for Health Education (1997). *Standards for the preparation of graduate-level health educators.*

Speller, V., Parish, R., Davison, H., & Zilnyk, A. (2012). Developing consensus on the CompHP professional standards for health promotion in Europe. *Health Education & Behavior, 39*(6), 663–671.

Taub, A., Birch, D. A., Auld, M. E., Lysoby, L., & King, L. R. (2009). Strengthening quality assurance in health education: Recent milestones and future directions. *Health Promotion Practice, 10*(2), 192–200.

US News and World Report. (2012). 7 Critical Steps to Find the Right Grad School. http://www.usnews.com/education/best-graduate-schools/articles/2012/04/06/7-critical-steps-to-find-the-right-grad-school

World Health Organization. (n.d.). *Track 1: Community Empowerment.* Retrieved December 3, 2020, from https://www.who.int/teams/health-promotion/enhanced-wellbeing/seventh-global-conference/community-empowerment

CHAPTER 7

The Settings for Health Education/Promotion

CHAPTER OBJECTIVES

After reading this chapter and answering the questions at the end, you should be able to:

- Identify the four major settings in which health education specialists are employed.
- Describe the major responsibilities for health education specialists in the four major settings.
- Discuss the advantages and disadvantages of the four major settings.
- Explain the qualifications and major responsibilities of health education specialists working in colleges and universities.
- Identify a variety of "nontraditional" settings in which health education specialists may be employed.
- State several action steps that can be taken to help procure one's first job in health education/promotion.

Today, most Americans live a healthier and longer life than ever before. Despite this fact, it is clear that many, if not most, Americans are not living at their optimal level of health. Hereditary, environmental, societal, and behavioral factors predispose too many U.S. citizens to disease, suffering, disability, and premature death. Health education specialists are professionally trained to help individuals and communities reduce their health risks. According to the U.S. Department of Labor Bureau of Labor Statistics (2020a), there were 58,590 health education specialists employed in the United States in 2019 earning a median annual wage of $55,220 or a median hourly wage of $26.55. The job outlook for 2019–2029 is for health education and community health worker positions to grow at a rate of 13%, which is considered much faster growth than for the average profession. The average growth rate for all occupations is 4% (U.S. Department of Labor Bureau of Labor Statistics, 2020b).

The challenge for health education specialists is to help people reduce their risk for disease and death and increase the probability of a long, happy, and productive life. To meet this challenge, health education specialists conduct programs in a variety of settings (Society for Public Health Education [SOPHE], n.d.). The use of multiple settings is important because it allows health education specialists to reach the greatest number of people in the most convenient, efficient, and effective ways possible. A comprehensive listing of settings and specific job titles is available through the National Commission for Health Education Credentialing (NCHEC, n.d.-a). Although settings differ, "The concept of a 'generic role' common to all health educators, regardless of work setting, emerged and formed the basis for the credentialing process for health education specialists" (National Commission for Health Education Credentialing, n.d.-b). While the goals of health education/promotion and the competencies needed to carry out the responsibilities are nearly the same in all settings, the actual duties of a specific job may differ greatly from setting to setting. For example, some positions may involve more assessing and planning while others may involve more research and evaluation, and still others may involve direct education of individuals and groups.

Professional preparation programs in health education/promotion should prepare students to meet the various competencies and subcompetencies of a health education specialist and thus prepare students for employment in one or more of four major settings. These settings are schools, hospitals/clinics, public/community health agencies, and business/industry. On obtaining a terminal degree, students from any of these settings may seek employment as college or university health education faculty. In addition, health education specialists can work in a variety of nontraditional employment areas.

This chapter discusses each of the four major settings for health education/promotion. After a short introduction to the setting, a description of one day in the career of a health education specialist from that particular setting is presented. This is designed to give the reader a general idea of what a workday is like. Because of the great diversity in duties from one health education specialist to another, even within the same setting, it is impossible to say that this is a typical day. For most health education specialists, there is no such thing

as a typical day. In this edition of the text, the authors have added information at the end of the "A Day in the Career of…" about how a health education specialist's role might have changed with the COVID-19 pandemic. It demonstrates how quickly job responsibilities can change and the flexibility a health education specialist needs to be successful in a given position. Following this description is a section that describes additional responsibilities that might be assigned to health education specialists in the setting. Again, this is not intended to be an exhaustive list but rather to further the reader's understanding of job responsibilities in that setting. Finally, each section ends with a listing of some advantages and disadvantages for that setting. As students become interested in one or more settings, they are encouraged to contact, interview, and job shadow health education specialists working in those settings.

School Health Education/Promotion

School health is more than just the health educator teaching in the classroom, although that is certainly a very important component. School health also involves a physically and socially healthy environment, health services such as nursing and athletic training, a good nutrition program that provides healthy and appetizing meals, physical education and athletics, programs to promote the health of faculty/staff, counseling and psychological services, and community buy in and involvement (American School Health Association, n.d.). **School health education/ promotion instruction**, as the name implies, primarily involves instructing school-age children about health and health-related behaviors. The initial impetus for school health stemmed from the terrible epidemics of the 1800s and the efforts of the Women's Christian Temperance Movement to promote abstinence from alcohol in the early

1900s. Many states mandated school health education/promotion to inform students about these health hazards.

Unfortunately, these mandates have seldom been strictly enforced. Furthermore, teachers have often been underqualified, with only an academic minor or a few elective courses to prepare them for the health classroom. Undergraduate majors specifically in health education have declined. Frequently, those teaching health education hold a dual certification in health education and physical education with the majority of their professional preparation being in physical education. As a result of poor teacher preparation and schools focusing on test scores vs. the whole child, the quality of school health programs has often been compromised (Doombrowski & Mallare, 2020).

Despite these limitations, the potential for school districts and health instruction programs in particular to impact students is tremendous. "Research has shown that when health education is delivered effectively in schools, students show improvements in health as well as key academic outcomes" (SOPHE, 2020). Jalloh (2007) noted that "school-based health education is an opportunity waiting to be taken advantage of; an opportunity for you to discover the best way to influence positive health-related change in the lives of youth and to maximize the use of some education dollars to achieve synergistic health and education goals" (p. 18). It is easier and more effective to establish healthy behaviors in childhood than it is to change unhealthy behaviors in adulthood. The goal of health education/promotion in schools is to help students adopt and maintain healthy behaviors (Joint Committee on National Health Education Standards, 2007). Each school day provides the opportunity to reach 50.7 million public school students and 5.7 million private school students. The 98,158 schools in the United States (National Center for Educational Statistics, n.d.) should provide a laboratory where students can eat healthy foods, participate in physical activity,

and learn how to take care of their health and well-being. The results of a recent comprehensive literature review found, "Schools can improve the health and learning of students by supporting opportunities to learn about and practice healthy behaviors, providing school health services, creating safe and positive school environments, and engaging families and community" (Michael, Merlo, Basch, et al., 2015, p. 740).

The sophistication of school health education/promotion instruction has increased dramatically over the years. Today's school health education specialist needs to be well trained and prepared to deliver a comprehensive and demanding curriculum. Comparing the 1922 "Rules of Good Health" with the 2007 National Health Education Standards (Joint Committee on National Health Education Standards, 2007) clearly illustrates this point (see **Tables 7.1** and **7.2**).

When the school health education/promotion component is made part of a broader, district-wide approach known as the **Whole School, Whole Community, Whole Child Model (WSCC)**, the potential to impact students in a positive way is even greater as is the alignment between student health and educational outcomes (Lewallen, Hunt, Potts-Datema et al., 2015, Birch, Goekler, Auld, et al., 2019). The WSCC Model is based on the original work of Allensworth

---

Table 7.1 Rules of Good Health—1922

1. Take a full bath more than once a week.
2. Brush teeth at least once a day.
3. Sleep long hours with window open.
4. Drink as much milk as possible, but no coffee or tea.
5. Eat some vegetables or fruit every day.
6. Drink at least four glasses of water a day.
7. Play part of every day outdoors.
8. Have a bowel movement every morning.

Reproduced from Reaney, B. C. (1922). Rules of the health game. In *Milk and our school children*. U.S. Government Publishing Office.

Table 7.2 National Health Education Standards

1. Students will comprehend concepts related to health promotion and disease prevention to enhance health.
2. Students will analyze the influence of family, peers, culture, media, technology, and other factors on health behaviors.
3. Students will demonstrate the ability to access valid information and products and services to enhance health.
4. Students will demonstrate the ability to use interpersonal communication skills to enhance health and avoid or reduce health risks.
5. Students will demonstrate the ability to use decision-making skills to enhance health.
6. Students will demonstrate the ability to use goal-setting skills to enhance health.
7. Students will demonstrate the ability to practice health-enhancing behaviors and avoid or reduce health risks.
8. Students will demonstrate the ability to advocate for personal, family, and community health.

Reproduced from The American Cancer Society. (2007). *National health education standards: Achieving excellence* (2nd ed.). SHAPE America.

and Kolbe (1987), who were the first to envision a comprehensive and coordinated school health program. They called this **coordinated school health**. They defined it as

> an integrated set of planned, sequential, school-affiliated strategies, activities, and services designed to promote the optimal physical, emotional, social, and educational development of students. The program involves and is supportive of families and is determined by the local community based on community needs, resources, standards and requirements. It is coordinated by a multidisciplinary team and accountable to the community for program quality and effectiveness. (p. 60)

The new WSCC Model focuses on student health and learning, addresses critical education and health outcomes, encourages collaborations, and engages community resources (Lewallen et al., 2015).

A health education specialist choosing to work in the school setting will find a challenging and rewarding career. Given the number of school districts in the United States, it is obvious that a large number of people teach health education/promotion in the schools.

Unfortunately, many of these people are not health education specialists. Some school districts have used biology, physical education, home economics or family life, and consumer science teachers to teach health. Even when certified health education teachers are employed, they may only have a minor in health education/promotion and are not fully prepared. A further problem confounding the employment situation in the schools is that the requirement for health education/promotion is usually less than for other academic subjects. Students typically need only one or two semesters of health education instruction to graduate from high school, whereas they probably are required to complete several years of English, math, or science. With such a minimal requirement for health education, the number of health teachers needed and the resulting demand for health teachers are lower than in other teaching fields. The bottom line is that, in many parts of the country, it is difficult to obtain a job in school health.

Those students who are really committed to being outstanding school health teachers, however, should not be deterred from this career path. With time, dedication, networking, and perseverance, those who really want to teach health in the schools can usually find employment. Substitute teaching, coaching, and volunteering are good ways to make one-self known in a school district and increase the likelihood of eventual employment. Students are encouraged to talk to their own professors to determine the job market for school health education/promotion in their area.

Beyond teaching in the classroom, the school health education specialist should also take a leadership role in advocating for and the development of school health policy. Policies are written statements that guide the school district related to many health issues. They may take the form of laws, mandates, rules, regulations, standards, resolutions or guidelines (McKenzie et al., 2018). For example, a school district may have policies related to tobacco use on school property, the food and snack items available in the cafeteria (see **Figure 7.1**), safety measures, violence, suicide, staff wellness programs, community advisory committees, and many more issues. Furthermore, once policy is developed, it needs to be carefully implemented and then monitored. Policy work is not easy, but it is extremely important for a school district. It is often the policy work that provides the most visibility to a coordinated school health education program and individual school health education specialists. When school boards, administrators, and the community know about and are proud of the health education program, that program is a success.

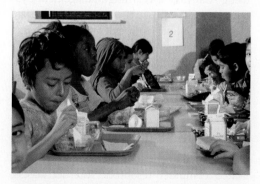

Figure 7.1 Food service is one component of a coordinated school health program.

© David Buffington/Photodisc/Getty Images.

A Day in the Career of a School Health Education Specialist

The alarm goes off at 5:45 AM, and Ms. Bell's (she/her/hers) day starts. Ms. Bell teaches seventh- and eighth-grade health at a junior high school in a suburban school district. After going through the normal morning routine, she arrives at the school building around 7:00 AM. There is a half-hour before homeroom, so she picks up her mail and duplicates a test that she prepared the night before for her eighth-grade health class. She then heads for her homeroom to meet the students. Essentially, homeroom involves administrative responsibilities and a considerable amount of paperwork.

In homeroom, she takes attendance, gets a lunch count, listens to announcements over the loudspeaker, and collects money from a fruit sale fundraiser. The fruit sale is being conducted by the PTA to raise money for new computers in the school. The PTA used to sell candy, but because of a new district policy that Ms. Bell and the WSCC Health team advocated for, candy sales are no longer allowed as fundraisers. Selling candy to raise money is counterproductive to the health message the school is trying to promote.

At 7:45 AM, the first period starts. This school has eight 50-minute periods, with only four minutes between periods. In the first three periods, Ms. Bell teaches seventh-grade health. Today's lesson is on refusal skills related to alcohol and drug use. Ms. Bell has written three scenarios that students could find themselves in. The scenarios are open ended, so after each one, Ms. Bell leads a discussion on how to use refusal skills to get out of a bad situation. She then asks students to role-play the situations to gain further practice in using refusal skills. Unfortunately, only two of her three classes will get this lesson today. The second-period class is one day behind because of an assembly that was held a week ago. Ms. Bell has to find a way to catch this group up with the rest of the classes.

Ms. Bell's fourth period is divided in half. During the first half, she has lunch-room duty. It is her responsibility to monitor the lunch room while students are eating. This is a noisy and somewhat stressful duty. In today's lunch room, two boys become unruly and nearly get into a fight. She sends them to the office for discipline, but the situation is still upsetting.

The second half of fourth period is Ms. Bell's lunch time. She usually has 25 minutes to eat lunch and relax before fifth period begins. Today; however, she must use part of that time to drop by the office for a follow-up discussion with the assistant principal concerning the incident with the two boys in the lunch room.

In fifth period, Ms. Bell teaches eighth-grade health. Today is a test day. While the students are taking their test, Ms. Bell works at her computer to update the online webpage that lists student assignments for the week. She must keep her online webpage up-to-date so that parents can be constantly informed of what is happening in the class and what assignments their children have due.

Sixth period is Ms. Bell's planning period. Today, she tries to make a phone call to the parents of one of her students who is having problems in health class, but no one is home. She then grades the test papers from her previous class and records the grades. She averages the grades and starts to develop interim reports for the fifth-period class, but she runs out of time. Seventh and eighth periods are also eighth-grade health classes. While students take their tests, Ms. Bell grades papers from the previous classes and works on developing her interim reports. She must develop an interim report for each student, which is then distributed to the parents.

School ends for the students at 2:57 PM. After monitoring the hall while students leave the building, Ms. Bell hurries to the cafeteria for the monthly teachers' meeting. General information and announcements are presented by the principal. The meeting ends at 4:00 PM.

In addition to her teaching responsibilities, Ms. Bell coaches the junior high girls' volleyball team. Practice usually goes from 3:15 PM to 5:00 PM. Today's practice will go from 4:00 PM to 5:30 PM because of the teachers' meeting. After practice, Ms. Bell waits until the last girl leaves the locker room, then returns to her classroom to prepare for the next day's classes. She leaves the school at around 6:00 PM.

After dinner and her family responsibilities, Ms. Bell spends 20 minutes on the phone with the student's parents who were not at home earlier in the day. She then finishes grading the tests she gave in class and continues working on interim reports. It will take her at least one more evening to finish the interims. At 11:00 PM, she turns off the light and goes to bed. Tomorrow will start again at 5:45 AM.

March 16, 2020

All of Ms. Bell's teaching responsibilities changed in just one day. On March 16, 2020, her school was scheduled to reopen following a week-long spring break. Unfortunately, COVID-19 was on the rise, and all schools in the state were closed. Suddenly, Ms. Bell had to change all of her lessons to an online learning format. Having never taught online and having only taken one online course herself, she was at a loss as to how to do this. Fortunately, her school district had been using "Canvas," a Learning Management System that takes all requirements of a physical classroom online. Both she and her students were familiar with this system and the district provided additional in-service training. Still it was very difficult to go from a face-to-face format to 100% online learning. She felt like she was constantly on her computer answering student questions that could come in any time of the day or night. In addition, she was very worried about some of her students who lacked computer resources, Internet access, and motivation. She and the guidance counselors had to follow up with students who did not submit course assignments and had essentially lost contact with the school. This required additional hours for calling parents and troubleshooting student connectivity issues. Ms. Bell estimates that she spent two to three times more hours with the additional planning, grading, and student follow-up required during the pandemic.

Additional Responsibilities

In addition to the lesson planning, grading, parent meetings, disciplining, coaching, and the various administrative duties, teachers may have still more responsibilities. They may be involved in curriculum development, the review of materials for classroom use, the chaperoning of dances or other after-school activities, fundraising, and the advising of student groups such as yearbook, debate, or student council. Many teachers now keep active webpages that can be accessed by students and parents. These webpages may contain announcements, assignments, and grades or progress reports. Teachers need to be responsive to their email accounts because parent, student, and school district communication is often conducted in this manner. School health education specialists should also be active members of their professional organizations such as the American School Health Association and/or the Society for Public Health Education. This allows them to network with other health education specialists and to stay up to date in the field. Finally, school health education specialists should be strong advocates for health and health education/promotion (see Practitioner's Perspective). They must make certain that fellow faculty, administrators, school boards, and the community as a whole are aware of the unique contributions of a school health program. (See **Table 7.3**.)

Practitioner's Perspective

School Health Education: Amy Abriani

CURRENT POSITION: 7th grade Health/Wellness Teacher
Westfield Middle School
Westfield, IN

EMPLOYER: Westfield Washington Schools

DEGREE INFORMATION (UNIVERSITY AND SUCH): Bachelor of Science in Health Education (Ball State, 07')

Master of Art in Curriculum and Educational Technology (Ball State, 12')

How I obtained my job (If appropriate, describe past and current professional positions and how you came to hold the job you now hold):

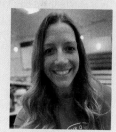

Courtesy of Amy Abriani.

I entered teaching during a tumultuous time in education. Most schools were facing a budget crisis and eliminating many teaching positions. The first on the chopping block were "specials" teachers, including Health and Physical Education (PE) teachers. My professors were clear that PE and Health teachers had to prove their worth. We could not teach a "roll out the ball" type of curriculum. There were actual skills that applied directly to life that needed to be taught and practiced within the health classroom—it shouldn't just be a movie viewing class. Making the class valuable was going to be the key to sustainability and employability.

I was lucky enough to land a part-time Health, part-time PE aid position in a tiny rural town where students in grades 5–12 were all under one roof and had special events like, "Bring Your Farm Animal to School Day," and "Ride Your Tractor to School Day." It was this position that allowed me to gain experience as a track coach, which is considered a valuable asset in our field.

(continues)

Practitioner's Perspective *(continued)*

School Health Education: Amy Abriani

Seeking full-time teaching work, I transitioned to a more urban setting. In a town devastated by a large factory shut down, I learned that teaching involved so many more skills than I had learned in college. I worked around some amazing educators who modeled how to truly step up and step in for students who had so many different needs. I was able to experience elementary, middle school, and high school teaching experiences. Middle school seemed to fit like my favorite pair of running shoes, and I actively sought to return to that level after moving through so many different teaching assignments.

I finally settled in close to the community where we had already started raising our family. I was ready to leave the long commutes behind and the economy was able to support more consistent teaching positions, again. I landed the dream spot here in Westfield as the 7th/8th grade Health/Wellness teacher.

Describe the duties of your current position: Westfield has created a Wellness program that includes classroom health lessons and PE lessons in two consecutive one year-long courses. During a typical year, each of the Health/Wellness teachers has between 150–170 students spread across six 45-minute classes. Students spend two full weeks in the classroom, then two in the gym and the pattern repeats. Our team of teachers has split the main health topics between the two grades, so students receive instruction on different content areas each year.

On a basic "teacher responsibilities" level, I am expected to plan curricula that are aligned with national and state standards. All grade level Wellness teachers implement the lessons at the same pace throughout the year. I attend two to five meetings a week related to professional growth and tracking our team of students. I act as a resource person as I share concerns with parents and administrators about student health. I evaluate student success, regularly, through assignments, discussions, projects, and checkpoint quizzes. I coach sports, sponsor clubs, and supervise dances.

On a challenging day, I report child abuse, suicidal thoughts, and runaway students. I listen to students unload about their parents during my lunch. I have meetings with the principal about parent concerns and the sex education curriculum. I must use great caution with my actions and words both at work and in public, as teachers are held to a higher "moral" standard and have more strict expectations regarding self-expression and political advocacy.

On the best days, I get to read parent emails that explain how our topic is being shared at home and how important it is. I help students achieve fitness goals after school. I get to see students grow and change for two very pivotal years of their lives. I get to laugh at the ridiculous things that students say and do nearly every hour. I get to work out during the workday. I get to teach the most important and applicable subject students learn all day.

How I utilize health education/promotion in my job: As a Health/Wellness teacher, I have an opportunity to build and strengthen foundations for healthy habits. My class is often the very first class students have taken that is completely dedicated to health. Many of the concepts are brand new, and it excites me to be able to introduce students to the information that could read straight out of a "user's manual" for the human body and mind. Students begin to explore basic health concepts and skills like positive communication, self-management, decision making, and advocacy. It is easy for them to understand the application to life and they can often utilize the skills right away. This answers the ever-present question for students at school during adolescence: "When am I ever going to use this?"

As a professional in the health education field, I have the responsibility to advocate for healthy policies within the school. This means being invested and involved in areas outside of my classroom. Forming a positive working relationship with administrators and community members is one way to help keep schools safe places to learn. In keeping close communication, we are able to give a 3-D perspective on why and how current practices exist, and our Health/Wellness teachers are able to help give input to be more health centered, when it applies.

What I like most about my job: There are so many things I truly enjoy about being a Health/Wellness teacher. Being able to play a significant role in shaping the future feels powerful, yet heavy. It is not easy to be so invested in other human beings, but it is incredibly rewarding to see their growth. I find it both exhausting and fulfilling to be around so many people each day, interacting with them on a personal level for 45 minutes at a time. The human connection component is by far the thing I like most about my job.

What I like least about my job: The aspects that I dislike about my job come and go. There is not one thing that I can pinpoint as a negative because most of the stresses are temporary. However, it is almost always the adults involved in education who cause the difficult times. This job requires a great deal of customer service. Finding the balance between keeping customers satisfied and teaching can be challenging.

What health education specialist responsibilities (assessing, planning, implementing, evaluating, resourcing, communicating, advocating) do you use in your position? As I stated, our team of Health/Wellness teachers works together to develop curricula and pacing that are developmentally appropriate for middle school aged children in our community. We use modeling and practicing to allow students to engage in learning. Most of our assessments come in the form of practical projects or culminating activities like advocacy assignments involving research or role plays. Our assessments encourage growth as they allow for feedback that can expand understanding and give students another chance to improve. Students get many opportunities to think through and apply the skills they learn. I use the responsibilities of health education specialists daily.

What recommendations do you have for current health education students who would like to eventually be school health educators: For those seeking employment in the health education field, I would encourage the consideration that my professors emphasized with me: Make your class valuable. Bring passion to your profession and remind others why it is important every day. Embody the understanding that taking care of our health is our obligation to ourselves and to our society. Being aware of the risks and precautions is our responsibility. Modeling these behaviors for our youth so they can see the long-term outcomes is critical. These are the principles that someone in this profession should take seriously, represent, and promote.

The role of the school health educator in the future: The school health educator of the future stays committed to the principles listed above. They continue to advocate for health-enhancing school environments and policies. There are unpredictable circumstances ahead, and health educators must keep the compass unwavering toward the priority of the health and safety of students, staff, community, and self.

Table 7.3 **Advantages and Disadvantages of Working in School Health Education/Promotion**

Advantages

- Health education specialists have the ability to work with young people during their developmental years.
- Health education specialists have the potential to prevent harmful health behaviors from forming instead of working with older people after such behaviors have been formed.
- Health education specialists have the opportunity to impact all students because health education/promotion is usually a required course.
- A graduate degree is not needed for entry-level employment.
- There is good job security.

(continues)

Table 7.3 **Advantages and Disadvantages of Working in School Health Education/Promotion**   *(continued)*

- Summer months are free and there are nice vacation periods in December and in the spring.
- Benefits are good.
- There is a multifaceted career ladder.
- There are typically good health and retirement benefit programs.

Disadvantages

- Good health education specialists usually spend many long hours at their job, including weekends and evenings.
- Health education specialists may have relatively low status in a school district compared with teachers of more traditional subjects such as math, science, and English.
- Pay is low compared with professionals in other fields but comparable with that of other health education specialists.
- Student discipline problems are often seen as a major disadvantage.
- Summer "free time" may be consumed with summer employment that is needed to compensate for the low salary or returning to college for additional required coursework.
- It is difficult dealing with conservative school boards, parents, and community groups when teaching controversial issues such as sex education and drug education.
- Resources may be limited to support the program.

Public or Community Health Education/ Promotion

Within the health education/promotion profession, there has been much discussion concerning the terms community health education/promotion and public health education/promotion. Some believe these two terms are synonymous whereas others feel there are unique differences between them. It is the opinion of the authors that the terms are more alike than different and that the field is gradually evolving to accept the term public health education/promotion. Both community health education/promotion and public health education/promotion students have similar skill sets, meet the competencies of the National Commission for Health Education Credentialing, and compete for similar jobs in departments of public health and community health agencies. A survey of professional preparation programs (Miller et al., 2010) found that 72.3% of respondents reported making modifications to their existing undergraduate health education/

promotion program or concentration within the past three years to take on a more public health focus. Sixty-three percent of the programs surveyed indicated they would seek accreditation as a public health education/promotion program when available whereas only 19% indicated they would not seek accreditation as a public health education/promotion program. For that reason, the authors use the term *public health education/promotion* to include both community health education/promotion and public health education/promotion programs.

Public health programs target individuals, local communities, states, and the nation. There is a reciprocal relationship between these various targets. Over the years, it has become clear that the health of a community is closely linked to the individual health of community members. Likewise, the collective behaviors, attitudes, and beliefs of everyone who lives in the community profoundly affect the community's health. Indeed, the underlying premise of *Healthy People 2030* was that the health of the individual is directly related to the health of the larger community, and that the health of every community in every state and territory determines the overall health status of the nation. Equity and inclusion for individuals and across society are important foci of *Healthy People 2030*. This explains why the vision for *Healthy People 2030* is "A society in which all people can achieve their full potential for health and well-being across the lifespan" (U.S. Department of Health and Human Services, n.d.).

The most likely sources of employment for public/community health education specialists are voluntary health agencies, community agencies, and public health departments. **Voluntary health agencies** are "nonprofit organizations created by concerned citizens to deal with a health need not met by governmental health agencies" (McKenzie et al., 2018, p. 49). "Their missions can be public education, professional education, patient education, research, direct services and support to or for people directly affected by a specific health or medical problem. They may also serve families, friends, or loved ones of those affected" (Daitz, 2007, p. 4). As their name implies, they rely heavily on volunteer help and donations. There are usually paid staff members who are responsible for administration, volunteer recruitment and coordination, program development, and fund-raising. Health education specialists are hired to plan, implement, and evaluate the education component of the agency's programs. They often, however, are involved in other aspects of the agency as well. Voluntary health agencies are usually nonprofits and are funded by such means as private donations, grants, fundraisers, and possibly United Way contributions. Examples of voluntary health agencies include the American Cancer Society (see **Figure 7.2**), American Heart Association,

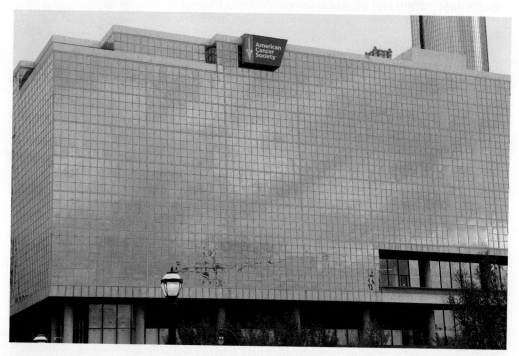

Figure 7.2 The American Cancer Society is a nationwide voluntary health organization dedicated to eliminating cancer as a major health problem by preventing cancer, saving lives from cancer, and diminishing suffering from cancer through research, education, advocacy, and service. Health education specialists often work for voluntary agencies such as the American Cancer Society.

and American Lung Association. Most of these large, well-known voluntary agencies have national, state, and local divisions.

In addition to the large national voluntary associations, there are many other nonprofit health-related organizations that provide a variety of services to the public. One such organization is Coastal Horizons Center, Inc., in Wilmington, N.C. See the following Practitioner's Perspective box for more information about working in such a program.

Public health agencies, or official governmental health agencies, are usually financed through public tax monies. Government has long been responsible for doing for the people as a whole what individuals cannot do for themselves. Thus, governments provide police protection, educational systems, clean air and water, and many other important services. Departments of public health, thus, are formed to coordinate and provide health services to a community. Health

---

Practitioner's Perspective

Teresa Mobley, BS

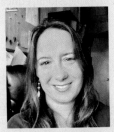

Courtesy of Teresa Mobley.

CURRENT POSITION/TITLE: Project Coordinator

EMPLOYER: Coastal Horizons Center, Inc., Wilmington, NC

MAJOR, INSTITUTION AND DEGREES: University of North Carolina at Wilmington, BS Public Health Studies with a Community Health Education Concentration

Describe your past and current professional positions and how you came to hold the job you now hold: I was fortunate to be hired by the organization I interned with during the last semester of my undergraduate public health program. My first role involved working on a grant (CURES) that focused on opioid prevention in my county (New Hanover, N.C.). I held the titles of Prevention Specialist and the New Hanover County Lock Your Meds Consultant. Lock Your Meds is a national campaign that promotes the importance of locking up household medications. I was responsible for creating, developing, and distributing valuable and innovative community resources such as a Physician toolkit (used to encourage physicians to have conversations with their patients about medication safety) and Medication Disposal Location postcards and posters. When that grant ended, I transitioned to being a Site Coordinator for Brunswick and Pender counties (neighboring counties of New Hanover county) working on a grant (RCORP-Planning) that focused on planning the implementation of opioid and substance misuse prevention strategies. That grant also ended. I am currently serving as the Project Coordinator on another grant designed to implement opioid misuse prevention strategies in Brunswick and Pender counties.

Describe your current job requirements: Every day is different for me, which I love. Depending on the grant, and the day, I could be doing any of the following:

- Creating a community resource to be distributed to focus populations or in focus areas ("Population of focus" or "Focus Population" is the most current term for "Population of need" or "Communities in need")
- Providing community outreach (which can include providing resources to community members or presenting at a community event)
- Conducting focus groups or key informant interviews
- Collecting and compiling data
- Assisting with writing a grant application

■ Meeting with the Rural Counties Opioid Response Program (RCORP) Consortium that I helped create and am currently in charge of maintaining

Generally, in a nutshell, I do community outreach, establish new community partnerships and strengthen existing ones, collect and compile data, work with local coalitions, tasks forces and consortiums, and assist with grant writing.

Describe what you like most about your position. Pros: My favorite part of the job is providing resources to individuals and communities. I am fortunate enough to be able to do this for both individuals and focused populations in my community, as well as neighboring communities. Being able to physically see and understand how a resource I'm providing is going to help improve someone's life, and possibly the lives of others, is a tremendously gratifying feeling that drives me to both continue and enjoy the work I do.

Describe what you like least about your position. Cons: To put it simply, the thing I like least about my job/position is the limitation on who and how many I can help. Working for a nonprofit organization that is primarily grant funded restricts me to specific populations and locations, and determines what services and resources I can and cannot provide.

What health education responsibilities do you use in your position? I utilize at least one health education responsibility for my job on a daily basis. Over a period of perhaps a month, I will have used all of the eight responsibilities and most of the associated competencies. I'm constantly conducting assessments at either a community or focus population level, and I'm always planning and implementing strategies to improve communities' quality of life in some regard (and searching for funding to implement those strategies). Furthermore, I'm always collecting and compiling data, some of which includes information that is used for planning, implementation, and evaluation. I am always using communication skills and advocating for my community, agency, and profession. I certainly try to always practice ethical behavior and try to be professional in all of my activities.

Recommendations for those preparing to be health education specialists: I don't have too much in the way of recommendations other than trying to practice the following on a daily basis: "Always be positive, proactive, and kind." I know that's brief and may come off as mildly cliché or corny, but it's extremely important to practice and be all of those things when a student or when working in the public health field, especially with focus populations.

departments may be organized by the city, county, state, or federal government. They operate primarily with paid staff and typically provide health education/promotion services as part of their total program. They may also seek grants and hire health education specialists on grant funds. Public health agencies are known for their bureaucracies, protocols, policies, and procedures. It often takes considerable time to accomplish tasks, and work often needs to be reviewed and approved by higher-level administrators. On the positive side, public health agencies often work with the groups of people most in need of health services and offer good benefit packages for employees (Hall, 2007). **Table 7.4** contains a partial list of agencies that have programs for which public health education specialists may be employed.

More diversity in terms of job responsibilities exists in the public/community health education/promotion settings than in the other major settings in which health education specialists are employed. This is as a result of the large number of community and public health agencies that exist and the vast differences in their missions, goals, and objectives. In some agencies, health education specialists serve administrative functions such as coordinating volunteers, budgeting, fundraising, program planning, and serving as liaisons to other agencies and groups. They often use

Table 7.4 Possible Sources of Employment in Public/Community Health Education/Promotion

State, local, city health departments

U.S. Public Health Service

U.S. Food and Drug Administration

U.S. or state departments of agriculture

U.S. or state departments of transportation

County extension services

U.S. Department of Health and Human Services

U.S. Centers for Disease Control and Prevention

National Institutes of Health

Environmental Protection Agency (EPA)

Health Resources and Services Administration (HRSA)

Substance Abuse and Mental Health Services Administration (SAMHSA)

Indian Health Service

U.S. or state penal institutions

Voluntary health agencies

Private health agencies/foundations

population-based strategies such as advocating for laws, policies, rules, and regulations that impact health. In other public/community agencies, the health education specialist may be more involved in direct program delivery to the clientele of that agency and/or the community at large. Most frequently; however, health education specialists are involved in a little bit of everything.

A Day in the Career of a Community Health Education Specialist

Mr. Hernandez (he/him/his) is a certified health education specialist (CHES) working for the county health department. He arrives at the health department around 8:30 in the morning. He spends a half hour looking through his emails, listening to his voice mails and going through his paper mail. Today at 9:00 is the weekly staff meeting that he must attend. This is run by the Health Commissioner and includes all staff working at the health department. At each staff meeting, Mr. Hernandez is expected to give a brief, five-minute report on what is happening in the health education division. At this meeting, he also learns what is happening in the other divisions of the health department. It is not unusual for staff in one division to assist staff in another division with projects or initiatives that they may have.

After the staff meeting, Mr. Hernandez has a couple of hours before lunch to respond to his emails and voice messages and work on a new grant proposal to fund a health education program for seasonal migrant workers. At 12:00, Mr. Hernandez breaks for lunch. He usually eats lunch at his desk while reading journal articles from *Health Promotion Practice*. This is one of the journals published by SOPHE, of which Mr. Hernandez is a member. He finds that many of the articles in this journal relate directly to his work and often provide ideas for new initiatives or for how he can better do his job.

At 1:00, Mr. Hernandez has a meeting scheduled with a group of bicycling enthusiasts and bicycle shop owners regarding the development of a biking safety program for the county. Data have shown that the number of bicycle accidents in this county is higher than for other counties in the state. This group will consider measures that may be taken to modify this problem and examine possible grants to fund the program.

At 2:00, Mr. Hernandez has a meeting with a local newspaper reporter. The reporter is doing a story on food poisoning during the summer months and how to prevent it. Mr. Hernandez only had one nutrition course in college, and this is not his area of expertise. He spent considerable time yesterday afternoon researching food poisoning and calling a dietician friend at the local hospital to confirm the information he will give the reporter. At 2:30, Mr. Hernandez heads over to the high school for a 3:00 meeting. He is part of the "Health Team" in the school district, and they are in the process of trying to develop and have approved a policy that soft drinks and candy cannot be sold in the lunchroom when school lunches are being served. This is controversial as some students oppose the policy and the vending machine company is lobbying against it. Today's meeting is to develop the actual wording for the policy that will be presented to the school board and to brainstorm other community organizations and groups that might provide additional support for the proposed policy.

At 4:00, when the school meeting ends, Mr Hernandez heads back to the health department to load his car with various health department pamphlets and displays. The local mall is having a health fair from 5:00 to 9:00 this evening. He, along with many other community organizations, will be there to display their materials and answer questions the public may have about health issues or health department services. Mr. Hernandez frequently has to work evenings and weekends as part of his job. He does receive comp time for the hours he works beyond the normal work week, which allows him to take some additional days off during the year.

March 16, 2020

Mr. Hernandez's job suddenly changed. The health department had been following the COVID-19 outbreak for about a month, but now the state has decided to shut down all schools, business activity and travel, except for essential workers, to help prevent further spread of the disease. He has been asked to serve on both the governor's state-level advisory council and the advisory council for the local county health department. This entails daily meetings of both groups as they closely follow the spread of the disease and try to determine future actions for state and local governments. Mr. Hernandez

communicates daily with concerned citizens, business owners, school personnel, medical personnel, and fellow public health professionals. He must read everything he can about the disease from professional publications and government entities such as the CDC and NIH. Twice a week he develops a press release that is distributed to various media outlets updating them on what is happening with the virus. Most of the initiatives he had been working on prior to COVID have been put on hold indefinitely.

Additional Duties

Mr. Hernandez is actually one of three health education specialists working at the health department. The other two health education specialists are working on grants. One is working on a grant to improve safety issues for elderly residents. This involves educating these residents on how to prevent falls and the importance of smoke and carbon monoxide detectors in their homes. The grant also provides financial resources to install safety features in bathrooms and to purchase smoke and carbon monoxide detectors for those who cannot afford these improvements. The other health educator is working on a grant to help the county and its residents prepare for a potential disaster such as an earthquake, hurricane, tornado, or terrorist attack. This grant will last for just one year, and then the health education specialist will have to find another funding source or will need to seek other employment.

Mr. Hernandez is an actual employee of the county health department. His position is funded by tax dollars and his job is not dependent on grants. In addition to his previously described work, Mr. Hernandez is the information/public relations officer for the health department. He is responsible for responding to questions called into the health department by county residents. Whenever a health-related news story breaks, local residents will often call the health department with questions. Recently, he has been addressing many questions about COVID-19. Furthermore, Mr. Hernandez is also the person who interfaces with the media when they have questions. As a result, he is often on the TV or radio speaking about health issues.

As can be seen from the example above, public/community health education specialists are involved in numerous and varied activities (see Practitioner's Perspective). Planning, implementing, and evaluating programs and events are major tasks, but, in conducting these tasks, health education specialists get involved in grant writing, fundraising, coalition building, committee work, budgeting, general administration, public speaking, volunteer recruitment, policy development, media relations, advocacy, and more. Furthermore, they must be ready to respond to any public health emergency as with the COVID-19 pandemic (see **Table 7.5**).

Practitioner's Perspective

Kailynn Mitchell, MPH

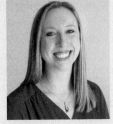

CURRENT POSITION/TITLE: Hepatitis C Surveillance and Outreach Specialist

EMPLOYER: University of Wisconsin State Lab of Hygiene/Wisconsin Department of Health Services Division of Public Health Communicable Disease Harm Reduction Section (UW Contractor for DHS)

DEGREE HELD/INSTITUTION ATTENDED/GRADUATION YEAR: BS Community Health Education, University of Wisconsin - La Crosse, 2012

Minor Professional and Organizational Communications

Master of Public Health, Medical College of Wisconsin, 2017

Courtesy of Kailynn Mitchell.

How I obtained my job: I was working in the Wisconsin Immunization Program on a two-year CDC grant using a quality improvement program called AFIX to improve the statewide vaccination rates of adolescents and adults. The final grant year was ending and unfortunately there was no opportunity for a funding extension for the AFIX positions. Also, the Wisconsin Immunization Program was unable to provide any positions besides an LTE (Limited-term employment, part-time position) due to limitations of the grant funding. So I started applying to other public health jobs in the area. At the time when I was looking for a new public health position, it just so happened that the Wisconsin Hepatitis C program was hiring for a surveillance and outreach specialist. This position would be located in the same office building that I was working in but on a different floor. After two rounds of interviews, I was offered the job for their newly created surveillance and outreach specialist position in the hepatitis C program. I was fortunate to have an easy transition to a different office space in the building and still work on projects with colleagues in the Wisconsin Immunization Program.

Job responsibilities and how I utilize the health education competencies in my job:

- Support preparing and writing CDC grants for the Wisconsin hepatitis C program.
- Implement, administer, and evaluate hepatitis C CDC grant objectives and activities.
- Develop, update, and implement protocols, guidance, and policies for the hepatitis C program.
- Collaborate with the HIV, Immunization, and Opioid programs to advance prevention and elimination strategies for hepatitis C.
- Work with hepatitis C epidemiologist to identify trends and gaps in services and outcomes among people who inject drugs, tribal communities, and people born from 1945–1965.

- Conduct active and passive hepatitis C virus (HCV) case surveillance in the Wisconsin Electronic Disease Surveillance System (WEDSS) for the state of Wisconsin.
- Process HCV-related laboratory data.
- Deliver educational site visits to healthcare providers about the need to screen and treat adults for HCV.
- Provide technical assistance to local health department public health nurses and healthcare providers on reporting HCV cases to the department of public health in addition to HCV rapid testing sites.
- Assess, communicate, and promote local and statewide HCV data to the public and community partners.
- Attend and present as a health educator at statewide and national conferences and summits on HCV.

What I like most about my job: I like that I get to utilize many different public health education specialist responsibilities, competencies and sub-competencies every day that I work on hepatitis C prevention, surveillance, harm reduction, treatment and care projects. I am able to work on data management and surveillance in the Wisconsin Electronic Disease Surveillance System (WEDSS) while assisting the hepatitis C epidemiologist and/or the local health department nurses and healthcare systems or reference laboratories. I get to work with community-based organizations, federally qualified health centers, tribal health centers, harm reduction organizations, county health departments, Department of Corrections (DOC), Division of Care and Treatment Services (DCTS), Division of Medicaid Services (DMS), Wisconsin Immunization Program, and many other service providers across the state. By being a public servant, I take pride in knowing that I help make change at the population level and individual patient level. My work focuses on a communicable disease that is curable and I am excited about the prospect of leading hepatitis C statewide elimination planning efforts in the next five years of our CDC grant. Working at the state public health department, I am energized by the level of collaboration that my colleagues and I strive for and that we all have a passion to improve the health of everyone living in Wisconsin.

What I like least about my job: Unstable and inconsistent funding from the federal government can make it hard to make progress on ending the HIV epidemic and eliminating hepatitis C in our state and country. This instability can lead to staffing shortages or burnout when there are too many competing public health priorities but not enough resources. Communities that we provide public health services to may not always trust us or see us as a credible resource of apolitical scientific information and guidance. Traditionally, federal and state government public health programs have worked in silos. This is changing but in my opinion, it may not be changing fast enough to address the people's need for holistic, well-rounded health services.

Recommendations for those preparing to become a health education specialist: Get your undergraduate and graduate degrees from accredited public health programs. Participate in national or statewide public health organizations and chapters to network with fellow colleagues and learn about new training opportunities available in your area or online. Continue to be a lifelong learner and take training, courses, and certificate programs in public health professional development-based skills. For example, over the past five years, I have found that I really enjoy leading and providing training to adults so I earned a certificate at my local university to provide me the latest information on how to facilitate training for adult learners. Next year, I plan to earn a project management certificate to increase my knowledge and abilities to organize and administer grant activities, coalition meetings, and a statewide elimination plan. Stay connected to your peers and professors from undergraduate and graduate school via social media or by phone or email. Seek opportunities to volunteer or take a part-time position to see which areas of public health you like most and in which you want to pursue a career. Don't be afraid to try new things and move around, there is no "set" career path in Public Health. Be flexible, adaptable, and always be open to new and exciting opportunities to use your health education specialist skills.

Table 7.5 Advantages and Disadvantages of Working in Public/Community Health Education/Promotion

Advantages

- Job responsibilities are highly varied and changing.
- There is a strong emphasis on prevention.
- There is usually a high community profile.
- Health education specialists work with multiple groups of people.
- There is a high degree of self-satisfaction.
- These positions typically offer good benefit packages.
- These positions typically allow flex time when working evenings or weekends.

Disadvantages

- Pay may be low, particularly in voluntary agencies.
- When hired directly by a community or public health agency, job security tends to be good. In such situations, the health education specialist is said to be employed on **hard money**. Sometimes, however, these agencies hire health education specialists on money secured through grants, which is known as **soft money**. In these situations, positions are terminated when grant funding is discontinued, so job security can be a concern.
- Relying heavily on volunteers can be frustrating. Although most volunteers are great, some do not demonstrate the same level of commitment as a paid employee might.
- There never seems to be enough money to run all of the programs that need to be offered in the way they should be offered.
- These positions often require irregular hours that may include evenings and weekends.
- There is a lot of bureaucracy in public health agencies.

Work-Site Health Education/Promotion

In describing WorkSite Health Promotion programs, the Centers for Disease Control and Prevention (CDC) refers to them as "a coordinated and comprehensive set of strategies which include programs, policies, benefits, environmental supports, and links to the surrounding community designed to meet the health and safety needs of all employees" (CDC, n.d.-b). Certainly, the workplace and the health of workers are closely related. Worksites should not only protect the safety of employees but should also provide employees with opportunities to enhance their overall health and well-being. Since the mid-1970s, business and industry in the United States have been offering worksite health promotion programs for their employees. Why are health education specialists interested in working in these settings? Why are worksites interested in offering these programs? Why are employees interested in participating in such programs?

For health education specialists, worksite wellness programs offer an additional setting for them to reach segments of the population that are not easily accessed through traditional community health programs. Program participants typically have to be at their work setting on a daily basis; thus, creating a situation where health education specialists can have regular and in-depth interactions with the participants. The worksite setting is conducive to incentive programs, participant recognition, and regular individualized feedback and support.

For employers, there are numerous potential benefits. The tangible benefits include reduced sick leave absenteeism, reduced use of health benefits, reduced workers' compensation costs, reduced injuries, and reduced presenteeism losses (losses resulting from poor productivity from those employees who are present). Beyond the tangible benefits, there are also intangible benefits including improved employee morale, increased employee loyalty, less organizational conflict, a more productive workforce, and improved employee decision-making ability (Edward Lowe Foundation, n.d.; CDC, n.d.-b).

For employees, the convenience of having health and fitness programs available at the worksite is a major advantage. Participation in these programs can improve health status, which decreases the risk of disease and may lead to enhanced self-image and self-esteem. Participating in such programs with fellow employees provides enhanced social support, reinforcement to change behaviors, and may increase motivation. In the United States, annual healthcare expenditures reached 3.8 trillion dollars in 2019 or an average of $11,582 for every man, woman, and child living in the United States. Overall, healthcare expenditures accounted for 17.7% of the gross domestic product in the United States (Centers for Medicare & Medicaid Services, 2020). Just as points of reference, a total of $253 billion was spent on health care in 1980; $714 billion was spent in 1990; and in 2010, the amount spent was $2.6 trillion. Approximately one-fourth of these healthcare costs are picked up by business and industry (Fronstin & Roebuck, 2015a). Starbucks, for example, pays more for its U.S. employees' health insurance each year than it does for coffee (Rubleski, 2007). Can worksite health promotion programs reduce these costs? According to the Wellness Councils of America (2020), "Employee well-being programs work. Not all of them, of course, but those that are high quality and evidence based do produce measurable and meaningful results"

Goetzel and Pronk (2010) conducted a systematic review of 51 worksite health promotion studies. They found that certain health behaviors, biometric measures, and financial outcomes could be influenced through worksite health promotion programs although the effect sizes for these improvements were modest compared with clinical interventions. The impact, however, of modest changes when applied to large groups of people combined with the relatively low cost of worksite programs compared with clinical interventions confirmed their value. This is especially true as many worksite programs are considered primary prevention. They assist workers to improve their diets, increase physical activity, manage stress, quit smoking, get flu shots, etc. They went on to say that such programs

> "may achieve long-lasting population-based health improvements at a low cost. Further, it was observed that health promotion interventions delivered at the worksite can be efficiently and cost-effectively provided, especially when company leadership, norms, culture, and policies are aligned to support adoption of healthy habits and prevention practices." (p. S224)

Health promotion programs at worksites differ greatly from site to site (Chenoweth, 2011; Fronstin & Roebuck, 2015b). Some are extensive, include elaborate facilities, and are conducted by full-time staff members hired by the company; others are minimal programs that may include only a brown bag lunch speaker's program or a discount at the local YMCA or health club (Chenoweth, 2011). **Figure 7.3** shows the percentage of companies offering different programs by company size. There is also a wide variety of health promotion activities that can be offered at any site. For a list of worksite health promotion activities, see **Table 7.6**.

The proportion of employers who provide worksite health promotion programs has increased over the years, especially among larger employers. Despite these increased numbers, more needs to be done. Many of

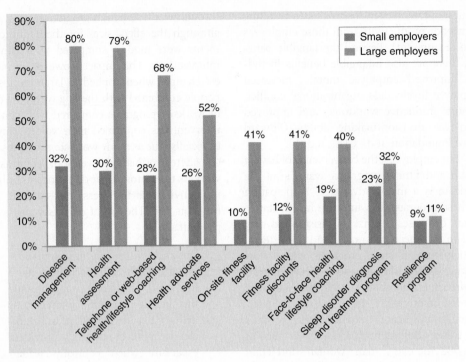

Figure 7.3 Use of Specific Health Management Programs by Firm Size 2013.

Reproduced from Fronstin, P., & Roebuck, M. C. (2015). Financial incentives, workplace wellness program participation, and utilization of health care services and spending. *EBRI Issue Brief, 417,* 1–23. https://www.ebri.org/docs/default-source/ebri-issue-brief/ebri_ib_417.pdf

Table 7.6 **Worksite Health Promotion Activities**

Smoking cessation	Cancer risk awareness	Lending libraries
Stress management		Physical examinations
	Cardiovascular risk awareness	
Weight loss		Smoke-free policies
Exercise/physical fitness	Skin cancer screenings	Counseling hotlines
Nutrition	Flu shots	Hypertension screenings
Safety	Health fairs	HIV/AIDS prevention
First aid & CPR	Bulletin boards	Paycheck stuffers
Mammography screenings	Newsletters	Website development

these large employers have only minimal health promotion offerings. Furthermore, the majority of U.S. employees work in small and medium-sized companies that are much less likely to offer comprehensive health promotion programs. Certain types of employers, such as

retailers, seldom offer health promotion programs, and any employer with a high rate of workforce turnover, like restaurants, has little motivation to offer health promotion programs.

The CDC is highly supportive of worksite health programs. They have developed a

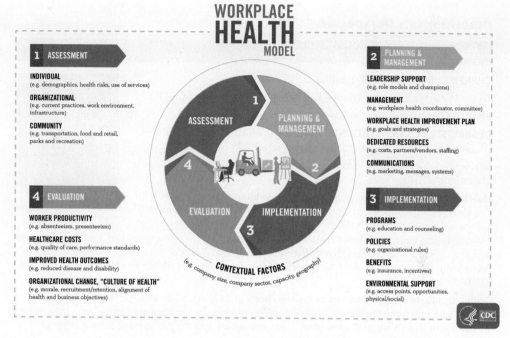

Figure 7.4 Workplace Health Model.

Reproduced from Centers for Disease Control and Prevention. (2016). *Workplace health model.* https://www.cdc.gov/workplacehealthpromotion/model

model that describes the necessary steps of a successful workplace health program (See **Figure 7.4**). The model identifies four steps: 1) Assessment, 2) Planning and Management, 3) Implementation, and 4) Evaluation (CDC, n.d.-b).

These four steps align closely with the responsibilities of a health education specialist and confirm the importance of having a certified health education specialist to conduct worksite programs.

Worksites can offer tangible incentives for employees to participate in health promotion programs. Even with incentives, questions exist regarding the ability of worksite programs to attract employees who are less well and at higher risk of health issues. In other words, do only the healthy and highly motivated employees participate? One recent study specifically designed to determine the impact of financial incentives concluded, ". . . financial incentives—on the order of $240 per employee per year—were successful at encouraging

widespread participation in this employer's workplace wellness program . . . these incentives brought in less-healthy individuals—those arguably in most need of the program" (Fronstin & Roebuck, 2015a, p. 19).

Although positions exist in the worksite health promotion setting that are strictly health education/promotion, more frequently, expertise in exercise testing and prescription is also required. This is because many worksite health promotion programs are centered around a fitness center. It is often the fitness center that is the most visible aspect of a worksite health promotion program and attracts many employees to health promotion activities. Therefore, skills related to exercise are important, and these skills are not part of the competencies required by a health education specialist. As a result, health education specialists preparing for employment in worksite health promotion should strongly consider a minor or second major in exercise science (see Practitioner's Perspective). Peabody and Linnan (2007)

Practitioner's Perspective

Alana Wall

CURRENT POSITION/TITLE: Health Fitness Professional

Toyota Motor Manufacturing Kentucky, Fitness Facility, Georgetown - KY

EMPLOYER: Health Fitness, A Trustmark Company

DEGREE(S) HELD/INSTITUTION(S) ATTENDED/GRADUATION YEAR(S):

BS Exercise Science, Morehead State University, 2014

MS Health Education and Promotion (Community Health Focus), University of Cincinnati, 2015

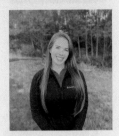

Courtesy of Alana Wall.

How I obtained my job: I completed a Corporate Internship with Health Fitness in Georgetown, KY, prior to the senior year of my undergraduate program. I am originally from Georgetown, KY, and Toyota Motor Manufacturing Kentucky Fitness (TMMK Fitness) was where I personally worked out for many years and where my passion for Health and Wellness blossomed. I was ecstatic to have this opportunity with Health Fitness because of the rapport I built with not only the TMMK Fitness staff but also the TMMK Fitness members.

During Graduate School, I worked at the University of Cincinnati Campus Recreation Center. I accepted a part-time position at the Campus Recreation Center after graduation until the position with Health Fitness came open. I was made aware of the job opening from a program manager at TMMK Fitness.

To apply for the Health Fitness Professional position, I submitted a resume through the Health Fitness website and completed a survey that asked a series of questions to determine my expectations of the position. The interview process consisted of a phone call followed by a face-to-face interview. The phone interview included previous work history questions, my opportunities for growth within the Health and Fitness industry, as well as my work ethic and previous work experiences. I was also asked to respond to some possible scenarios that might come up in the work environment.

Job responsibilities: My typical day as a Health Fitness Professional consists of personal training (where I incorporate Spectrum Fitness Methodology and Fusionetics Movement Efficiency Screenings), leading group exercise classes, incentive program planning, social media coordination and data analysis, and a variety of business-related administrative tasks along with working the reception desk and monitoring the fitness floor. First and foremost, we are committed to our members and they come first. This helps us not only with retention but also creates a feeling of community.

Incentive Program planning consists of coordinating and leading a variety of program-specific health improvement initiatives & promotions. I research health & fitness educational topics, identify appropriate participant educational materials and conduct health education seminars/presentations including What's What Seminars on a variety of health topics. I do not have my CHES. It is not a requirement for me to hold this certification. TMMK Fitness is considered a fitness-only site within the Health Fitness company. However, a CHES could be beneficial to those who work in one of Health Fitness's Health/Injury Prevention and Treatment sites.

Is working in this position what you thought it would be? I knew what to expect within this position due to my previous work experience as an intern at TMMK Fitness; however, as the fitness industry continues to grow, so does the opportunity for training and development. My position is entry level, but it is a great steppingstone for future career opportunities in management, health coaching, and administration. I get to work with other knowledgeable fitness and health professionals who support each other to grow in the profession. It is all about teamwork! HealthFitness has over

200 sites across the United States, which gives me plenty of opportunities to grow, network, and advance within the company.

Certifications: When working in corporate health/fitness, there are a number of available certifications that can make one more marketable and valuable to the organization. Since my site is considered a fitness-only site, I have achieved the following certifications:

ACE Certified Personal Trainer

AFAA Certified Group Exercise Instructor

ACE Health Coach

Biomechanics Method Corrective Exercise Specialist

Box n' Burn Academy—Level 1

Currently Pursuing ACE Nutrition Specialist

What I like most about my job: At a corporate level, there is a lot of opportunity and variety in my position. Not only do I build rapport and meaningful relationships with the members, but there are numerous opportunities to be involved with the Toyota corporate facility where I can grow and develop in other areas that assist the business. Over the past five years of working at TMMK Fitness, not only have I grown as a Personal Trainer and Group Exercise Instructor, but I have been able to develop stronger marketing skills, initiate incentive programs, utilize social media, and help introduce a virtual experience for our members that includes online group exercise classes and other education material!

What I like least about my job: By nature, working for a corporate facility as a contractor means you are always at the mercy of the client. Many aspects of my position such as facility hours, staffing, budgeting, resource allocation, and other impactful decisions are made by the client with little input from us professionals at the site level. Being a fully staffed 24-hour facility means working hours that may not be one's first choice for an undetermined amount of time. However, there is some flexibility within my set schedule to accommodate personal training appointments along with other various tasks.

Recommendations for those preparing to become a work-site health education specialist: Don't be afraid to ask for help and build a network! There are so many great resources, such as your professors, counselors, and other professionals who can give you insight to your future as a health education specialist. Find a mentor who you can learn from and who can help you identify what fuels your passion in health education. Find the ideal internship during your undergraduate and/or graduate school career. A good internship can help you obtain future employment and can assist with your overall career development.

recommend that those wanting careers in the worksite setting consider getting two degrees: one a more generalist degree (e.g., health education, public health, or health promotion) and the second a specialist degree (e.g., exercise physiology, nutrition science, nursing, or athletic training). They indicate that it does not matter which degree is the undergraduate and which is the graduate but that an individual with both a generalist and a specialist degree "will have many more options than someone with two degrees in either field" (Peabody & Linnan, 2007, p. 31). Beyond

specialty expertise, a master's degree is also required for many entry-level health education/promotion positions in business and industry. In addition to the Certified Health Education Specialist (CHES) or Master Certified Health Education Specialist (MCHES) credential, certifications more specific to exercise are available from the American College of Sports Medicine and may be required at some worksite settings. Certifications for specific aspects of worksite health promotion, such as aerobic dance, wellness coaching, first aid, and cardiopulmonary resuscitation (CPR), and for smoking cessation instructors are also available and encouraged. In general, the more degrees, certifications, and credentials one has, the better one will compete for worksite health promotion positions.

A Day in the Career of a Worksite Health Education Specialist

The day begins early for Alisa (she/her/hers). The fitness center opens promptly at 5:00 AM so that employees who start work at 6:00 AM have time to work out before beginning their shift. Alisa has to be there at 4:45 AM. to open the doors, turn on the lights, and greet the first members. The first two hours of her day are spent "working the floor." This means she greets members as they enter the facility; walks around the machines, providing instruction where needed; chats with the members; answers health-related questions; and basically makes everyone feel important and welcome. By 7:00 AM, all the shift workers have left the fitness facility and, by 9:00 AM, the managerial employees have cleared out.

From 9:00 AM to 11:00 AM is a slow time in the center. A few retired employees and spouses use the machines, but this is basically the time for Alisa to get other tasks done. She begins by laundering the dirty towels and folding those that come out of the dryer. Next, she provides the routine maintenance to the machines. This involves cleaning them with disinfectant and applying a lubricant to the moving parts. Once this is completed, Alisa has about an hour to work at her desk. Today, she is writing an article on the different types of dietary fats, to be included in the Wellness Center newsletter she publishes each month. The newsletter is distributed to all active employees and retirees of the company. Alisa is always amazed at how important writing skills are to her position in worksite health promotion.

Between 11:00 AM and 12:15 PM, Alisa teaches two aerobics classes for the employees. The first is a beginners' class for new

members. The second is supposed to be a more advanced class. Unfortunately, many of the shift employees have no choice in their lunch time, so Alisa ends up with some very advanced members in the beginners' class and some beginners in the advanced class. This is frustrating and could be avoided if there were another fitness center employee. There are, however, only two employees in the center, and Rob (he/him/his), the other health education specialist, must work the floor with the lunch crowd while Alisa teaches. Alisa is going to pursue the possibility of hiring a part-time aerobics instructor just for the lunch hours. This would allow her to offer a beginning and an advanced class at each time slot.

From 12:15 PM to 1:00 PM, Alisa runs an ongoing weigh loss support group for employees. All participants bring a brown bag lunch that is supposed to contain food appropriate for a weight-loss diet. They weigh in weekly, and Alisa provides each participant with a voluntary body composition (fat vs. lean) analysis every three months. At least twice a week, Alisa prepares a 20-minute lecture on a weight-loss topic or invites a guest speaker from the community. The same issue concerning lunch breaks also impacts the weight loss support class. Some employees who take a lunch break from 11:00–12:00 are not able to participate.

At 1:00 PM, the employees are back at their work stations, and there is again a quiet time in the health promotion center. Alisa spends the next hour eating lunch at her desk and working on a new incentive program for employees to join the health promotion center that will be offered next month. She has to develop all the brochures, promotional material, and registration forms and arrange for the purchase of incentive items.

At 2:00 PM, she has a meeting with upper management of the company. She has been advocating for the company to establish a no-smoking policy for the past five years. Two years ago, the company did restrict smoking to specified smoking areas, which was a major accomplishment. Today she will present a proposal to phase out all smoking over a one-year period. Alisa would be responsible for offering several smoking cessation classes over the 12-month period before the no-smoking policy takes effect. She has already decided that her next advocacy effort will be to have more healthy alternatives available in the vending machines, snack rooms, and cafeteria. She has begun a literature review to learn what other companies have done to improve the nutrition of their employees.

By 2:30 PM, she is back in the health promotion center. The second-shift employees are in the center now ahead of their shifts, so Alisa is again working the floor. Today, she has to do initial fitness assessments on three new employees. This involves running the employees through a standardized series of tests. Based on the results of these tests and each employee's fitness objectives, she prescribes an individualized exercise program for each employee. She then takes the employees through the fitness center and teaches them how to use the equipment and maintain a record of their progress.

By 3:30 PM, Alisa is finished with the assessments. Because she had the early shift, opening the facility, she is finished for the day. Rob, who came in later, will stay and close the facility at 8:00 PM.

March 16, 2020

The company and the fitness center were closed down due to COVID-19 and employees who could work from home were instructed to do so. Unfortunately, many of the shift workers had to be either laid off or furloughed as their work could not take place from home. Rob also was furloughed as there was not enough work for two health education specialists with the fitness center closed. Upper management talked with Alisa and asked her to offer as much of her program as possible online. They recognized the need for health and fitness programming during this stressful time. Alisa developed a series of exercise videos

that were shared with employees over the company website. She also initiated a Zoom meeting with those who were in her weight control class twice a week. Furthermore, she developed a weekly newsletter that presented health information and discussed COVID-19, what was known and unknown about the disease, and how employees could best protect themselves and others. Alisa spent part of each day reading and staying current on the pandemic. She was also asked to be a member of the company's COVID-19 Committee, which had the responsibility for establishing protocol for when employees would be allowed to return to work.

Additional Responsibilities

The responsibilities involved in working in a corporate health promotion center are many and varied. In some facilities, maintaining records such as who is using the center, which programs are most popular, fitness assessment results, and health profiles are major tasks. Fortunately, there are software programs available to assist with this. There are always many little things that need to be done, such as the creation and updating of bulletin boards, equipment maintenance, and towel distribution and laundering. In many cases, annual health fairs, company-wide health screenings, and flu shot/COVID-19 vaccination programs are the responsibility of the health promotion staff. In addition, advocating for population-based, corporate-wide policies, rules, and regulations to enhance the health of employees is important. These policies, rules, or regulations may relate to tobacco use, food service, safety, violence, stress, and so forth.

Being a health education specialist in a worksite setting is not easy. It is imperative that worksite health education professionals stay up to date with health information and the operational processes of running a worksite program. Plus, they must always be willing to flex and adapt programs as was demanded during the COVID pandemic. As noted by the American College of Sports Medicine (2003), "the worksite health promotion professional needs to have a good handle on where to find the information, knowledge, resources, and expertise that are needed to access the underlying foundations on which programs are built, the operational processes that allow programs to flourish, and the motivation to continually keep a heads-up attitude toward new and innovative strategies that allow well-established programs to maintain their cutting edge" (p. xi). See **Table 7.7** for a listing of the advantages and disadvantages of employment in worksite health education/promotion.

Those who combine health education/promotion with a fitness background may find employment in settings beyond the business world. See **Table 7.8** for a partial listing of employment opportunities for those with both health education/promotion and exercise training.

Table 7.7 Advantages and Disadvantages of Working in Worksite Health Promotion

Advantages

- It affords excellent opportunities for prevention.
- It provides access to individuals who may not participate in community programs.
- Health education specialists work with multiple and diverse groups of people, including everyone from upper management to shift workers.
- Most health education specialists in the corporate setting enjoy their positions and report a high degree of job satisfaction.
- Pay is usually higher than in other health education settings. Benefits are usually good, but they vary considerably from employer to employer.
- Health education specialists have access to fitness facilities for personal use.

Disadvantages

- Hours are long and irregular. To cover employees on all shifts in a company may necessitate health education specialists working hours early in the morning or late in the evening. It is not unusual to work more than eight hours a day.
- Upward mobility may be a problem. Typically, there are only one or two managerial positions in health promotion at any given worksite. This makes it difficult for health education specialists to move up. In addition, those holding managerial positions as directors of health and fitness have nowhere to move up in a company unless they are willing to get out of the health promotion field.
- Health promotion programs and fitness centers often seem to be low on a company's priority list. Such programs are often the first to receive budget cuts in difficult times and often seem to be short of the staff necessary to run optimal programs.
- Some companies subcontract their health promotion and fitness programs to outside vendors. Some of these outside vendors hire part-time health education specialists, pay lower wages, and provide few or no benefits.
- Health education specialists have strong pressure to be extremely fit and be healthy role models for other employees.

Table 7.8 Employment Opportunities in Health Education/Promotion with an Emphasis in Exercise and Fitness

Corporations, business, and industry corporate/industrial parks	Outside commercial vendors that provide programs to worksites
YMCAs/YWCAs	Entrepreneurial enterprises (aerobics studios, consulting, club owner, personal training)
Private health and fitness clubs	

Table 7.8 **Employment Opportunities in Health Education/Promotion with an Emphasis in Exercise and Fitness** *(continued)*

Special-population clubs (women, elderly, etc.)	Fitness product/service companies (sales and marketing)
Community parks & recreation programs	Condos and apartment complexes
Colleges/universities	Hotels
Hospitals	Spas
Sports medicine centers	Resorts and cruise lines
Insurance companies that offer health education/promotion programs to their corporate clients	

Health Education/ Promotion in Healthcare Settings

Positions are available for health education specialists in a variety of **healthcare settings**, including clinics, hospitals, and managed care organizations (McKenzie et al., 2017). "Typically in the medical care field, health education specialists serve as administrators, directors, managers, and coordinators, supporting and consulting on health education programs and services" (Totzkay-Sitar & Cornett, 2007, p. 8). Health education specialists have also been used in healthcare settings to provide patient education (Byrd et al., 2007). For example, a patient is diagnosed with heart disease or an increased risk for heart disease. That patient is then referred to the health education specialist for information about exercise, nutrition, weight control, stress management, smoking cessation, and so on. This could involve one-on-one education or counseling sessions with the patient, or it might involve group programs in which multiple patients receive the same program at the same time (NCHEC & SOPHE, 2020).

In hospitals and other healthcare settings, health education specialists have also been hired to direct health and fitness programs for company employees, much the same as in other worksite settings (NCHEC & SOPHE, 2020) (see **Figure 7.5**). Sometimes, these programs are also open as an outreach service to community members. Other times, health education specialists are responsible for developing and conducting health and fitness programs specifically designed for community members through fitness facilities that are affiliated with the hospital (see Practitioner's Perspective).

Unfortunately, patient education has not emerged as a major source of employment for health education specialists. Although it seems like an ideal activity for health education specialists, third-party reimbursement is not provided by health insurance companies to cover a health education specialist. Third-party reimbursement refers to the system whereby healthcare providers can submit their bills to the patient's insurance company for reimbursement (McKenzie, Pinger and Seabert, 2018). Thus, patient education does not happen or it may be done by nurses who can also serve other functions in the healthcare setting that are reimbursable. Although health insurance companies are certainly concerned about reducing healthcare costs, their strategies to date have been more short term. The impact of health promotion and education programs may not be seen for years, and cause-and-effect relationships are difficult to establish. Therefore, without the availability of third-party payment, there is no financial incentive for hospitals, clinics, and private practice physicians to offer health promotion and education services to their patients.

In response to this problem, SOPHE has made third-party reimbursement one of its

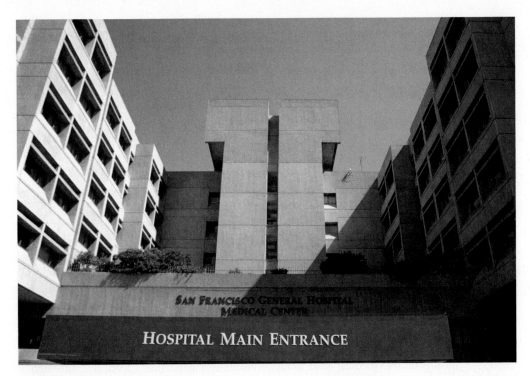

Figure 7.5 Hospitals employ health education specialists to provide programs for employees, patients, or the community at large.

© Robert Clay/Alamy Stock Photo.

Practitioner's Perspective

Patient Educator: Heather Rhodes, BS, CHES

CURRENT POSITION/TITLE: Health Educator

EMPLOYER: IU Health Ball Memorial Family Medicine Residency Center

DEGREE/INSTITUTION/YEAR: BS Ball State University, 2007

MAJOR: Health Science

Job responsibilities: My job as the Health Educator for the Family Medicine Residency Center includes a wide range of responsibilities. I receive referrals from our resident physicians to educate clinic patients about a number of health topics, such as diabetes management, healthy nutrition, smoking cessation, and weight loss. All of our family medicine residents are responsible for completing a set number of community

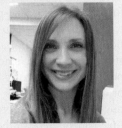

Courtesy of Heather Rhodes.

service hours throughout their residency, and I serve as the coordinator for all community outreach activities. I also serve as the coordinator for our Reach Out and Read program, a program that offers free books to children ages six months to five years during their well-child visits. I am very involved in the community and serve on a number of local boards and councils that all promote health and wellness as well as provide education to the community. I am responsible for displaying timely and appropriate health information on 26 bulletin boards throughout the clinic. I offer group smoking cessation classes in the community and also serve as a resource for the IU Health Ball Memorial Cancer Center by providing one-on-one cessation to their patients. I serve as the supervisor for a number of interns, both health education and administrative, who spend time at our facility. In addition, I have recently started conducting intake and education sessions with our newly pregnant patients in which I gather all pertinent information for their doctor and educate them about what to expect throughout pregnancy.

How I obtained my job: I stayed in touch with my internship supervisor after graduation, and they shared that the job was available. I was familiar with the position as I had shadowed the previous Health Educator as a part of curriculum requirements for one of my health science classes, and they had offered me an internship there as well. The job required a four-year degree as well as a CHES certification, and I possessed both. I felt that it was the perfect fit because my favorite part of my internship was the one-on-one education that I was able to give during health screenings. My previous job was telephone-based health coaching, which made me realize that I really desired to work with patients face to face. I had the valuable health coaching experience, which I feel made me a great candidate for the position.

What I like most about my job: I love the fact that I get to try and help people and make a difference in their lives on a daily basis. I also really enjoy the variety that my job provides. I am given a great deal of freedom to be creative and expand my position in new ways. Another thing I appreciate about my job is the positive and family-oriented work environment. Everyone is passionate about helping others, and we all work as a team to provide our patients with the best care possible.

What I like least about my job: The biggest challenge of my job and what I sometimes like least is the fact that I am the only educator in the facility. There are no other health education specialists to bounce ideas off of and collaborate with. As a result, I have to wear many hats and try to be available in all areas as much as possible. I love having the variety, but because my job provides a little more flexibility, I am given a wide variety of extra tasks that others may not have the ability to complete due to more rigid schedules.

How my work relates to the responsibilities and competencies of a health education specialist: As part of my job, I am constantly assessing the needs of my patients on an individual basis. I am assessing their learning levels as well as readiness to change so that I can really tailor information to the patient in a way that will make it most valuable for them. On a larger scale, I have had several opportunities to partner with outside agencies to provide health education/promotion programs for the community. In each instance, we work together to assess needs, plan, implement, and evaluate our programs. I serve as a resource person within our clinic and help residents find appropriate services, information, organizations, etc., that can meet the needs of their patients. I also serve as a resource for the community by participating in health fairs as well as local boards and councils.

Recommendations for those preparing to be health education specialists: For those who are preparing to be health education specialists, I would encourage you to make the most of your health science classes and learn all you can. Your classes will help prepare you for the CHES exam and will provide you with the necessary framework to start your career successfully. I also think it is always beneficial to take every opportunity to gain practical experience with program planning and health education through volunteering, research, and part-time work. Work on building your knowledge base about chronic disease management, nutrition, and other important health and wellness topics. Choose wisely when picking your internship site as this will really help you determine your desired career path after graduation. It will give you valuable hands-on experience and will either confirm that you are on the right path or can help you find a new direction.

The role of health education specialist in the future: I think that the sky is the limit when it comes to the role of the health education specialist in the future. Over the last eight years, my career has continued to evolve and grow. I think that opportunities will expand beyond the typical clinical and

(continues)

major advocacy issues. Another positive development occurred in 2020 when the American Medical Association recognized NCHEC Certified Health Education Specialists to use the new Category III CPT (Current Procedural Terminology) codes (Lysoby, 2021). This would allow some reimbursement to health education specialists.

Of all healthcare settings, health maintenance organizations (HMOs) have been most receptive to hiring health education specialists. The first HMOs were established in the 1970s as a result of federal money that was made available to help with start-up costs and to study the effectiveness of this healthcare delivery mechanism. In essence, patients belonging to an HMO pay one set fee for all of their medical services in a given year. It, therefore, benefits the HMO to provide preventive health services and health education/promotion programs to keep their patients healthy. The fewer services a patient uses, the greater the cost benefit to the HMO. In the initial HMO legislation, one of the criteria for establishing an HMO was providing health education/promotion. Unfortunately, there were no stipulations on the professional preparation of the health education/promotion provider. Often, nurses or other individuals with little or no health education/promotion preparation or experience were given the responsibility of providing health education/promotion programs. As a result, some HMOs have developed outstanding health education/

promotion programs with health education specialists, whereas others do very little.

There is, however, reason to be optimistic about future employment opportunities in healthcare settings for health education specialists. The Health Promoting Hospitals Network (HPH), initiated by the World Health Organization (WHO), functions to incorporate more health promotion and education programs in hospitals worldwide (The International Network of Health Promoting Hospitals and Health Services, 2016). With changes in the U.S. medical care system rapidly occurring, the increased emphasis on cost-cutting measures, and movement toward more managed care, it is likely that prevention will take a higher profile in the future. As these changes occur, health education specialists will be the best prepared professionals to assume responsibility for helping individuals adopt healthy lifestyles.

A Day in the Career of a Healthcare Setting Health Education Specialist

Mary's (she/her/hers) day begins at 8:30 AM, when she arrives at the hospital, picks up her mail, and proceeds to her office where she reviews her emails and phone messages. She is the only health education specialist employed by this large metropolitan hospital, but she does have a secretary/assistant who works closely with her to carry out the duties of the position.

At 9:00 AM, Mary has to attend the weekly staff meeting. This is a meeting with all department heads at the hospital. Much of the agenda does not concern Mary directly, but it is important for her to know what is going on in all departments. At today's meeting, it was decided to have an open house for the public to see the newly renovated obstetrics wing of the hospital. Mary is given the responsibility of planning and advertising this event.

At 10:00 AM, Mary has an appointment with the administrative head of the Cardiac Rehabilitation Program at the hospital. The purpose of the meeting is to begin planning the development of two brochures that will eventually be distributed to all cardiac rehabilitation patients and will be posted on the hospital education website that Mary maintains. One brochure will be on stress-management strategies and the other on different types of dietary fat. They brainstorm ideas, and Mary agrees to develop a rough draft of the content of the brochures for the administrative head to review prior to their next meeting. They will also discuss graphics, layout, and production at the next meeting.

At 11:00 AM, Mary leaves the hospital to drive to one of the local malls. The mall has decided to conduct a three-day health fair, and the hospital has agreed to be a co-sponsor of the event. Today is a planning meeting for all of the agencies and businesses that will participate. In addition to serving on the planning committee, Mary is responsible for setting up the hospital's display and coordinating nurses and physicians to work in several screening stations. During the health fair, Mary will be at the hospital's booth all day, handing out materials, answering questions, and promoting the hospital's community outreach health promotion programs.

After lunch, Mary returns to the hospital at around 1:00 PM and spends the next two hours working on the hospital's health and wellness newsletter. As a public service and to promote the hospital, Mary is responsible for developing a newsletter every other month that is mailed to all households in the hospital's immediate service area. Each edition of the newsletter features one department in the hospital and contains several additional articles about health and wellness. Mary writes much of each newsletter, using information she obtains from the Internet and from a variety of health journals and newsletters to which she subscribes. She designs and formats the newsletter with a desktop publishing program she has on her computer. She marvels at how important good writing skills are to her position.

At 3:00 PM, Mary leads a weight-loss support group for hospital employees. Most of the participants are nurses and housekeeping staff from either the first or second shift. At each session, participants weigh in, share their experiences over the previous week, and listen to a 20-minute presentation designed to enhance their weight-loss program. Mary is responsible for each week's presentation. In addition, she provides participants with healthy recipes, exercise tips, motivational incentives, and recognition awards. The weight loss support group also has a website that Mary maintains where additional recipes and information on weight loss are posted. In the future, Mary plans to expand the website and develop an online evidence-based weight-loss program that will be made available to the entire community.

After class, Mary returns phone calls, answers emails, and ties up loose ends until it is time for her to go home at 5:00 PM. It is not unusual for Mary to take some work home in the evenings or on weekends. Tonight; however, Mary must return to the hospital at 7:30 PM to teach a stress-management class for the community. The stress class is part of the hospital's ongoing community outreach program. Each month, a different health topic is taught, and Mary is responsible for either teaching the class or lining up the instructor/speaker for the class.

March 16, 2020

As COVID-19 cases and deaths continued to increase, hospital routine drastically changed. Employees who could work from home were required to do so. Clinical staff focused all of their attention on COVID patients and any elective surgeries were canceled. Weekly staff meetings became daily staff meetings just to keep everyone informed about COVID and the hospital's response to it. All of Mary's current programs and initiatives were suspended and she was given other duties to meet the needs of the hospital. The hospital education website that Mary maintains became a major outlet for COVID-related information and Mary must update the site regularly. Stress management and exercise are very important for the highly stressed hospital employees so Mary develops a series of short exercise and stress management videos that can be utilized by employees during breaks or at home when time allows. Mary is also asked to assist the social worker in serving as an information conduit. She takes messages via phone or email from patients' loved ones who are not allowed in the hospital. She then relays those messages to the patients via their nurses. Mary is not allowed to have patient contact, but just being in the hospital on a regular basis causes her to worry about possibly contracting the disease and passing it on to her own family. This is a very sad and stressful time for Mary and she looks forward to getting back to her typical duties when the crisis is over.

Additional Responsibilities

Health education specialists working in healthcare settings are involved in numerous and varied activities. The actual responsibilities can differ greatly from one healthcare setting to another. Planning, implementing, and evaluating programs and events are certainly major tasks. Health education specialists may also be involved in grant writing, one-on-one or group patient education services, publicity, public relations, employee wellness activities, and various collaborative efforts with other hospital staff, community agencies, or departments of public health.

Administration is a major responsibility of many health education specialists working in hospitals. They are often hired as managers, directors, or coordinators of programs. Hospitals often adopt a "team" approach to health education/promotion, in which doctors, nurses, physical therapists, dieticians and other health specialists are all part of the team. Health education specialists plan and coordinate the programs and serve as resources for the other team members, who actually present the programs. In this type of position, the health education specialist provides little direct client service (Breckon et al., 1998). (See **Table 7.9**.)

Table 7.9 Advantages and Disadvantages of Working in a Healthcare Setting

Advantages

- Job responsibilities are highly varied and changing.
- There is increased credibility due to the healthcare connection.
- There is usually a high community profile.
- Health education specialists work with multiple groups of people.
- Wages and benefits are good.
- There is a high degree of self-satisfaction.

Disadvantages

- Health education/promotion may have low status and low priority within healthcare settings.
- Health education specialists must continually justify the program's value.
- Jobs are difficult to obtain.
- Turf issues over educational responsibilities can develop.
- Hours may be long and irregular.
- Some medical doctors may be difficult to work with.

Health Education/ Promotion in Colleges and Universities

Colleges and universities are another source of employment for health education specialists. Within the college setting, there are typically two types of positions that health education specialists hold. The first is an academic, or faculty, position, and the second is as a health education specialist in a student health service or wellness center.

As a faculty member, the health education specialist typically has three major responsibilities: teaching, community and professional service, and scholarly research (Preparing Future Faculty, n.d.). The amount of emphasis on each of these major responsibilities is dependent on the institution. In large research institutions, faculty may spend most of their time writing grants and conducting research. In smaller four-year colleges, teaching may be the major responsibility. In addition to the major responsibilities, faculty may be asked to advise students, serve on committees, coordinate or lead student groups, attend professional conferences, and accept administrative duties.

The minimum qualification for working as a faculty member in the college/university setting is usually a doctoral degree in health education/promotion or public health with a focus in health education. Although some junior colleges and small four-year schools may hire faculty with only a master's degree, most tenure-track positions require a doctorate. In addition, depending on the position for which one is applying, it may be necessary to have had prior experience or academic training in school health, public/community health, or worksite health promotion. Holding or being eligible for a CHES or MCHES credential is often listed as a preference or requirement for faculty positions.

For a health education specialist in a university health service or wellness center, the major responsibility is to plan, implement, and evaluate health education/promotion programs for program participants (see Practitioner's Perspective). In some universities, the program participants are students, whereas in others it is the faculty and staff. Often, both groups are included as program participants. In addition to program planning, the health education specialist may be responsible for maintaining a resource library; maintaining a

---

Practitioner's Perspective

University Wellness Center: Elizabeth D. Peeler, MSPH, CHES

CURRENT POSITION: Health Educator – Alcohol and Other Drugs

EMPLOYER: Emory University

DEGREE INFORMATION: Undergraduate: Appalachian State University (Bachelor of Science)

MAJOR: Cell/Molecular Biology

MINOR(S): Art History and Chemistry

GRADUATE: University of South Carolina (Master in Science of Public Health)

CONCENTRATION: Health Promotion, Education, and Behavior

How I got into health education: I stumbled my way into health education as a pre-med freshman at Appalachian State University. I applied to be a Wellness Peer Educator to show medical schools that I had the skills to communicate to patients on how to change their

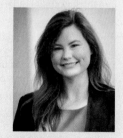

Courtesy of Elizabeth Peeler.

(continues)

Practitioner's Perspective *(continued)*

University Wellness Center: Elizabeth D. Peeler, MSPH, CHES

health behaviors to become healthier. Little did I know that by joining this organization I would change my career path from medicine to public health.

My current job responsibilities: As a health educator Emory University, I present to student groups in a number of different health topics, and plan, implement, create and review policies, and evaluate campus-wide events to promote better health and wellbeing especially around alcohol and other drugs. I assist in administering the American College Health Association – National College Health Assessment and other surveys to determine student health needs. Based on needs assessments and climate surveys, I am responsible for strategic planning within my office.

I collaborate with a number of offices and departments on campus to better serve the needs of our students. As such, I serve on a number of campus and community committees. I also engage with the outside community to build rapport and relationships to address any issues that may arise off-campus. As well, I participate in national professional organizations through conferences, coalitions, and committees to further health education and health promotion in higher education.

How I obtained my job: After I graduated with my master's, I accepted a position at Ball State University (BSU) as a health educator. After three years at BSU, I decided to apply to Emory University as a health educator focusing on alcohol and other drugs. I submitted my cover letter along with my curriculum vitae and list of references to the search committee for review. Emory University contacted me for a 30-minute phone interview followed by an in-person interview. I received the job offer two weeks after the in-person interview and happily accepted the position.

How I utilize health education/promotion in my job: I utilize a number of different theories and models in my programs. Most commonly, I use the Socio-Ecological Model, Transtheoretical Model, and Health Belief Model to inform my programming. I use process, impact, and outcome evaluations to measure behavior and culture change. Needs assessments and climate surveys are administered to help inform my programming on the current needs of students. I also use community and stakeholder engagement to organize and disseminate health promotion programming. I collect, analyze, and report data on my programs' reach and effectiveness to university administrators and community leaders.

What I like most about my job: There are so many things I love about my job, I cannot possibly mention them all. While there are definitely challenges working with college-aged students, their energy, enthusiasm, and creativity more than makes up for the challenges they present. Without students' input into programs, events, and initiatives, I would not be able to do my job. Students are the key stakeholders, and they must be fully engaged to change the climate and culture in a university.

I also enjoy working with different disciplines across campus to bring better programs and initiatives to students. By working collaboratively with different departments, I am able to ensure that I am approaching all needs of students. Some departments I have worked with include student life, residence life, campus police, dining services, and recreation services.

What I like least about my job: With any position in public health, there seems to be never enough resources to go around. This leads to stress in trying to figure out how to implement programs, but it also encourages creativity. Further, it can be incredibly frustrating to work on improving students' health but not see immediate changes in their behaviors. Behavior change is not instantaneous, and health educators must learn patience.

Recommendations for those preparing to be health education specialists: For future health education specialists, I suggest finding a mentor in their field of choice. I have been very lucky in finding a number of mentors in my field that have helped me immensely whether that has been professionally, academically, or even personally.

I also recommend completing observations, practicums, and internships in different settings. You may find that you prefer a clinical setting over an office setting or vice-versa. Interning is also a great networking opportunity to health better prepare you for the field.

Another important recommendation that often gets overlooked for health education specialists is the importance of research. The fundamentals of research help immensely when reading the literature to help in developing cutting edge, evidence-based programs. Research is also vital when trying to justify the importance of a needed resource or program.

The role of health education specialists in the future: Based on my experience as a health educator, future health education specialists are going to be utilized more in clinical settings to change health behavior than they currently do. Health coaching will become a part of the clinical experience for patients who need to change health behaviors for a healthier and more productive life. Health education specialists are also going to be utilized more in administrator roles to better address the needs of the community.

website; one-on-one advising with students; developing and coordinating a peer-education program; speaking to residence hall, fraternity, and sorority groups; conducting incentive programs; and planning special events.

International Opportunities

Health education/promotion specialists may wish to consider working in global health for all or a portion of their careers. There is great need for professionals with health education/promotion skills in many low- and middle-income countries. These positions often require special dedication because the living and working conditions may be more challenging than those experienced in the United States. For those so inclined, however, the rewards in terms of personal satisfaction and accomplishment can be tremendous. Furthermore, the experience gained by planning, implementing, and evaluating health promotion and education programs in foreign countries can be invaluable to one's professional development (see Practitioner's Perspective).

Working in developing countries often requires the health education specialist to examine different health problems and to try different approaches. For example, instead of helping people reduce high-fat, high-cholesterol diets, as in the United States, the health education specialist may be helping people deal with problems of starvation, malnutrition, and parasitic and bacterial infections. Instead of dealing with heart disease and lung cancer, the health education specialist in a developing country may be facing schistosomiasis, diarrhea, and ascariasis and tapeworm infections.

Consider the case of Sofia. Sofia was working as a community health education specialist for the health department in a rural community of about 2,000 people in a developing country. The water source for this community consisted of several large ponds. These ponds were the only source of drinking water and were also used for bathing, clothes washing, and care of animals. Many people were getting sick with severe diarrhea, and there had been several deaths among the elderly and very young. To alleviate this problem, it was decided to develop an educational campaign to get people to boil their water before consumption. Sofia was given the responsibility for developing this campaign. There were no local newspapers or radio stations and no

Practitioner's Perspective

Nontraditional health education/promotion positions (including global health): Janet Kamiri

How I obtained my job (If appropriate, describe past and current professional positions and how you came to hold the job you now hold):
After completing my undergraduate degree in school health education, I started my career as a health and physical education teacher in a large public-school system. I loved being a classroom teacher and enjoyed working with students across many grade levels. However, I wanted to focus on the health education component so I left the traditional classroom setting and transitioned into a role as a traveling adolescent sexual health educator for a nonprofit youth health education agency. I enjoyed working in health education and promotion in a new way and decided to pursue a Master of Public Health (MPH) degree. After receiving my MPH and honing my program development, implementation, and evaluation skills, I shifted directions and worked at a disease-specific voluntary health organization. This experience helped me realize that my passion work lies in holistically improving the health of individuals. I started seeking out a role that would allow me to look at health from the perspective of both individual behaviors and the systems and factors that influence those behaviors. Ultimately, I obtained my current position as the Director of Health and Wellness at the Indianapolis Urban League.

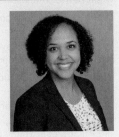

Courtesy of Janet Kamiri.

Describe the duties of your current position: In my role as the Director of Health and Wellness, I manage the health and wellness team (staff and interns) and programs of the Indianapolis Urban League. Many of the health and wellness initiatives are grant-funded and it is my responsibility to ensure our programs are high quality and meet our funders' requirements and expectations. Therefore, I am responsible for grant reporting as well as seeking out new funding sources for future programming.

A primary responsibility of my position is developing new programming to grow the scope of work in the health and wellness department. This allows me to work collaboratively and cross-functionally with other program areas including college and career readiness and workforce development, to plan and implement programming that addresses multiple dimensions of health. I also participate in several coalitions that are working to reduce health disparities in the Indianapolis area.

My global health experience: Global health is a broad field that encompasses many different disciplines. It is a collaborative field that promotes health equity. What I think is most important in global health is centering the experiences and knowledge of the local population. My first exposure to global health work was through a study abroad program in western Kenya. On this trip, I visited schools and health centers. While I had learned about social determinants of health and health disparities within and between countries prior to this trip, this experience gave me a real-life context for my textbook learning. While working on my MPH, I also took many courses with a focus on global health. I had hoped to pursue a career in global health; however, I found it challenging to secure a position because there are so many qualified candidates around the world who possess local expertise and knowledge. However, even though I was not able to secure a paid position, I have continued to dedicate time to volunteering every year at a school holiday day camp that I co-founded in Kenya. I use my skills and knowledge in health education and promotion to plan and implement health-based education programming for youth. This programming is done in partnership with volunteers and other organizations from around the world and from the local community in Kenya.

What health education specialist responsibilities do you use in your position? In your global health work? I use principles of health education and promotion in my job on a daily basis. At the Indianapolis Urban League, my role is focused on planning, implementing, and evaluating health education programs. Some of the programs we implement, such as smoking cessation classes, are evidence-based programs that I make small adjustments to in order to best serve the program participants. Other programs, like our Family, Food, and Fitness program, were developed in house and it is my responsibility to implement the programs and evaluate their efficacy and determine whether to continue, change, or eliminate the programs. I also develop new programs based on organizational goals and the needs of the community. I also serve as a resource person. My colleagues from other departments often call on me to help them link their program participants with health resources from various social service organizations to securing health insurance.

In my global health work, I also use principles of health education and promotion even though the work is not entirely on health education. Assessing needs in global health is critically important. As someone working in a new culture, it is most important to first know the community before trying to plan a program or intervention to solve a problem.

What I like most about my work as a health education specialist: In my work as a health education specialist, I am constantly able to be creative in addressing health disparities and improving health outcomes. While every position I have held has been different, there have been consistent themes across each role. In every role, I have worked collaboratively with my colleagues as well as with individuals from other organizations or sectors. I also really enjoy that the work is truly impactful. The impact is often seen in post-program empirical evaluation data, but it is also seen throughout the program execution in the anecdotal stories participants share about how their lives are healthier after participating in an event or program.

What I like least about my work as a health education specialist: The responsibility I like least about my work as a health education specialist is convincing others why a particular program is important. There are so many competing priorities that a big part of health education is convincing funders and policy makers that health education, promotion, and care is valuable and necessary. This is why advocacy is such an important skill to develop.

What recommendations/advice do you have for those preparing to be health education specialists: For those preparing to be health education specialists, I think one of the most important things you can do is talk to people who are doing work you find interesting or inspiring. Ask them about their career paths and then ask them to connect you with others. Whenever you can, attend workshops and conferences. I find that when I attend conferences, I learn many new things, and perhaps more importantly, I leave feeling re-energized and committed to my career path.

If you're interested in global health specifically, networking becomes even more critical to success. Study abroad if you can and try to approach any international experience from a position of humility and genuine curiosity. Recognize that locals will always be the experts in the needs of their own community. Use your knowledge and skills to support good work.

Future considerations for health education specialists/role of health education specialists in the future: I see the availability of roles for health education specialists continuing to grow in the coming years. The COVID-19 pandemic has really highlighted the need for public health professionals who can not only understand and interpret information but who can also communicate that information out to the general public. Health education specialists will be needed to continue to plan and implement programs to address the increasing rates of obesity and other chronic illnesses and to address changing patterns of behavior such as decreasing cigarette use and increasing e-cigarette use. As more people recognize the impact of social determinants on health outcomes, health education specialists will also be uniquely positioned to address systemic barriers to high levels of health through their training in not only planning and implementing health education but also in communicating and advocating for change.

billboards, and many of the people could not read. After consulting with local leaders, it was decided that the best way to spread the information would be through word of mouth using a "mobile communication system." This was accomplished by hooking up an old stereo system to a car battery and driving around the community, broadcasting information about the importance of boiling water. In addition, Sofia set up several demonstrations around the community about how to boil water effectively. These sessions were also advertised via the "mobile communication system."

As can be seen from Sofia's experience, health education specialists working in foreign countries must be able to develop creative, innovative programs to solve identified health problems. Most often, these programs must be low-cost, easily developed and implemented, acceptable to the social and cultural norms of the community, and available to all aspects of the public. It is imperative that these programs be developed in conjunction with the local people being served. It is also helpful when programs are sponsored by organizations seen as credible by the priority population.

One of the best ways to begin a career in international health is to volunteer with the Peace Corps. Health education/promotion professionals are in demand by the Peace Corps, and students should begin the application process early in their senior year. Many colleges and universities are visited by Peace Corps recruiters every year, and talking to one of these Peace Corps volunteers is a good place to start. Faculty members on your campus may have been former Peace Corps volunteers and talking to these individuals can provide valuable insight into the Peace Corps experience. Some colleges and universities have developed Peace Corps Prep Programs, which provide students with a certificate upon completion of a specific set of classes and an approved internship experience. Students completing the Peace Corps Prep Program are not guaranteed entry into the Peace Corps, but they are given strong consideration.

There are many advantages to volunteering with the Peace Corps. The Peace Corps provides volunteers with some of the best language and technical training in the world. Each Peace Corps volunteer is granted a monthly allowance for housing, food, clothing, and miscellaneous expenses. Free dental and medical care are provided, as well as free transportation to the placement setting and 24 vacation days per year. Deferment of federal student loans is also possible while serving in the Peace Corps. After completing the two-year experience, volunteers are given a postservice readjustment allowance of $10,000. They are also given preference for federal jobs and have enhanced scholarship and assistantship opportunities at many major colleges and universities (Peace Corps, n.d.). In addition, a successful Peace Corps experience may serve as a steppingstone to paid positions in other international health organizations (see **Table 7.10**).

The CDC is expanding its presence overseas. This may create future opportunities for health education specialists. The "CDC strives to find well-qualified, talented people to help CDC improve health and save lives around the world. Global public health is a field where you can make a difference!" (CDC, n.d.-a).

Table 7.10 International Health Organizations

National Council for International Health

American Association for World Health

World Health Organization (WHO)

Joint United Nations Program on HIV and AIDS (UNAIDS)

Pan American Health Organization

U.S. Agency for International Development (U.S.A.I.D.)

Foundations such as the Bill and Melinda Gates Foundation

Nongovernmental organizations such as Save the Children

CDC Coordinating Office for Global Health

Nontraditional Health Education/Promotion Positions

In addition to the traditional settings for health education/promotion that have been described in this chapter, there are a variety of nontraditional jobs that health education specialists may wish to consider. These positions may or may not carry the title of health education specialist. In some cases, they require the health education specialist to use the skills and competencies in different or unique ways. Furthermore, it is often necessary for health education specialists to sell themselves to get these positions because the persons doing the hiring may be unfamiliar with the skills and training of a health education specialist.

Given health education specialists' knowledge of health and fitness, sales positions related to health and fitness products are a real possibility. Pharmacy sales, fitness equipment sales, and the sales of health-related textbooks are all areas in which health education specialists have found employment. Life and health insurance are two additional options to consider in the area of sales.

By emphasizing the communication competencies that are part of the professional training in health education/promotion, the health education specialist may seek employment in journalism, TV, or radio. Television stations often have a regular health or medical reporter who does feature stories on health-related issues. Newspapers may have a health column that could and should be written by a health education specialist. Writing articles for health-related websites or actually developing websites for health-related organizations are other possibilities. Again, it is necessary for health education specialists to sell themselves to obtain these positions. Taking elective classes or minors in media, communications, and journalism and doing one's internship in these settings also may assist those interested in this career field.

Health education specialists should always be alert to unique job opportunities, many of which may not even carry the title of health education specialist. One health education specialist, for example, was hired by a state mental hospital as a "Teacher II." His job was to provide drug education to patients who had a history of drug problems and sex education to patients who had a history of sex problems. The remainder of his work schedule involved tutoring patients in math and science who were studying to obtain their high school general equivalency diploma.

Landing That First Job

At first, it may seem unusual to discuss landing one's first job in an introductory text, but it is never too early to consider the issue of future employment. There are several actions students can take during their college years to enhance their chances of obtaining employment. By following the suggestions made in this section, a student will be far ahead of those who wait until the end of their degree program to address these issues.

No matter what the setting in which a health education specialist hopes to eventually work, landing the first job can be a frustrating experience. Students often find themselves in a dilemma. Employers want their new employees to have had "experience," but where are students supposed to get experience if they can't get hired? There are several possible answers to this question. One way to gain experience is to obtain part-time or summer employment in one's preferred health education/promotion setting. Typically, there are many more students looking for this type of employment than there are employment situations. Should such an opportunity be available, however, it is an excellent way to gain experience before graduation. Another way to obtain experience is to volunteer time in the chosen health education/promotion setting. Most professional health education specialists working in the field are more than willing to accept and use the volunteer time of health education/promotion students. In addition to experience, volunteering also begins the important process of **networking**. Networking involves establishing and maintaining a wide range of contacts in the field that may be of help when looking for a job and in carrying out one's job responsibilities once hired.

Many health education/promotion programs now offer **service learning** opportunities to their students (Cleary et al., 1998). The "Learn by doing" approach to training is common in public health and provides benefits for both the students and the community organizations being served (Wigington et al., 2017). Organized service learning opportunities provide course credit for students to work with a community agency to meet an identified community need. For example, university students helped elderly residents of a low socioeconomic area of the city to develop community vegetable gardens. Not only did they help with cultivation, planting, and harvesting, but they also provided education messages about healthy diet.

This service learning experience provided hands-on, practical, real-world experience that students could not obtain from the classroom. Service learning can also be beneficial in broadening one's professional network, which is so important in the health education/promotion field. Take advantage of as many service learning opportunities as possible. The experience and networking gained through service learning can give new health education/promotion professionals a tremendous advantage in the job market.

Carefully planning internships and practicums can help students obtain their first professional position (see Practitioner's Perspective). Required field experiences are

Practitioner's Perspective

Monica Sarp

DEGREE HELD/INSTITUTION ATTENDED/GRADUATION YEAR: BS Health Sciences, The Ohio State University, May 2019

MINOR: Business

Certified Health Education Specialist (CHES), 2019

MPH Health Behavior and Health Promotion, The Ohio State University. Anticipated graduation May 2022

Internship Organization: The Society for Public Health Education (SOPHE)

Internship Placement: I found the SOPHE internship online when I was researching career opportunities in public health. I decided to apply to SOPHE because I was impressed by the broad scope of their internship program and I wanted to gain experience in different disciplines of public health. I was also very interested in the opportunity to work in the nation's capital and learn more about health policy.

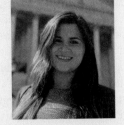

Courtesy of Monica Sarp.

Although I learned about the internship while I was still an undergraduate student, I decided to wait until I finished my degree to pursue this opportunity. Shortly after graduating from OSU in May of 2019 and passing my Certified Health Education Specialist exam, I applied to the SOPHE Internship for the fall semester. The application consisted of a cover letter, resume, sample of work, and Internship Application Form. I gave myself plenty of time to complete these items and I made sure to include my experience in public health and health care, including previous employment, internships, volunteer positions, and relevant coursework. I submitted my application in May and had a phone interview in June. I was offered the position in early July, and my internship began in September.

Internship Description: As a SOPHE Intern, I was able to participate in a wide variety of opportunities. The SOPHE Internship program is designed to reflect the CHES competencies as outlined by NCHEC and SOPHE. SOPHE has multiple focus areas, and interns are encouraged to gain experience in each area. I found this approach very helpful, as I was able to identify aspects of each field that I enjoyed and did not enjoy. This helped me narrow my focus within the field of public health and health education.

Although the responsibilities of a SOPHE intern can vary based on the organization's current projects, as well as your personal strengths and interests, overarching responsibilities include assisting with planning for the SOPHE Advocacy Summit and SOPHE National Conference, helping team members with ongoing projects, attending briefings about important health policies, organizing a health education webinar, and facilitating a staff presentation about a discipline in which you are experienced. The highlight of my SOPHE experience was participating in policy and advocacy-related events, such as the SOPHE Advocacy Summit. The Advocacy Summit is an annual event where SOPHE members convene in Washington, D.C., to advocate for legislation addressing public health issues. Members gather to learn about a designated public health issue, discuss how to be an effective advocate, and meet with legislators to advocate for proposed solutions.

I was lucky to be mentored by two individuals while at SOPHE. The Director of Communications took me under her wing, shared her wisdom and experience in communications, and allowed me to practice and hone my skills in health communication. We worked together to craft infographics, flyers, emails, and social media posts to appeal to SOPHE's target audience. The skills I gained in health communication have been very helpful in my graduate education, and will be applicable in any setting as a Health Education Specialist. Another important mentorship was the guidance from the Internship Program Director and Manager of Professional Development. She organized the internship, including the application process, and served as an important resource throughout the entire program. She made sure to check in with interns frequently to see how we were doing and if we needed any assistance. I appreciate the guidance from these talented individuals, both during the internship period and throughout the following year.

Internship Pros: Something I really enjoyed about the internship was the supportive environment. The SOPHE staff members made sure to include interns at every opportunity, whether it was attending a briefing on the Hill or sitting in on a conference call. I appreciated that staff members treated interns as equals, gave us key responsibilities, and allowed us to control our own schedule and priorities. This was very helpful to my professional development and self-efficacy as a recent graduate.

Internship Cons: One difficult aspect of the internship, as with any internship in Washington, D.C., was affording the high cost of living. Interns receive a small stipend, so it was very important to create a budget for my time in D.C. Although it was challenging at times, I believe the experience was worth it and has paid off tremendously in the long run.

Importance of the Internship Experience: The SOPHE internship was very important to my professional development as a health education specialist. I was able to apply health education concepts in a variety of settings, as well as gain experience applying the Certified Health Education Specialist competencies. During the internship, I was able to participate in multiple webinars and trainings that counted toward my CHES continuing education (CE) requirements. One experience that was particularly helpful in this respect was the opportunity to organize and host a SOPHE Webinar for CHES CE credit. The webinar I planned and hosted discussed strategies to implement and evaluate workplace wellness programs. When creating this webinar, I tailored the content

(continues)

Practitioner's Perspective *(continued)*

Monica Sarp

to meet identified areas of responsibility and competencies as outlined by NCHEC and SOPHE. This was helpful to me as a new Certified Health Education Specialist because it allowed me to understand and appreciate the process of creating CE opportunities.

Interning at SOPHE was an important step in my career path. The internship allowed me to explore different disciplines and settings in which Health Education Specialists can work. This was important to me because it helped me narrow my area of interest before beginning graduate school. The most interesting aspect I was able to observe was policymaking. I enjoyed attending policy briefings and witnessing the incredible effort and interdisciplinary collaboration required to create and enact health policy.

This experience has also been a strong asset for my academic career. Completing the internship shortly after graduation was a great opportunity to synthesize what I learned during my undergraduate career and during my training as a Certified Health Education Specialist. Not only did the internship strengthen my graduate school application but I was able to gain valuable experience that I can draw from during my graduate program.

Recommendations for those preparing to be health education specialists: If you are considering a career as a health education specialist, I strongly recommend making connections with your professors. Participating in class and attending office hours will help you build positive relationships. In addition to learning more about the course material, you can learn about your professor's career path, ask them for advice about your own career, and ask them if they have any contacts working in your desired field. I also strongly recommend finding a mentor. This person could be one of your professors, a supervisor, or simply someone whose career you admire. My mentor was one of my undergraduate professors—not only did she inspire me to become a Certified Health Education Specialist, she also gave me valuable advice for applying to the SOPHE internship and for applying to graduate school.

Another piece of advice I have is to get involved during your undergraduate program. One of my favorite experiences during college was volunteering at The Ohio State University Student Wellness Center as a Wellness Coach and Wellness Ambassador. Both of these roles were invaluable to me as I began my career in health education. Not only was I able to build my health education skills under the direction of a skilled supervisor but I also got to make an impact on my fellow Buckeyes.

When searching for an internship or job opportunity, I encourage you to keep an open mind and pursue opportunities that may be different from your previous experience. I recommend getting involved in a variety of experiences within your field—even if you think you know exactly what you want your future position to be, it is useful to gain experience in all disciplines of public health. Health education specialists can work in multiple settings, and it is important to understand and appreciate the function of each discipline.

Lastly, I recommend that you keep the "big picture" in mind. Treat every experience as an opportunity to grow—whether it is through classroom learning, building skills, or networking.

often the best way to obtain practical experience in one's chosen setting. Students should consider what they would like to be doing five years after graduation and select an experience that closely matches that goal. Frequently, students are hired by the agency after completing their practicum or internship experience.

In addition to obtaining experience, students should strive to obtain an excellent academic record. When there is heavy competition for an open position, one of the first strategies in making hiring decisions is to examine grade point average. This is not to say that the person with the highest grade point average is always the best person or will always get the job. But, when there are 50 applications for one job, grade point average is an easy way to begin limiting the field.

Develop a well-organized, professional-looking portfolio. A **portfolio** is a collection of evidence that enables students to demonstrate mastery of desired course or program outcomes/competencies. In health education/promotion, the responsibilities, competencies, and subcompetencies should be emphasized. Many health education/promotion programs now require portfolios as part of their professional preparation programs. With today's advancements in technology, electronic portfolios, or e-portfolios, is the preferred format for portfolio development (Crowell & Calamidas, 2016). Even if the portfolio is not required, students should develop a portfolio on their own. Thompson and Bybee (2004) note that a portfolio is a "living document that is ever-changing with the increasing depth of knowledge and experience of the individual" (p. 52). They go on to identify five basic elements that should be included in any portfolio: (1) table of contents, (2) résumé, (3) education and credentials, (4) samples of work, and (5) references. The samples of work could include such exhibits as student papers or course projects, audio or video of students giving a presentation, analyses of student work by professors or outside reviewers, student goal statements, reflections, and summaries (Cleary & Birch, 1996, 1997). Another way to design the portfolio is to structure it around the NCHEC health education specialist competencies. Essentially, exhibits are included in the portfolio for each competency. Imagine the impact on a prospective employer when a new health education specialist provides a well-developed, attractive e-portfolio that clearly demonstrates health education responsibilities and competencies.

Your résumé is extremely important in obtaining your first job. The résumé is your advertisement for yourself. It is the first item of yours that most prospective employers will see. It will create a first and lasting impression of you. What you include in the résumé and how you present the information may make a difference in whether or not you are hired. You should start now to involve yourself in experiences that will look good on your résumé. As you develop your résumé, make sure that there are no spelling or grammatical errors. One former student actually lost a job opportunity because of three spelling errors on her résumé.

It is important to be specific and detailed without being too long winded when developing the resume. On the resume, people often state generalities about themselves such as being a team player, results oriented, having a strong work ethic or excellent communication skills. Going one step further to explain what you mean by these general characteristics and providing an example will help make your resume stand out. For example if you are trying to sell yourself as being "results oriented," describe a problem you solved that created the desired results. If you say you are a "team player," give examples of team projects you worked on that were successful. If you describe yourself as having a "strong work ethic," explain what having a strong work ethic means to you and how your work ethic has helped you to be successful in previous endeavors. When employers are reading numerous job applicant resumes, it is little things like these that help separate your resume from others.

Beyond the portfolio and résumé, consider what certifications are going to be important in landing your first job and carefully plan to make sure they are awarded either before graduation or as soon after graduation as possible. All professional health education specialists should pursue the CHES and MCHES credentials. In the future, this may be a prerequisite for many health promotion and education positions. Other certifications should be obtained depending on work setting and need.

Get to know your faculty. They are a great source of information about jobs and how to compete for them successfully. Often, employers contact faculty directly, asking for the names of students who might be interested in a particular position. But unless a faculty member knows a student by name and knows that the student is in the job market, there is little the faculty member can do.

Most colleges and universities have placement centers that provide a variety of services to students, including help in developing an effective resume. They may also assist by maintaining a list of job openings, providing workshops or handouts on interviewing skills, and establishing reference files for students. The placement center at the University of North Carolina Wilmington provides in-depth trainings for students on how to use LinkedIn to help land a job. It would be a good idea to contact the placement center at your university well before graduation to determine when and how to access its services.

A final suggestion is to join one or more of the health education professional associations (see Chapter 8). Employers are typically impressed when they see that a young professional has chosen to become a member of a professional association and perhaps has attended one or more professional meetings. "Professional meetings and conferences are filled with opportunities. . . . Where else can you find hundreds, even thousands, of education professionals from all over the world coming together to share cutting-edge knowledge through presentations, sessions, workshops, socials, and other events, than at professional meetings and conferences?" (Dixon-Terry, 2004, p. 16). If your campus

has a student health association or a chapter of Eta Sigma Gamma, the professional health education/promotion honorary, try to get involved. Eta Sigma Gamma recognizes high academic achievement, provides opportunities to obtain valuable leadership experience, and allows students to plan, implement, and evaluate various service projects and social activities. Eta Sigma Gamma recognition awards are presented at the SOPHE National Conference each year.

In addition to the aforementioned suggestions, one caution is in order. Be careful what you place on social networking websites such as Facebook and Twitter. Prospective employers are savvy and often will look online to see what additional information they can find about you. "Susan Masterson, a recruiter with TeamHealth in Knoxville, TN, said, using social networking sites is a strategy that anyone in recruiting, whether it be physicians or otherwise, needs to incorporate in their plan. It's here. It's here to stay" (Dolan, 2009). Health education/promotion internship site supervisors have even looked online before accepting a student for internship. One author of this text actually received a letter from a prospective employer indicating that they had not hired the author's student because of offensive content they found online. Furthermore, they admonished the program to caution students about what they include online. Students posting questionable information online seems to be a somewhat common practice. According to an *AMNews* article, in one study, 60% of U.S. medical schools surveyed reported incidents of students posting unprofessional content online (Dolan, 2009). What is questionable content is difficult to define. Certainly pictures involving sex, alcohol, or drugs are not appropriate, but anything that causes doubt should be removed. Students should restrict who can be friends and can access their information as much as possible. It is also a good idea for students to do an online search of themselves to see what information they can find and eliminate anything that may be offensive.

Students who follow the aforementioned suggestions will be better positioned to obtain initial employment in the health promotion and education profession. This is a good time to be a health education specialist, and the future looks even brighter than the present.

Excelling in Your Health Education/ Promotion Career

Landing a job is merely the first step in becoming a successful health education specialist. Once you have the job, it is critical that you excel in the job. This is important for two reasons. First, you must excel to demonstrate that you are an important and contributing member of the organization that hired you and to enhance your career potential. Second, you need to excel to help further the health education/promotion profession. Your work reflects on all health education specialists and may determine whether your organization or other organizations will hire more health education specialists in the future.

What does it take to excel in health education/promotion? Obviously, one must demonstrate the ability to meet the competencies and subcompetencies of a health education specialist, but one must also meet the standards of a good employee. Numerous authors writing about careers in health education/promotion have elaborated on what is needed to excel as an employee in a health education/promotion position. In talking about how to excel in a voluntary health agency position, one author wrote, "Completing your tasks and projects on time, under budget, and with minimum problems is your

most obvious goal, but do not underestimate the value of attitude, spirit, and the ability to work under pressure and with difficult people. A positive, can-do attitude, a willingness to learn new and different skills on the job, and the ability to work in an environment that values teamwork is a 'must'" (Daitz, 2007, pp. 5–6). Other authors writing about working in health and medical care note, "Being successful means meeting and exceeding the expectations of the job and showing initiative in achieving organizational goals" (Totzkay-Sitar & Cornett, 2007, pp. 9–10). In discussing federal health education/promotion positions, Howze (2007) said, "With any job, success requires continually showing how you add value to the organization. For example, many federal agencies are struggling to find workers with language skills, so consider becoming fluent in a second language" (p. 13). And finally, if you are trying to excel in a public health department position. "Become known as a high achiever/performer and a good team player. Make a positive and lasting impression on your supervisor as well as upper level managers with whom you may have contact through your assignments. Anticipate what needs to be done" (Hall, 2007, p. 17). The following Practitioner's Perspective box discusses what one employer of health education specialists looks for in the interview and hiring process.

The aforementioned quotes clearly indicate that, regardless of the setting, you must go beyond simply meeting the minimum expectations of the job to be a good employee and a good health education specialist. To excel, you must go the extra mile and do the unexpected as well as the expected. You need to be a good "people person," demonstrate a positive attitude, and be willing to learn and take on new tasks. These are the things that will separate you from other employees and establish you as a truly outstanding health education specialist.

Practitioner's Perspective

Theresa Blanco, MCHES

CURRENT POSITION: Chief Planning and Development Officer

EMPLOYER: Shasta Community Health Center

DEGREE/INSTITUTION: California State University, Chico, BS; Simpson University, MA

MAJOR: Health Education/Education

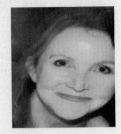

Courtesy of Theresa Blanco.

My employment history: I began my health education career at Tehama County Health Services Agency, Public Health (PH). I was hired as a Program Coordinator for the HIV/AIDS Prevention Program. I knew it would be a challenging program to manage in a conservative rural community. However, I hit the ground running, and within 18 months, I had presented in every school, juvenile hall, jail, and drug & alcohol group in the county. I collaborated with a small but innovative HIV/AIDS Awareness Coalition, and we managed to launch a needle exchange program and bring two World AIDS Day quilts to our little community.

Through this work and my collaborations, I learned how to engage an audience, tailor classes to the specific needs of a diverse group and teach in various ways that create awareness and respect around difficult topics. My assignments grew, as well as the variety of health education I delivered. I effectively managed five to seven programs simultaneously. Many classes were done in English or Spanish and included outreach to migrant worker camps.

I stayed with PH for 10 years, and during that time, I worked with many professional health educators, which provided me with a tremendous amount of growth and experience. This is the reason I hire qualified Health Education Specialists today. I know what they can do.

In 2011, I left PH to work as a Patient Educator at Shasta Community Health Center. I learned that the challenges in a clinic are very different; however, I was promoted to Manager of Patient Education & Health Promotion Services within a year. The following year, I had an official department with six outreach & education staff. Our goal was to serve as many of our 37,000 patients as possible. We hosted a variety of services, classes, and one-on-one coaching sessions. We even implemented a successful employee wellness program.

To keep our skills fresh, we met regularly to apply health education models and theories to our practice. My team had a high level of health literacy knowledge and trained our clinic staff. This improved the quality of our patient communications as well as the educational materials we distributed.

My current job responsibilities: In 2019, I took the position of Chief Planning and Development Officer. I am responsible for writing and managing over 11 million in grant dollars for our organization. I also oversee our scope of services to ensure they are included in our federal medical malpractice insurance. In addition, I work with key personnel to create and manage our organization's strategic plan.

How I develop a job description: I begin with the organization's standard template. I then create a list of essential job functions, required certifications, education, and experience. I correlate this with the Eight Areas of Responsibility of a Health Education Specialist. A final review is completed by HR and senior management before it is posted.

What I look for in reviewing applications: I review educational background, certifications (CHES/MCHES), and experience (*in school or in the field*). I track and compare each candidates' qualifications. This allows me to narrow down candidates who will be selected for preinterview testing.

What I look for in an interview: I observe communication styles, examples of past projects, adaptability, stamina, innovation, and a willingness to learn. A rubric is used to score target areas. Those who reference health education models, theories, or practice stand out.

Recommendations for health education specialist looking for employment: Degreed health education specialists are master planners, organizers, and problem-solvers. This is a unique, rewarding career that is not easily understood by other professionals. Take time, be proud, and share your qualifications through various means. Don't be afraid to branch out in related fields that interest you. Health education specialists can be great quality improvement staff. Study and practice potential interview questions and connect with others in the field. When you are interviewed, make sure you are familiar with the organization's mission and values. Bring it up—*it will impress, and* always send a thank you note. The field is growing; be a part of the evolution.

Summary

There are many settings in which a health education specialist can seek employment. In this chapter, we have discussed in detail health education/promotion positions in schools, public/community health agencies, worksites, healthcare facilities, colleges and universities, and international settings. In addition, we have examined the potential for employment in nontraditional settings and have considered what introductory-level, undergraduate students can do to help themselves obtain their first job. Finally, we discussed what it takes to be successful in a health education/promotion position.

Review Questions

1. Identify four major settings and two nontraditional settings in which health education specialists are employed.
2. Compare and contrast the roles and responsibilities of health education specialists working in schools, public and community health agencies, worksites, and healthcare facilities. How are all of these settings similar? How are they different?
3. What is the difference between a position funded with hard money and a position funded with soft money? Which position is preferable and why?
4. Explain why it might be said that health education/promotion has never reached its real potential in the healthcare setting. What factors have kept health education/promotion positions at a minimal level in this setting?
5. What is networking and why is it important in health education/promotion?
6. What can introductory-level health education/promotion students do now that might help them land their first job after graduation?
7. Summarize the impact COVID-19 has had on the health education specialists working in one of the major employment settings.

Case Study

Marla (she/her/hers) has a BS degree in health education/promotion and is CHES certified. For the past five years, since graduating from college, she has been working as a health education specialist for a private vendor who then contracts with companies to offer health education/promotion and fitness services to their employees. During this time, the vendor has placed her at three different corporations. All three corporations have been extremely satisfied with her services and the vendor/employer has also given her positive evaluations.

Marla has started to question her long-term potential with this company. She feels that her $30,000 annual salary is too low, and she gets no retirement, dental, vision, or pharmacy benefits. With her current employer, there is no opportunity for promotion, and raises are small and infrequent. She has two specific goals for the future. One, she wants to continue working in health education/promotion, but she is open to working in any setting. Two, she wants to earn a higher salary and have better benefits. If you were advising Marla, identify options you could suggest. What things could she do to make herself more marketable? What additional education or professional development does she need? What does she need to do in terms of networking? What types of positions and settings should she be considering? Outline a plan for Marla in the next 12 to 24 months that will help her to realize the two goals she has established.

Critical Thinking Questions

1. Select any health education/promotion setting and give specific examples of how a health education specialist working in that setting would need to use all eight responsibilities of a health education specialist (i.e., when thinking about assessment at the worksite setting, a health education specialist might have to assess the health needs of employees, assess the current health behaviors of employees, assess how responsive employees would be to a given health promotion program, assess upper management support for a given program, etc.).

2. If you were in a position to hire a new health education specialist, what qualities, traits, and experiences would you look for in making your hiring decision? Compare this with the qualities, traits, and experiences you currently possess. Make a list of things you could do to enhance your marketability prior to graduation.

3. How has COVID-19 impacted the health education profession? What evidence do you have to support your contentions?

4. What responsibilities, competencies, and subcompetencies of a health education specialist would be especially helpful when confronted with a crisis such as the COVID-19 pandemic?

Activities

1. Select the one setting you think you would most like to work in. Develop a short essay describing why you prefer this setting to other health education/promotion settings and what you think you will need to do to land a job in that setting.

2. Visit a health education/promotion professional who works in the setting in which you would most like to be employed. Develop a job description for this person's position that explains the qualifications and responsibilities needed for the job.

3. Examine the online classified ads of a major-city Sunday newspaper as well as any online employment sites you can find. Identify jobs that specifically ask for a health education specialist. Next, look through the same classified ads/job listings and identify jobs that do not specify a health education specialist but

require competencies and skills similar to those of a health education specialist. Compare your results with others in the class.

4. Interview someone who is responsible for hiring health education specialists. Find out what that person looks for in a letter of application, a resume, and a personal interview.

5. Contact the placement office at your institution. Determine what services it offers and when these services should be accessed.

Weblinks

1. **http://www.bls.gov**

   U.S. Bureau of Labor Statistics

   Go to this website and run a search for "health education specialists." Review the various documents you find to determine workforce size, average salaries, states with most health education specialists employed, states with highest average salaries, metropolitan areas with highest average salaries, and other important information about health education specialists.

2. **http://www.peacecorps.gov**

   Peace Corps

   This website provides information about the Peace Corps, what volunteers do, where the Peace Corps is active, benefits of Peace Corps service, how to become a Peace Corps volunteer, and much more.

3. **http://www.welcoa.org**

   Wellness Council of America

   The Free Resources section of this site indexes a number of free worksite health promotion resources, including COVID-19 resources, which can be easily downloaded in PDF format.

4. **https://www.cdc.gov/workplacehealth promotion/index.html**

   Centers for Disease Control and Prevention's Workplace Health Promotion

   This page provides access to a number of resources to help one plan, implement, and evaluate worksite wellness programs. There is also a worksite health scorecard to help employers assess their worksite program.

5. **http://www.cjhp.org**

   Californian Journal of Health Promotion

   Use the Past Issues section to access Volume 5, Issue 2, of the *Californian Journal of Health Promotion* and specifically an article written by Byrd, Hoke, and Gottlieb titled "Integrating Health Education into Clinical Settings." This is an excellent article that describes a successful use of health education specialists in a clinical setting.

6. **http://www.cjhp.org**

   Californian Journal of Health Promotion

   Use the Past Issues section to access Volume 2, Issue 1, of the *Californian Journal of Health Promotion* and specifically an article by Eleanor Dixon Terry titled "Attending Professional Health Education Meetings: What's In It for the Student and New Professional." This is an excellent article with good advice for students or new professionals attending their first professional health education/promotion meeting.

7. **http://www.acha.org**

   American College Health Association

   Click on "Resources" and under this section, click on the "Publications" section of the website, go to the

"Guidelines, Recommendations, and White Papers" area. There, you can download a document titled "Guidelines for Hiring Health Promotion Professionals in Higher Education." Compare yourself to the guidelines and recommendations presented in this document. While this document was designed specifically for health education specialists working in college or university wellness programs, many of these guidelines and recommendations would be appropriate for employers in other settings.

8. **https://www.nchec.org/guide-to-health -education-careers**

   National Commission for Health Education Credentialing

   This page is a guide to health education careers. It describes the health education specialist and provides a comprehensive list of the jobs that health education specialists may hold. Furthermore, it provides information on how to become a health education specialist.

9. **https://www.sophe.org/wp-content /uploads/2018/01/SOPHE -Qualifications-of-Health-Educators _adopted9aug2017.pdf**

   Society for Public Health Education

   This Resolution, adopted by the Society for Public Health Education, clearly articulates the practice of health education and the qualifications of a health education specialist. It provides strong justification for hiring health education specialists and should be provided to any prospective employer seeking to hire a health educator.

References

Allensworth, D. D., & Kolbe, L. J. (1987). The comprehensive school health program: Exploring an expanded concept. *Journal of School Health, 57*(10), 409–412. https://doi.org/10.1111/j.1746-1561.1987 .tb03183.x

American College of Sports Medicine. (2003). *ACSM's worksite health promotion manual.* Human Kinetics.

American School Health Association. (2020). *What is school health?* Retrieved December 22, 2020, from http://www.ashaweb.org/about/what-is-school-health

Breckon, J., Harvey, J. R., & Lancaster, R. B. (1998). *Community health education: Settings, roles, and skills for the 21st century.* Aspen Publishers.

Birch, D. A., Goekler, S., Auld, M. E., Lohrmann, D. K., & Lyde, A. (2019). Quality assurance in teaching K-12 health education: Paving a new path forward. *Health Promotion Practice, 20*(6), 845–857. https://doi .org/10.1177/1524839919868167

Byrd, T. L., Hoke, M. M., & Gottlieb, N. H. (2007). Integrating health education into clinical settings. *Californian Journal of Health Promotion, 5*(2), 18–28.

Centers for Disease Control and Prevention. (n.d.-a). *Global health jobs and opportunities.* Retrieved January 5, 2021, from http://www.cdc.gov/global health/employment/

Centers for Disease Control and Prevention. (n.d.-b). *Workplace health model.* Retrieved December 30, 2020, from https://www.cdc.gov/workplacehealth promotion/model/

Centers for Medicare & Medicaid Services. (2020). *National health expenditure data: Historical.* https:// www.cms.gov/research-statistics-data-and-systems /statistics-trends-and-reports/nationalhealthexpend data/nationalhealthaccountshistorical.html

Chenoweth, D. H. (2011). *Worksite health promotion* (3rd ed.). Human Kinetics.

Cleary, M. J., & Birch, D. A. (1996). Using portfolios for assessment in the college personal health course. *Journal of Health Education, 27*(2), 92–96.

Cleary, M. J., & Birch, D. A. (1997). How prospective school health education specialists can build a portfolio to communicate professional expertise. *Journal of School Health, 67*(6), 228–231.

Cleary, M. J., Kaiser-Drobney, A. E., Ubbes, V. E., Stuhldreher, W. L., & Birch, D. A. (1998). Service learning in the "third sector": Implications for professional preparation. *Journal of Health Education, 29*(5), 304–311.

Crowell, T., & Calamidas, E. (2016). Assessing public health majors through the use of e-portfolios. *Journal of the Scholarship of Teaching and Learning, 16*(4), 62–74. https://doi.org/10.14434/josotl.v16i4.19370

Daitz, S. J. (2007). Health education careers at nonprofit voluntary health agencies. *Health Education Monograph, 24*(1), 4–6.

Dixon-Terry, E. (2004). Attending professional health education meetings: What's in it for the student and new professional? *Californian Journal of Health Promotion, 2*(1), 16–21.

Dolan, P. L. (2009). Social media behavior could threaten your reputation, job prospects. *American Medical News.* https://amednews.com/article/20091012/business/310129997/2

Dombrowski, R .D. & Mallare, J. (2020). Environmental scan of health education teacher preparation programs 2020. Report prepared for the Society for Public Health Education. https://www.sophe.org/professional-preparation/teacher-preparation/

Edward Lowe Foundation. (n.d.). Working well together: Promoting health in the workplace. Retrieved December 31, 2020, from, https://edwardlowe.org/working-well-together-promoting-health-in-the-workplace-2/

Fronstin, P., & Roebuck, M. C. (2015a). Financial incentives and workplace wellness program participation. *Employee Benefit Research Institute, Issue Brief #412.*

Fronstin, P., & Roebuck, M. C. (2015b). Financial incentives, workplace wellness program participation, and utilization of health care services and spending. *Employee Benefit Research Institute, Issue Brief #417.*

Goetzel, R. Z., & Pronk, N. P. (2010). Worksite Health Promotion: How much do we really know about what works. *American Journal of Preventive Medicine, 38*(2S), S223–S225.

Hall, J. Y. (2007). Entering and navigating a health education career in the local public sector. *The Health Education Monograph, 24*(1), 15–17.

Howze, E. H. (2007). Health education jobs in the federal government. *The Health Education Monograph, 24*(1), 11–14.

International Network of Health Promoting Hospitals & Health Services. (2016). Development. Retrieved April 16, 2016, from http://www.hphnet.org/index.php?option=com_content&view=article&id=22&Itemid=4

Jalloh, M. G. (2007). Health education careers in schools. *The Health Education Monograph, 24*(1), 18–22.

Joint Committee on National Health Education Standards (JCNHES). (2007). *National Health Education Standards: Achieving Excellence* (2nd ed.). American Cancer Society.

Lewallen, T. C., Hunt, H., Potts-Datema, W., Zaza, S., & Giles, W. (2015). The Whole School, Whole Commuity, Whole Child Model: A new approach for improving educational attainment and healthy development for students. *Journal of School Health, 85*(11), 729–739.

Lysoby, L. (2021). Embracing challenge while moving forward. *National Commission for Health Education Credentialing Bulletin, Winter 2021,* 2. https://assets.speakcdn.com/assets/2251/final_bulletinwinter_jan2021.pdf

McKenzie, J. F., Neiger, B. L., & Thackeray, R. (2017). *Planning, implementing, & evaluating health promotion programs* (7th ed.). Pearson Education.

McKenzie, J. F., Pinger, R. R., and Seabert (2018). *An introduction to community and public health* (9th ed.). Jones & Bartlett Learning.

Michael, S. L., Merlo, C. L., Basch, C. E., Wentzel, K. R., & Wechsler, H. (2015). Critical connections: Health and academics. *Journal of School Health, 85*(11), 740–758.

Miller, B., Birch, D., & Cottrell, R. R. (2010). Current status and future plans for undergraduate public/community health education program accreditation. *American Journal of Health Education, 41*(5), 301–307.

National Center for Educational Statistics. (n.d.). *Back to school statistics.* Retrieved December 22, 2020, from https://nces.ed.gov/fastfacts/display.asp?id=372#PK12_enrollment

National Commission for Health Education Credentialing (n.d.-a). *Guide to health education careers.* Retrieved January 15, 2021 from, https://www.nchec.org/guide-to-health-education-careers

National Commission for Health Education Credentialing (n.d.-b). *Health education job analysis projects—Role Delineation Project.* Retrieved December 22, 2020, from https://www.nchec.org/HESPA

National Commission for Health Education Credentialing & Society for Public Health Education. (2020). *A competency-based framework for health education specialists—2020.* Author.

Peabody, K. L., & Linnan, L. A. (2007). Careers in worksite health promotion. *The Health Education Monograph, 24*(1), 29–32.

Peace Corps. (n.d.). Peace Corps: *Financial Benefits?* Retrieved January 5, 2021, from http://www.peacecorps.gov/volunteer/learn/whyvol/

Preparing Future Faculty. (n.d.). *Faculty roles and responsibilities.* Retrieved January 5, 2021, from http://www.preparing-faculty.org/PFFWeb.Roles.htm

Rubleski, J. (2007). Embracing workplace wellness. *Absolute Advantage, 6*(5), 30–33.

Society for Public Health Education. (n.d.). *Health education specialist.* Retrieved December 22, 2020, from: https://www.sophe.org/careerhub/health-education-profession/

Society for Public Health Education. (2020). *Environmental scan of health education teacher preparation programs.* https://www.sophe.org/resources/he-environmental-scan-report/

Thompson, S. E., & Bybee, R. F. (2004). Professional portfolios for health education specialists and other allied health professionals. *Californian Journal of Health Promotion, 2*(1), 52–55.

Totzkay-Sitar, C., & Cornett, S. (2007). Health education options in health and medical care. *The Health Education Monograph, 24*(1), 7–10.

U.S. Department of Health and Human Services. (n.d.). *Healthy People 2030 Framework.* Retrieved

December 28, 2020, from https://health.gov/healthy people/about/healthy-people-2030-framework

U.S. Department of Labor Bureau of Labor Statistics. (2020a). *Occupational Employment and Wages, May 2019*. Retrieved December 22, 2020, from https://www.bls.gov/oes/current/oes211091.htm#ind

U.S. Department of Labor Bureau of Labor Statistics. (2020b). *Occupational Outlook Handbook*. Retrieved December 22, 2020, from https://www.bls.gov/ooh /community-and-social-service/health-educators.htm

Wellness Council of America. (2020). *Employee Wellbeing Works When Done the Right Way*. Retrieved December 31, 2020, from, https://www.welcoa.org/blog/employee -wellbeing-works-when-done-the-right-way/

Wigington, C. J., Sobelson, R. K., Duncan, H. L., & Young, A. C. (2017). Service learning in public health: Exploring the benefit to host agencies in CDC's Public Health Associate Program. *Journal of Public Health Management Practice, 23*(5), 434–438. doi: 10.1097 /PHH.0000000000000523

Agencies, Associations, and Organizations Associated with Health Education/Promotion

CHAPTER OBJECTIVES

After reading this chapter and answering the questions at the end, you should be able to:

- Define each of the following terms and give several examples of each: *governmental health agency*, *quasi-governmental health agency*, and *nongovernmental health agency*.
- Briefly describe the levels of governmental agencies and provide several examples of each.
- List and explain the four primary activities of most voluntary health agencies.
- Explain the purpose of a professional association/organization.
- Identify the benefits derived from membership in a professional organization.
- Identify the primary professional associations/organizations and coalitions associated with health education/promotion.
- Describe the process by which a person can become a member of a professional association/organization.
- Describe what the National Commission for Health Education Credentialing, Inc. is and its mission and purpose.

There are many health agencies, associations, and organizations with which health education specialists interact. Most of these agencies/associations/organizations were created to help promote, protect, and maintain the health of individuals, families, and communities. For many health education specialists, these agencies/associations/organizations will be places of employment. These groups regularly hire health education specialists to plan, implement, evaluate, and coordinate their educational efforts. Health education specialists not employed by these groups will find them to be valuable sources of up-to-date information and materials. This chapter classifies the agencies/associations/organizations into three major categories: governmental, quasi-governmental, and nongovernmental.

Because information on most of these agencies/associations/organizations that support the efforts of health education/promotion is accessible throughout the Internet and because this text was written primarily as an introduction to the profession, the primary emphasis of this chapter is on the professional health education associations/organizations.

Governmental Health Agencies

Governmental health agencies are health agencies that have authority for certain duties or tasks outlined by the governmental bodies that oversee them. For example, a **local health department (LHD)** has the authority to protect, promote, and enhance the health of people living in a specific geographic area. Authority is given by the county, city, or township government that oversees the local health department. Governmental agencies, which are primarily funded by tax dollars (they may also charge fees for services rendered) and managed by government employees, exist at four governmental levels: international, national, state, and local (city and county). **Table 8.1** provides examples of governmental agencies and their governing bodies.

Table 8.1 Governmental Agencies and Their Governing Bodies

Level/Agency	Governing Body
International Level	
World Health Organization (WHO)	United Nations (UN)
Pan American Health Organization (PAHO)	An independent agency
National Level	
Centers for Disease Control and Prevention (CDC)	U.S. government, Department of Health and Human Services (HHS)
Food and Drug Administration (FDA)	U.S. government, Department of Health and Human Services (HHS)
State Level	
State health department	Individual state governments
State environmental protection agency	Individual state governments
Local Level	
Local health department (LHD)	City, county, or township governments
Local school district	Local school boards

Quasi-Governmental Health Agencies

Quasi-governmental health agencies (see **Figure 8.1**) are so named because they possess characteristics of both governmental health agencies and nongovernmental agencies. They obtain their funding from a variety of sources, including community fundraising efforts such as the United Way, special allocations from government bodies, fees for services rendered, and donations. They carry out tasks that are often thought of as services of governmental agencies, yet they operate independently of governmental supervision.

Probably the best known quasi-governmental health agency is the **American Red Cross (ARC)**. Clara Barton founded it in 1881 as an outgrowth of her work during the Civil War. Today, the ARC has several "official" responsibilities given to it by the federal government, such as providing relief to victims of natural disasters (Disaster Services) and serving as the liaison between members of the active armed forces and their families during family emergencies (Services to the Armed Forces and Veterans). The ARC also provides many nongovernmental services such as its blood drives and safety services classes such as water safety, first aid, and CPR.

Nongovernmental Health Agencies

Nongovernmental health agencies operate, for the most part, free from governmental interference as long as they comply with the Internal Revenue Service's guidelines for their tax status. They are primarily funded by private donations, or, as is the case with professional and service groups, membership fees. The nongovernmental agencies can be categorized into the following subgroups: voluntary, philanthropic, service, religious, and professional.

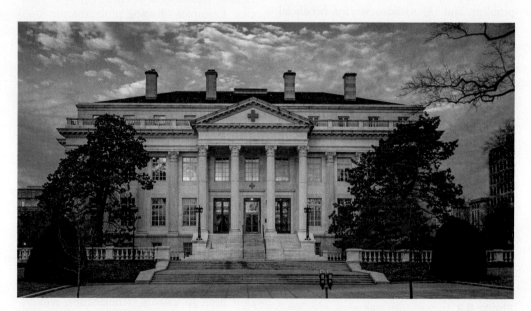

Figure 8.1 The American Red Cross is one of the best examples of a quasi-governmental agency.

© RozenskiP/Shutterstock.

Voluntary Health Agencies

Voluntary health agencies (see **Figure 8.2**) are some of the most visible health agencies in a community. Voluntary health agencies are a U.S. creation and grew out of unmet needs in communities. When governmental or quasi-governmental agencies were not in place to meet the needs of communities, interested citizens came together to form voluntary agencies. Such was the case with the American Cancer Society, the American Heart Association, the American Lung Association, and the Alzheimer's Association. The number of voluntary agencies seems endless, with agencies for about every disease and part of the body impacted by a disease or an illness. Most voluntary agencies have four primary purposes: (1) raise money to fund research and their programs, (2) provide education to both professionals and the public, (3) provide service to individuals and families affected by the disease or health problem, and (4) to advocate for beneficial policies, laws, and regulations that impact the work of the agency and in turn the people it is trying to help. Some of these organizations obtain their money from community fundraising efforts like the United Way, but most raise their money through writing successful grant proposals, carrying out specific special events (e.g., danceathons and golf outings),

Figure 8.2 Through their education, advocacy and research efforts, the American Lung Association touches the lives of more than 20 million Americans each year.

Courtesy of the American Lung Association.

conducting direct-mail campaigns, and other means of receiving donations.

Philanthropic Foundations

Philanthropic foundations play an important role by funding programs and research on the prevention, control, and treatment of diseases and other health problems. *Philanthropy* means "altruistic concern for human welfare and advancement, usually manifested by donations of money, property, or work to needy persons, by endowment of institutions of learning and hospitals, and by generosity to other socially useful purposes" (Random House, 2020, ¶ 1). Although many philanthropic foundations accept charitable contributions, they differ from voluntary health agencies in two primary ways. First, they were created with an endowment and, thus, do not have to raise money. Second, they are able to finance long-term projects that may be too expensive or risky to be funded by other agencies. Examples of some philanthropic foundations that have supported work by health education specialists are the Ford Foundation, the Robert Wood Johnson Foundation, and the Rockefeller Foundation.

The health education has one foundation, the **Foundation for the Advancement of Health Education (FAHE)**. FAHE is a nonprofit foundation founded in 1992 by past presidents and past executive directors of the American Association for Health Education (AAHE). As the AAHE organizational structure no longer exists, FAHE has expanded its collaborations and mission in order to "advance the health education profession with a social justice and equity perspective by supporting students, the workforce, and leaders in the field" (FAHE, n.d., ¶ 2). They fulfill their mission through awards, scholarships, and fellowships which are presented at the annual conference of the Society for Public Health Education (SOPHE) (see below for more information on SOPHE).

Service, Fraternal, and Religious Groups

Many different service, fraternal, and religious groups have also been important to health education specialists. Even though none of these groups has the primary purpose of enhancing the health of a community, they often get involved in health-related projects. Health education specialists commonly interact with these groups as part of community coalitions or when they are seeking resources to fund or enhance their programs. Examples of service and fraternal groups (and their health-related projects) include Rotary International (worldwide polio eradication), Lions (Lions Quest and preservation of sight), Shriners (children's hospitals), and American Legion (community recreation programs).

Religious groups also have contributed to the work of health education specialists' projects, both on a global level (e.g., the Protestants' One Great Hour of Sharing, the Catholic Relief Services, and the United Jewish Appeal Federation) and on a local level (e.g., food pantries, sleeping rooms, and soup kitchens).

Professional Health Associations/ Organizations

As noted earlier, the primary focus of this chapter is the professional health associations/organizations. The mission of **professional health associations/organizations** is to promote the high standards of professional practice for their respective profession, thereby improving the health of society by improving the people in the profession. The mission is carried out by advocating for the profession; keeping the members up to date via the publication of professional journals, books, and newsletters; and providing the members with an avenue to come together at professional meetings (see **Figure 8.3**). At these meetings, members have the opportunity to share and hear the new research findings, network with

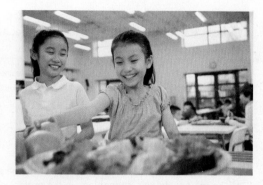

Figure 8.3 The American School Health Association focuses on the health of the school-aged child.
© XiXinXing/Alamy Stock Photo.

fellow professionals, and find out more about the latest equipment and published materials in the field. In addition, professional associations/organizations provide their members with benefits such as continuing education opportunities, networking, participation in tax-deferred annuity programs, discounts (annual national conventions, professional development sessions, publications), job placement, and a variety of other associated items (see **Box 8.1**).

Professional associations/organizations are member driven and composed, for the most part, of professionals who have completed specialized education and training and who are eligible for certification/licensure in their respective professions. These associations/organizations are funded primarily by membership dues, but it is becoming more common for them to seek grant funds (*soft money*) to help promote their missions. Most of these associations/organizations hire staff for day-to-day operations, but the officers are usually elected professionals.

In the remaining portions of this chapter, we present information on the national professional associations/organizations that help promote the health education/promotion profession. The reader should also be aware that many of these national associations/organizations have affiliates and

Box 8.1 Benefits of Joining a Professional Association/Organization as a Student Member

- Opportunity to interact, collaborate, and network with other professionals in the profession
- Opportunity to meet and interact with health education/promotion students and faculty from other colleges and universities
- Develop professional colleagues
- Have a professional identity
- Professional guidance and mentoring
- Leadership development
- Learn more about how the profession and the association/organization operate
- Keep up to date on happenings in the profession and new health information
- Opportunity to participate in the association's/organization's listservs, webinars, and learning communities
- Advocacy alerts and updates
- Opportunity to grow professionally and personally while being supported and encouraged by others
- Be exposed to current research and pedagogy of the profession through meeting attendance and reading the publications of the association/organization
- Make professional contacts for future practicums, internships, or jobs
- Get connected to job banks and internship opportunities
- Opportunity to make a presentation at a professional meeting
- Opportunity to serve the profession through an association/organization
- Discounted registration fees for professional meetings and publications
- If certified, opportunity to earn continuing education contact hours (CECHs) for recertification of the Certified Health Education Specialist and Master Certified Health Education Specialist credentials and other licensures

Data from Society for Public Health Education. (n.d.-c). *Our mission.* Retrieved June 28, 2021, from https://www.sophe.org/about/mission; Young, K. J., & Boling, W. (2004). Improving the quality of professional life: Benefits of health education and promotion association membership. *California Journal of Health Promotion,* 2(1), 39–44. http://www.cjhp.org/Volume2_2004/Issue1-TEXTONLY/39-44-young.pdf

other related groups at the regional and/or state level. For example, the American Public Health Association is a national organization, but there are also state associations such as the Ohio Public Health Association or the Indiana Public Health Association. In addition, there are also some state-only organizations that are not affiliated with any national organization. (Ask your instructor if there are any such organizations in your state.) Often, it is these regional or state affiliates/organizations that health education/promotion students become members of first because of their proximity to campus, opportunities to get involved in the professional organization, less-expensive membership dues, and local networking benefits.

Table 8.2 contains information about the following organizations.

American Public Health Association

The **American Public Health Association (APHA)** "champions the health of all people and all communities" (APHA, n.d.-a, ¶ 2). APHA was founded in 1872 when scientific advances were helping discover the causes of communicable diseases. The mission of APHA is to "[i]mprove the health of the public and achieve equity in health status" (APHA, n.d.-a, ¶ 3). The association works toward this mission by bringing together the public health disciplines to collaborate on priority issues,

Table 8.2 **Information About Key Professional Associations/Organizations**

The American Academy of Health Behavior 17 Indian Creek Drive Rudolph, OH 43462 *Telephone*: 419/760-6020 *Internet*: http://www.aahb.org/	**International Union for Health Promotion and Education (IUHPE)** c/o Santé publique France 12 rue du Val d'Osne 94415 Saint-Maurice France *Email*: iuhpe@iuhpe.org *Internet*: http://www.iuhpe.org
American College Health Association (ACHA) 8455 Colesville Road, Suite 740 Silver Spring, MD 20910 *Telephone*: 410/859-1500 *Email*: contact@acha.org *Internet*: http://www.acha.org	**National Wellness Institute, Inc. (NWI)** 1300 College Court PO Box 827 Stevens Point, WI 54481 *Telephone*: 715/342-2969 *Email*: nwi@nationalwellness.org *Internet*: http://www.nationalwellness.org
American Public Health Association (APHA) 800 I Street, NW Washington, DC 20001 *Telephone*: 202/777-APHA (2742) *Email*: membership.mail@apha.org *Internet*: http://www.apha.org	**Society for Public Health Education (SOPHE)** 10 G Street, NE, Suite 605 Washington, DC 20002 *Telephone*: 202/408-9804 *Email*: info@sophe.org *Internet*: http://www.sophe.org
American School Health Association (ASHA) *Telephone*: 202/854-1721 *Email*: info@ashaweb.org *Internet*: http://www.ashaweb.org	**Society of Health and Physical Educators (SHAPE America)** PO Box 225 Annapolis Junction, MD 20701 *Telephone*: 800/213-7193 *Email*: askmembership@shapeamerica.org *Internet*: http://www.shapeamerica.org/
Eta Sigma Gamma (ESG) 4319 West Clara Lane, PMB #285 Muncie, IN 47304 *Telephone*: 765/372-8189 *Email*: nationaloffice@etasigmagamma.org *Internet*: http://www.etasigmagamma.org	

publishing research and reports to improve public health science, providing a collective voice to advocate for laws and regulations that will advance public health while encouraging equity and access to care (APHA, n.d.-c).

Membership in APHA is a community of professionals, students, and retired health professionals, as well as agencies and voluntary organizations engaged in public health work. APHA currently has about 25,000 members, which includes organizational members, Caucuses, and affiliated state and regional health association members (Asin, A., personal communication, November 17, 2020). Once individuals become members, they have the opportunity to join one of the subgroups

of the organization—called Sections. The 32 Sections "represent major public health disciplines or public health programs. These Sections allow members with shared interests to come together to develop scientific program content and policy papers in their areas of interest or fields of practice, and they provide for professional and social networking, career development and mentoring" (APHA, n.d.-b, ¶ 2). Members can engage in a Section based on their area of work, such as health administration, or the area of emphasis of their work, such as food and nutrition.

The primary publication of APHA is the *American Journal of Public Health* (*AJPH*). This peer-reviewed journal is published monthly and is dedicated to the publication of original work in public health research, research methods, and program evaluation. The *AJPH* regularly includes editorials and commentaries and serves as a forum for health policy analysis. The association also publishes *The Nation's Health* 10 times per year. This newspaper includes reporting on current and proposed legislation, policy issues, news of actions within the federal agencies and Congress, or global issues. The publication also includes association and section news, job openings, and information on upcoming conferences. In addition to the *AJPH* and *The Nation's Health*, APHA also publishes books and other media on a variety of public health topics. Examples include *Racism: Science & Tools for the Public Health Professional* (Ford, Griffith, Bruce, & Gilbert) and the recent publication *Climate Change, Health and Equity: A Guide for Local Health Departments* (Harrison, Buckley & North). Additionally, members receive *Inside Public Health*, a monthly update highlighting member-only offers, events, and updates (APHA, n.d.-d).

There are other professional health associations that have a more focused mission. Some of those include the American College Health Association (ACHA), the American School Health Association (ASHA) (see **Figure 8.4**), the National Wellness

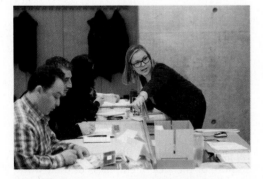

Figure 8.4 Annual professional conventions are an important benefit of membership in a professional organization.

© Klaus-Dietmar Gabbert/picture alliance/Getty Images.

Institute, Inc. (NWI), the SOPHE, the American Academy of Health Behavior, and SHAPE America (Society of Health and Physical Educators).

American College Health Association

The **American College Health Association (ACHA)** was founded originally as the American Student Health Association in 1920. In 1948, the name of the association was changed to its current name. ACHA's mission is to "serve as the principal leadership organization for advancing the health of college students and campus communities through advocacy, education, and research." (ACHA, n.d.-a, ¶ 2). The association has three distinct types of memberships. One is for institutions of higher education. Currently, there are more than 700 such members. ACHA also serves nearly 5,500 individual members who are interested in college health—that is, the health of college students. Included among the members are administrators, physicians and physicians' assistants, nurses and nurse practitioners, health education specialists, pharmacists, dentists, support staff who care for this special group of young adults, and students who are dedicated to health promotion on their campus. Most of these individual members are associated with the health service facilities on their respective campuses. The third type of membership is called sustaining members. This group is made up of nonprofit organizations and corporations "interested in being more connected with the college health field" (ACHA, n.d.-c).

Like some of the other associations/organizations, ACHA also has affiliates across the United States. ACHA is divided into 11 affiliates, each providing regional leadership and annual meeting opportunities. ACHA members receive concurrent membership in the affiliate organization at no additional cost (ACHA, n.d.-d). In addition, ACHA has nine membership sections, which are defined by the disciplines of college health. The Health Promotion Section was formed in 1958.

ACHA publishes several newsletters, numerous health information brochures, and other special publications. The members-only digital newsletter, *College Health and Wellness in Action*, is available online at the Association's website. The professional journal of the ACHA is the *Journal of American College Health*, which is published bimonthly and is the only journal devoted entirely to the health of college students. The journal publishes articles encompassing many areas of college health, "including clinical and preventive medicine, health promotion, environmental health and safety, nursing assessment, interventions, and management, pharmacy, and sports medicine. The journal regularly publishes major articles on student behaviors, mental health and health care policies, and includes a section for discussion of controversial issues" (ACHA, n.d.-b, ¶ 1).

American School Health Association

The **American School Health Association (ASHA)** began on October 27, 1927, as the American Association of School Physicians. The organization began to use its current name in 1936 (ASHA, n.d.-a). The mission of ASHA "is to transform all schools into places where every student learns and thrives" (ASHA, n.d.-a, ¶ 3).

Membership in the association comprises individuals and organizations, including schools and school districts that are supportive of an alignment with the advancement of school health programs and the mission of ASHA. ASHA is a multidisciplinary organization with nearly 650 members. Included in its membership are administrators, counselors, dieticians, nutritionists, health education specialists, physical educators, psychologists, school health coordinators, school nurses, school physicians, and social workers. ASHA members are provided a host of networking

and professional development opportunities in the following four broad areas that impact school health: administration, coordination and leadership; programs and services; research and emerging issues; and teaching and learning (Celis, K., personal communication, November 18, 2020).

The *Journal of School Health* (JOSH), which is published 12 times a year, is the primary publication of the ASHA. The journal is recognized widely and "is committed to communicating information regarding the role of schools, school personnel, or the school environment in facilitating optimal growth and development of children and youth" (ASHA, n.d.-b, ¶ 1). The readership of the journal "includes researchers, school administrators, . . . educators, nurses, physicians, dentists, psychologists [and] counselors, social workers, nutritionists, dietitians, and other health professionals . . . . These individuals work cooperatively with parents and the community to achieve the common goal of providing youths with programs, services, and environment" needed to promote health and to improve learning (ASHA, n.d.-b).

National Wellness Institute, Inc.

The **National Wellness Institute (NWI)**, founded in 1977, was formed around the Six Dimensions of Wellness model: intellectual, emotional, social, spiritual, occupational, and physical. The founders believed that by balancing these six dimensions and actively seeking to improve them, they could improve their overall well-being (NWI, n.d.-b). The mission of NWI "is enrich the lives and careers of wellness professionals" (NWI, n.d-b, "Our Mission"). The mission is accomplished by

- Serving as the global professional network for connecting to all disciplines of wellness

- Providing education and training that promotes life-long learning
- Identifying and representing inclusive whole-person professional standards and competencies (NWI, n.d.-b, "Our Mission")

Joining NWI provides a connection with over 10,000 community members (Miller, K., personal communication, November 19, 2020). There are three types of memberships in NWI: individual, organizational, and student. The organizational membership allows five individuals at the same location to receive full NWI benefits. With each type of membership, there is regular membership and the option to include a subscription to the *American Journal of Health Promotion* (NWI, n.d.-a). One of the most visible components of the NWI is its National Wellness Conference. The conference is open to members and nonmembers alike and is a unique conference because it is a week of immersion into a wellness experience.

Society for Public Health Education

The Society for Public Health Educators (SOPHE), founded in 1950, promotes healthy behaviors, healthy communities, and healthy environments through its membership, local chapters, and various partnerships. In 1969, the organization changed its name to the **Society for Public Health Education (SOPHE)**. The mission of SOPHE's strategic plan for 2021–2025 is "supporting leaders in health education and promotion to advance healthy and equitable communities across the globe" (SOPHE, n.d.-c, ¶ 1). At the national and local levels, SOPHE's membership includes nearly 4,000 professionals from throughout the United States and many international countries. Members work in a variety of places, including K–12 schools, universities, healthcare settings, worksites, voluntary organizations, and local/state/federal government agencies. There are currently 22 SOPHE chapters spanning over 25 states (SOPHE, n.d.-e, ¶ 1) (see Practitioner's Perspective). Like several of the other associations or organizations, SOPHE members have the opportunity to associate with one or more smaller working groups. In SOPHE, the smaller groups are called Communities of Practice (CoP). CoP allow members "who share a similar professional role or a passion about a health topic or an area of practice can exchange ideas, resources, research, or build solutions to common issues" (SOPHE, n.d.-a, ¶ 2). Additionally, the CoPs maintain listservs throughout the year to encourage dialogue and exchange (SOPHE, n.d.-a).

Practitioner's Perspective

Professional Association (Society For Public Health Education): Melissa E. Shelton

CURRENT POSITION/TITLE: Staff Analyst

EMPLOYER: Houston Health Department

DEGREE/INSTITUTION/YEAR: PhD, Walden University, 2017

MAJOR: Public Health

SPECIALIZATION: Community Health Education

MASTER CERTIFIED HEALTH EDUCATION SPECIALIST

Becoming a public health education professional: When I entered my public health profession, it began from a nontraditional approach; I initially started in an undergraduate program, and then I served active duty in the United States Navy (USN) as an enlisted medical specialist, also known as a hospital corpsman. I gained my experience in a public health role by providing health care and health education to Navy and Marine Corp military members and their families. While serving in the USN, I completed my undergraduate degree in resource management. I continued my education to earn a Master of Public Administration with a specialization in healthcare administration. During my time in the USN, I enjoyed being around and serving the public, which happens to be the military family. After completing my military obligation with the USN, I relocated to Houston, Texas. My first civilian professional job was with a local city health department in the Bureau of HIV/AIDS. My role as a community involvement coordinator involved coordinating, developing, and providing health education on HIV prevention to grades kindergarten through 12th grades and youth-related projects. The topic was challenging, but this experience increased my passion for public health. I wanted to keep growing professionally and obtain more experience in the public health education field. I received an opportunity to expand my skills by working in the private sector at a health maintenance organization (HMO) associated with a hospital system. My job as a Health Education/Texas Health Steps Coordinator with the HMO's Medicaid program allowed me to develop materials and provide health education and health promotion services and resources to women and children. The program's concept was similar to working in a governmental public health education program but in the private sector. During my career growth, I had an excellent opportunity to be commissioned as an Army Reserve officer and served in the medical service corp. I then continued my career with a local county health department as a health communication specialist in their public health preparedness program. This position entailed developing a public health preparedness communication plan that outlines how to outreach to a diverse community in the event of a disaster. The communication plan served as a standard operating procedure (SOP) that included various components such as health education, public information, outreach team, etc. This opportunity allowed me to grow to take additional courses at a local university. The health education courses help me qualify to take the certified health education specialist exam. I had another opportunity to be promoted to a health communications coordinator at the local county health department, which allows for breadth to work across the entire health department's divisions, such as environmental health. While previously working for a county health department, I was among the first to obtain my Master of Certified Health Education Specialist (MCHES) certification. I continued my education by pursuing a PhD in public health and specializing in community health from Walden University. Lastly, my career continues as a staff analyst with a local city health department working in program development and planning.

Serving in a professional association: A previous assistant director of health education for a county health department suggested joining and becoming involved in Society for Public Health Education. This discussion took place after my local county health department responded to the 2005 Hurricane Katrina event. Many of the residents from Louisiana had evacuated to Harris County/Houston, Texas, area for refuge. I had a fantastic opportunity to work in Harris County's Office of Emergency Management Unified Command Joint Information Center (JIC), composed of various agencies throughout Houston, Texas. Working in the JIC allowed me to see firsthand what was going on with the new residents who relocated temporarily to the Astrodome. Upon my observation and discussion with the new residents, I realized that a newsletter is necessary to keep everyone informed. During that time, I approached my supervisor about creating a newsletter that will inform, provide health education information, and updates to residents in the Astrodome. Several health education messages consisted of the importance of handwashing before eating, after eating, going to the bathroom, and changing a baby's diaper. The reason was to help reduced gastrointestinal problems that had occurred. After this event, I had my first opportunity to co-present with my assistant director in the health education division at the local county health department at the Society for Public Health Education (SOPHE). I honestly felt that

(continues)

Practitioner's Perspective   *(continued)*

Professional Association (Society For Public Health Education): Melissa E. Shelton

SOPHE was the place to be a member and become more involved as a member. I had the honor to be appointed and served as Co-Editor of SOPHE's News & Views. During my appointment, I had the opportunity to revise the newsletter guidelines, provide input on the format, and make recommendations to the editorial board about submitting articles. Also, I provided insight into how SOPHE members can tap into advanced leaders in the profession, highlighting professional development programs that emphasize global health issues and promote the health education advocacy summit by highlighting the use of social media platforms. I also had the opportunity to serve as a SOPHE Abstract Reviewer for the past two conferences. My growth was continued by serving on the Texas Society for Public Health Education (TSOPHE) board for five years. My first role as TSOPHE Secretary allowed me to learn TSOPHE's structure, goals, and how it falls within SOPHE's strategic plan. Upon being elected President-Elect and President, my goals were to enhance the profession by recruiting and mentoring students as members and assigning them projects with my health department. I also served as TSOPHE Communications Chair with the opportunity to redesign the TSOPHE newsletter to allow for TSOPHE members to be highlighted and have continuing education opportunities to be spotlighted.

Being able to serve in the SOPHE arena allowed me to grow tremendously professionally as I completed my PhD in public health and specialized in community health education. I had an excellent opportunity to humbly serve as the elected 2015 Student Trustee, which allowed me to bring 14 years of professional and student experiences to the table. As a PhD student, SOPHE allowed me to provide some unique perspectives on integrating academic pedagogy, research, and practice related to advancing health promotion, health education, and new public health. As the elected Student Trustee, I had the opportunity to work collaboratively with SOPHE to refine students' pathways to enter the evolving Health Education/Health Promotion profession. My goal was to facilitate my peers' development, encourage them to have an active voice, and advocate for the profession. My passion for health promotions and health education has continued to grow throughout my education and career journey.

Recommendation for those preparing to be public health education specialists: First, get involved in SOPHE and your local SOPHE chapter. Opportunities for personal growth are just more than going to work. If you want to serve in a leadership role, SOPHE is the best place to start. You can take the first step by joining SOPHE as a student and sign up for a committee of your interest. SOPHE allows you the opportunity to grow, learn group dynamics, strengthen leadership, and learn a new skill. Second, develop your brand through relationships with leaders and having a mentor who can guide your direction. Reach out to your university's professors who come from a diverse background and a wealth of information about the health education specialist field. And third, have an open mind. We are now working in an environment in which a health education specialist must be innovative and flexible. Check out the professional opportunities on SOPHE's website. You can access SOPHE's resources to obtain continuing education to enhance your skills and find out about internships and fellowships that will jump-start your career.

SOPHE has three premier peer-reviewed journals: *Health Education and Behavior, Health Promotion Practice*, and *Pedagogy in Health Promotion: The Scholarship of Teaching and Learning. Health Education and Behavior,* published bimonthly, is a well-respected journal that provides empirical research, case studies, program evaluations, and discussions of theories of health behavior and health status (SOPHE, n.d.-b). *Health Promotion*

Practice is a "peer-reviewed bi-monthly journal devoted to the practical application of health promotion and education" (SOPHE, n.d.-b, ¶ 3). *Pedagogy in Health Promotion: The Scholarship of Teaching and Learning* (PHP) is a quarterly journal focusing on such "areas as curriculum and course/program design, assessment, and administration relevant to teaching and learning" (SOPHE, n.d.-b, ¶ 4). Additionally, SOPHE members can keep current with the latest health education news through two newsletters, "News U Can Use" and "SOPHE News & Views" (SOPHE, n.d.-d).

Like several of the other associations/organizations, SOPHE holds an annual meeting that provides members and health education professionals with the opportunity to share and receive the most recent research findings, to earn continuing education contact hours, and to network with other professionals. The Advocacy Summit is another professional development opportunity that SOPHE supports. The Advocacy Summit provides an opportunity for health education specialists to receive training in advocacy techniques and apply their new knowledge on a trip to Capitol Hill in Washington, D.C., to discuss health-related issues with staffers from key legislative subcommittees and representatives of their congressional districts.

International Union for Health Promotion and Education

Though all of the professional associations/organizations noted already in this chapter have members from countries other than the United States, there is one professional association that is truly worldwide: the **International Union for Health Promotion and Education (IUHPE)**. There are over 2,000 members worldwide in approximately 150 countries. The IUHPE, founded in 1951 in Paris, is a global association with a mission "to promote global health and wellbeing and to contribute to the achievement of equity in health between and within countries of the

world" (IUHPE, n.d.-b, ¶ 4). IUHPE fulfills its mission by "building and operating an independent, global, professional network of people and institutions to encourage the free exchange of ideas, knowledge, know-how, experiences, and the development of relevant collaborative projects, both at global and regional levels" (IUHPE, n.d.-b, ¶ 5). Membership includes government bodies, including universities and institutes, nongovernmental organizations, and individuals across all continents working to advance public health. IUHPE is involved in advocacy efforts as well as capacity-building, policy development, and dissemination initiatives. The IUHPE has four priority areas: social determinants of health, health promotion in sustainable development, noncommunicable disease prevention and control, and health promotion systems. An obvious distinctiveness of IUHPE is its global reach in every continent (IUHPE, n.d.-c).

Every three years, IUHPE holds a World Conference on Health Promotion as well as regional conferences, which have become important gatherings of health promotion experts and practitioners worldwide. The next World Conference on Health Promotion is scheduled to be held in Québec, Canada, in May 2022. IUHPE has a "family" of journals. The official membership journal, which is published quarterly, is *Global Health Promotion* (formerly called *Promotion & Education*). "It is a multilingual journal that publishes authoritative peer-reviewed articles and practical information for a worldwide audience of professionals interested in health promotion and health education" (IUHPE, n.d.-a, ¶ 1). All IUHPE members receive *Global Health Promotion* and can purchase, at a reduced rate, any of the other five journals (*Critical Public Health, Health Promotion International, Health Education Research, International Journal of Mental Health Promotion*, or the *International Journal of Public Health*) published in association through collaborative agreements with their respective publisher (IUHPE, n.d.-d).

American Academy of Health Behavior™

The **American Academy of Health Behavior™ (AAHB)** is a professional organization unlike those presented so far in this chapter. Founded in 1997, the AAHB, or just The Academy, as it is referred to, is a society of researchers and scholars in the areas of health behavior, health education, and health promotion. The Academy "was created to improve the stature of health educators by supporting and promoting quality health behavior, health education, and health promotion research conducted by health educators" (Werch, 2000, p. 3). The mission of The Academy "is to serve as the 'research home' for health behavior scholars committed to excellence and diversity in research to improve the public's health" (AAHB, n.d.-b, ¶ 1).

Individuals must apply for membership in The Academy, and acceptance is based on one's area of academic preparation and level of scholarly activity. The specific qualifications for membership are listed on The Academy's website (see Table 8.2). Currently, The Academy has 200 members. The Academy publishes *Health Behavior Research,* a peer-reviewed open-access scholarly journal, four-times per year. *Health Behavior Research* is "dedicated to the translation of research to advance policy, program planning, and/or practice relevant to behavior change" (AAHB, n.d.-a, ¶ 2).

SHAPE America

SHAPE (Society of Health and Physical Educators) is the nation's largest membership organization of health and physical education professionals—from pre-K–12 educators to university professors. Their mission is to "advance professional practice and promote research related to health and physical education, physical activity, dance, and sport" (SHAPE America, n.d.-a, ¶ 4).

SHAPE America publishes four signature journals for professionals in health education, physical education, and related fields. The *American Journal of Health Education* (AJHE) is published six times a year and includes research findings, community learning strategies, and recent health promotion trends. The other journals that SHAPE America publishes are *Journal of Physical Education, Recreation & Dance* (JOPERD), *Strategies: A Journal for Physical and Sport Educators,* and *Research Quarterly for Exercise and Sport* (RQES) (SHAPE America, n.d.-b).

Professional development is one important membership benefit of SHAPE America. They offer workshops, webinars, online toolboxes for teachers and coaches, and various newsletters. A national convention brings nearly 5,000 health and physical education professionals together annually.

Eta Sigma Gamma

Founded in 1967, **Eta Sigma Gamma (ESG)** is the national health education honorary. The idea for the organization was born when three professors from Ball State University, Drs. William Bock, Warren E. Schaller, and Robert Synovitz, were on their way to a professional conference and were discussing the need for an honorary for the discipline. Their discussion led to the formation of the organization, which has had, from its beginning, the primary purpose of furthering the professional competence and dedication of individual members of the health education/promotion profession (ESG, 1991). The ideals of the honorary are symbolized in its seal. The seal (see **Figure 8.5**) "is divided into four equilateral triangles, each carrying a symbol. A lamp of learning is in the center triangle, surrounded by an open book representing teaching, a microscope signifying research, and an outstretched hand representing service. These three elements form the basic purposes of the organization and profession; teaching/education, research, and service. The unifying element of these purposes is symbolized by the lamp of learning, since it is through the learning

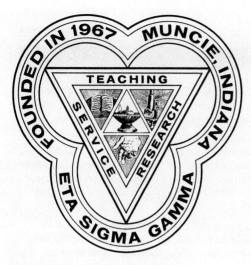

Figure 8.5 Seal of Eta Sigma Gamma.

Courtesy of Eta Sigma Gamma.

process that each purpose is achieved" (ESG, 1991, p. 2).

There have been 142 chapters installed on university/college campuses throughout the United States and more than 8,500 members, over 3,000 of whom are active members (J. Soules, personal communication, November 30, 2020). Chapters are awarded to colleges/universities based on a review and vote by the National Executive Committee of ESG on an application prepared by personnel at the petitioning college/university. From its beginnings, ESG has focused on the student members. Most individuals join the honorary when they are either undergraduate or graduate students. Membership is open to those who have a major or minor in health education and a grade point average equivalent to at least a *B–*. In fact, students can achieve membership only by affiliating through a collegiate chapter. Through their affiliation with the collegiate chapters, they are eligible to apply for the awards and scholarships of the honorary. Professionals who are active in the discipline of health education/promotion and holding a degree can affiliate through the Chapter-at-Large (ESG, 1991) (see Practitioner's Perspective).

Practitioner's Perspective

Eta Sigma Gamma: Alison Yelsma

CURRENT POSITION: President, Gamma Mu Chapter of Eta Sigma Gamma; Student ambassador, Western Michigan University College of Health and Human Services; Collegiate Champion, Society for Public Health Education

DEGREE/INSTITUTION: BS Public Health, anticipated December 2021, Western Michigan University

MAJOR: Bachelor of Science in Public Health

MINORS: Integrative Holistic Health and Wellness; Health Informatics and Information Management

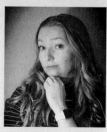

Courtesy of Alison Yelsma.

Becoming a public health major: Many people in my family work in the healthcare field and unsurprisingly, I also inherited the "empathy bone." After high school, I started my university years in a direct entry doctor of pharmacy program out of state. However, in my third semester, I experienced a myriad of health issues that led me to move back home with my parents. During that time, I also realized that pharmacy was not a good fit for me and I began exploring other paths in the health field. Throughout the various doctor's appointments, my mom would always remind me, in her typically optimistic fashion, that I could look at these experiences as field trips. After much reflection, I concluded that I did not see myself working in a patient/provider setting

(continues)

and was actually more concerned about the big picture and how things worked at the system level. I remembered how fascinating I had found our public health module in a first-year pharmacy course, so I decided that public health was exactly what I was looking for in my future career.

Getting involved in health education: Happily, I was accepted at Western Michigan University. I finished up my general education courses and prerequisites for the program that spring and summer at the local community college and joined the next cohort in the fall of that year as a junior at WMU. On the first day of the semester, in our biostatistics course, it was very reassuring to hear that many of my peers had started in other fields such as nursing and social work before finding public health.

One of the main reasons why I pursued health education is that I can continue studying science, a major passion of mine, as well as have plenty of time to be creative. It is refreshing to be in a field that challenges both sides of me. At the end of my junior year, I thought back on what subjects I enjoyed the most to narrow down what I would select as my minor, although it ended up being two. The first minor I selected was Integrative Holistic Health and Wellness. I love that health education takes a holistic approach to population health and am learning so much about the eight dimensions of wellness in these courses. Additionally, with the ever-increasing technological innovations and skillsets, I choose health informatics and information management as my second minor. It can be stressful to choose a minor and ultimately find your path in health education, but the best piece of advice I can offer in this area is to not compare yourself to others. So, follow what you are passionate and curious about. Health education is such a broad area and there is room for whatever skills and knowledge you have to share.

Why I decided to join Eta Sigma Gamma: Right away, I decided to join the Gamma Mu chapter of Eta Sigma Gamma, the national health education honorary. The organization embodies what I value (service, teaching, and research) and it has helped me decide who I want to become in health education—an aspiring researcher and professor. Some of my fondest college memories are planning events with other students and spending time with peers in my cohort and the senior cohort that I met in ESG!

My involvement in Eta Sigma Gamma: I was initiated in the fall of 2019, when I was a junior in my first semester at Western Michigan University. After participating in "Sober October" that year and going to the first few weekly meetings, I felt like I had found my people. Everyone enjoyed studying public health. They were nerds, like me, for social justice, advocacy, and putting into action what we were all learning about in health education courses. Later that fall, I assisted with the planning and implementing of the ESG booth on Health Literacy Day. In the spring, I assisted with the implementation of our "Love Your Selfie" event and with the planning of our "See a Need, Help a Need" COVID-19 fundraiser. Starting that spring, our ESG chapter developed a health communication plan based on social media posts for our university. This allowed us to use our peer influence to help educate other students on safe guidelines surrounding COVID-19. That spring, I was voted one of the "Outstanding New Initiates" for the 2019–2020 academic year and elected president for the 2020-2021 academic year.

Recommendations for those preparing to be health education specialists: The biggest recommendation I have for emerging health education specialists is to volunteer for as many events as you can to explore different areas. Also, do not ignore your previous experience in other fields or in classes that you might not think tie directly into health education—because they do. They all do. Public health is so interdisciplinary and everything can be relevant. Something else I want to share is please do not feel like you have to be locked into one thing, one population group, or even one health condition. Having a variety of interests is great and can lead to countless opportunities.

Future plans: My anticipated graduation date is in December of 2021 and I plan on going to grad school for MPH and PhD degrees. My main interests include epidemiology, chronic diseases, health literacy, and the social determinants of health. I hope to research and teach in those areas. Since I know it is important to have goals outside of academia, I also plan on taking teacher training to become a registered yoga instructor after completing my undergraduate degree and before I start grad school. I also plan to finish reading all of Macolm Galdwell's books. Be kind, stay humble and never stop learning!

ESG regularly produces three publications: its journal, *The Health Educator*; *The Health Education Monograph Series*; and "The Vision," an online newsletter. Each of these journals is distributed twice a year. Like the publications of the other associations/organizations, the journals include the current works of the professionals in the field. However, unlike the others, only individuals who are current members of ESG can write articles for *The Health Educator* and *The Health Education Monograph Series*. Another unusual characteristic of the publications of ESG is that one entire issue of the *Monograph Series* each year is composed of articles written only by student members. This is another indication that the honorary is concerned about the preservice professional.

Associations for Directors

There is one professional group that has ties to health education. Unlike all of the other professional groups discussed, membership in this organization is tied to one's employment. The individuals who belong are employees of their respective state/territorial/Indian Health Service departments of health or education. The **Society of State Leaders of Health and Physical Education** (the Society) was founded in 1926 and is "a professional association whose . . . members supervise and coordinate programs in health, physical education, and related fields of coordinated school health programs within state departments of education" (The Society, n.d.-a, ¶ 1). The mission of The Society is to use "advocacy, partnerships, professional development and resources

to build capacity of school health leaders to implement effective health education and physical education policies and practices that support success in school, work and life" (The Society, n.d.-b, "Our Mission").

Coalitions

Because of the large number of professional health education/promotion associations, there are times when there is a need to have a common voice for the profession. To help provide such a voice, coalitions of health associations/organizations have been created. The most prominent coalition is the Coalition of National Health Education Organizations, USA.

The **Coalition of National Health Education Organizations, USA (CNHEO)** is a nonprofit federation of organizations dedicated to advancing the health education/promotion profession. The coalition is composed of representatives (delegates and alternates) from eight national associations/organizations with identifiable health education specialist memberships and ongoing health education/promotion programs. The associations/organizations include the American College Health Association, American Public Health Association, American School Health Association, Eta Sigma Gamma, International Union for Health Promotion and Education, National Commission for Health Education Credentialing, Inc., Society for Public Health Education, and the Society of State Leaders of Health and Physical Education (CNHEO, n.d.-b).

CNHEO was formed on March 1, 1972, after a series of three meetings in 1971 and 1972 to determine the feasibility of such an organization. The primary mission of the coalition is "the mobilization of the resources of the Health Education Profession in order to expand and improve health education, regardless of the setting" (CNHEO, n.d.-a, ¶ 1).

The work of CNHEO is financed by funds obtained from coalition member organizations, public and private agencies, and contributions and gifts from individuals. Over the years, the working relationship of the member organizations has been outlined in the *Working Agreement of the CNHEO*. Also included in this document are the purposes of the coalition (CNHEO, 2021, "Purposes"):

1. To strengthen communications among the Member Organizations as well as between the health education/promotion profession and policymakers, other professions, and consumers.
2. To develop, implement, and evaluate a shared vision and strategic plan for health education/promotion.
3. To educate policy makers on the need for federal and state public policies that support healthy behaviors and healthy communities.
4. To collaborate on common documents, issues, problems, and concerns related to health education/promotion.
5. Increase the visibility of the health education/promotion profession and its member organizations.

Unlike the other organizations and groups discussed in this chapter, the CNHEO functions with no paid staff members or permanent location. "The CNHEO carries on business by means of email communication, monthly conference calls, and periodic face-to-face meetings during member organization conferences. Through these means it has made significant progress in addressing its purposes and priorities" (Capwell, 2004, p. 13). Since its inception, the CNHEO has operationalized its purposes in a number of ways, contributing to the growth of the profession. Below is a list of some of the recent

activities and accomplishments in which the CNHEO has been involved:

- Creation of position papers on topics of importance to the profession (e.g., preparation of elementary school teachers in the area of health education, and the strengthening of health education in the public health arena).
- Cosponsoring three invitational conferences in 1995 (NCHEC & CNHEO, 1996), 2002 (CNHEO, 2003), and 2016 to examine the status and future of the health education/promotion profession. These conferences led to the creation of goals and recommendations for the profession for the 21st century and commitments by member organizations to lead or assist in addressing the recommendations (CNHEO, 2003). (See Chapter 10 for more on the future of health education/promotion.)
- Creation of a unified "Code of Ethics for the Health Education Profession" (see Chapter 5 and Appendix A).

More information about CNHEO can be obtained by contacting the office of any of the member organizations or by logging on to the CNHEO website. The URL for this site is presented in the Weblinks at the end of the chapter.

Joining a Professional Health Association/ Organization

Becoming a member of a professional organization is not difficult. With the exception of a few of the associations/organizations previously noted (CNHEO, AAHB, ESG, and The Society), membership in a professional organization can be obtained by completing an application form (available from any of the organizations, included in many of the official publications, or found at the organization's website [see Table 8.2]) and sending the money with the desired length and category of membership (different rates apply to different types of membership—for example, student, professional, retired) to the association/organization of choice. Most individuals join a professional association/organization for a year at a time. Some associations, however, provide multiple-year memberships at a reduced rate or even a lifetime membership. In general, the cost of a membership in a state or regional association/organization is separate from and less than a membership in a national association/organization. If you are interested in joining a state or local association/organization, you can usually contact its national office to find out whom to contact locally.

The Certification Body of the Health Education/Promotion Profession: National Commission for Health Education Credentialing, Inc.

NCHEC (pronounced N-check) is unlike any other organization that has been discussed in this chapter. NCHEC is not a professional organization that health education specialists join, but rather the organization responsible for the individual credentialing of health education specialists; thus, it has no members. The history of the development of NCHEC was presented in Chapter 6, while the information presented here is to give the reader an understanding of how NCHEC operates.

"The mission of NCHEC is to enhance the professional practice of Health Education by promoting and sustaining a credentialed body of Health Education Specialists. To meet this mission, NCHEC certifies health education specialists, promotes professional development, and strengthens professional preparation and practice" (NCHEC, n.d.-b, ¶ 1). Four boards and the NCHEC staff carry out the work of NCHEC. The boards include the Board of Commissioners [BOC], the Division Board for Certification of Health Education Specialists, the Division Board of Professional Development, and the Division Board for Professional Preparation and Practice. The four boards meet monthly via conference calls and have one or two face-to-face meetings each year.

The BOC, which is composed of 11 commissioners, is the governing board and the board responsible for all NCHEC activities (NCHEC, n.d.-b). The three division boards address the three activities noted in NCHEC's mission statement: certification, professional development, and professional preparation. Those who either hold the CHES or the MCHES credential elect the directors and commissioners of the various boards, with the exception of one. The lone exception is the public member of the BOC, who is appointed by the BOC after a call for nominations. In addition, the elected directors and commissioners are volunteers and must hold an active CHES® or MCHES® credential (NCHEC, n.d.-b).

The primary responsibility of the Division Board for Certification of Health Education Specialists (DBCHES) is to maintain and evaluate the two certification examinations of NCHEC—the CHES® exam and the MCHES® exam. More specifically, DBCHES, which is currently composed of 11 directors, along with the guidance of Professional Examination Services (PES) ensures a periodic review and evaluation of certification and examination processes, recommends policies and procedures for administering the CHES® and MCHES® examinations, participates in item-writing workshops, and ensures that NCHEC's competency testing meets acceptable standards (NCHEC, n.d.-b).

The work of the Division Board for Professional Development (DBPD), which is composed of seven directors, is to oversee the recertification and annual renewal procedures (NCHEC, n.d.-b). "More specifically, the DBPD recommends policies and procedures related to the designation of continuing education providers, recertification, and the annual renewal of CHES®; recommends fees for recertification, annual renewal and provider designation; and assures that the processes are monitored and periodically evaluated" (NCHEC, n.d.-b, ¶ 6).

The Division Board for Professional Preparation and Practice (DBPPP), which is also composed of seven directors, is responsible for promoting professional preparation (NCHEC, n.d.-b). "More specifically, the DBPPP works with colleges, universities,

and accrediting agencies to improve professional preparation programs and promote best practices in health education settings; and monitors and updates the certification application and eligibility review process" (NCHEC, n.d.-b, ¶ 7).

The CHES® examination was given for the first time in 1990. The first MCHES® examination was offered in 2011. Both examinations are offered twice a year—one in April and one in October—at more than 125 locations throughout the United States. The examinations are each 165 questions long, and candidates have three hours to complete the exam. The eligibility criteria to take the examinations are presented in **Box 8.2**.

Box 8.2 Eligibility Criteria to Sit for the CHES® and MCHES® Examinations

CHES Examination

Eligibility to take the CHES® examination is based exclusively on academic qualifications. An individual is eligible to take the examination if they have the following:

A bachelor's, master's, or doctoral degree from an accredited institution of higher education; AND one of the following:

- An official transcript (including course titles) that clearly shows a major in health education (e.g., Health Education, Community Health Education, Public Health Education, School Health Education, etc.). Degree/major must explicitly be in a discipline of "Health Education." OR
- An official transcript that reflects at least 25 semester hours or 37 quarter hours of course work (with a grade "C" or better) with specific preparation addressing the Seven Areas of Responsibility and Competency for Health Education Specialists http://www .nchec.org/ches-exam-eligibility

MCHES® Exam Eligibility

The MCHES® exam eligibility includes both academic and experience requirements.

Exam Eligibility

For CHES®: A minimum of the past five (5) continuous years in active status as a CHES®.

For Non-CHES® or CHES® with fewer than five years active status AND five years of experience:

- A master's degree or higher in Health Education, Public Health Education, School Health Education, Community Health Education, etc.
- OR a Master's degree or higher with an academic transcript reflecting at least 25 semester hours (37 quarter hours) of course work in which the Seven Areas of Responsibility of Health Educators were addressed.
- Five (5) years of documented experience as a health education specialist.

To verify, applicants must submit:

1. Two verification forms from a current or past manager/supervisor, and/or a leader in a health education professional organization
2. A current curriculum vitae/résumé http:// www.nchec.org/mches-exam-eligibility

Data from The National Commission for Health Education Credentialing. (n.d.). *CHES® exam eligibility.* http://www.nchec.org/ches-exam-eligibility; and The National Commission for Health Education Credentialing. (n.d.). *MCHES® exam eligibility.* http://www.nchec.org/mches-exam-eligibility

NCHEC produces a number of different publications. The *NCHEC News* is NCHEC's newsletter for all CHES® and MCHES®. The newsletter is published three times a year and is mailed to each current certification holder. Past issues of the newsletter are available online at the NCHEC website (www.nchec.org/nchec-news-bulletins). NCHEC also publishes documents that are useful for those working in professional preparation programs, those offering continuing education opportunities, and those individuals preparing to take either the CHES® or the MCHES® examination.

Included in these publications are a companion guide for the examinations and the competency-based framework. This document was generated from the findings of the Health Education Specialists Practice Analysis (HESPA) project (NCHEC, n.d.-a).

More information about NCHEC can be obtained by contacting the NCHEC office, 1541 Alta Drive, Suite 303, Whitehall, PA 18052-5642, Phone: (484) 223-0770, Toll-Free: (888) 624-3248, Facsimile: (800) 813-0727 or by logging on to the NCHEC website. The URL for this site is presented in the Weblinks at the end of the chapter.

Summary

This chapter discussed the various health agencies, associations, and organizations with which the profession of health education/promotion interacts. The agencies/associations/organizations were presented in three major categories: governmental, quasi-governmental, and nongovernmental. The primary emphasis of the chapter was to present information about a subcategory of the nongovernmental associations/organizations, the professional associations/organizations. Those discussed included the American Academy of Health Behavior; the American Public Health Association; the American College Health Association; the American School Health Association; the National Wellness Institute, Inc.; the Society for Public Health Education; the Society of Health and Physical Educators; the International Union for Health Promotion and Education; Eta Sigma Gamma; and an association for directors (The Society of State Leaders of Health and Physical Education). Also, information about a coalition—the Coalition of National Health Education Organizations—and information on how to become a member of a professional association/organization was presented. The chapter concluded with an overview of the National Commission for Health Education Credentialing, Inc. and the eligibility criteria for taking the CHES® or MCHES® examination.

Review Questions

1. Define and explain the differences among the following types of agencies: *governmental health agency, quasi-governmental health agency,* and *nongovernmental health agency.*
2. At which levels do governmental agencies exist? Provide an example of an agency at each level.
3. What are the four primary activities of most voluntary health agencies? Give an example of each.
4. What are the purposes of a professional association/organization?
5. What are the benefits derived from membership in a professional association/organization? Why should students become members?
6. What is the oldest and largest professional health association in the United States?
7. Name two professional health associations/organizations that focus their efforts on work settings for

health education specialists. Name two other professional health associations/organizations that are not as focused on a work setting.

8. What is the name of the health education honorary? In general, where are the chapters of the honorary found?

9. What makes the AAHB different from the other professional organizations/associations presented in this chapter?

10. What is a coalition? Name one health education coalition. What is the primary purpose of this coalition? What are some of the recent activities of the coalition?

11. How does a person become a member of a professional organization?

12. What is the NCHEC? How is it different from the other organizations presented in the chapter?

Case Study

Zoyer (pronouns: they/them/theirs) has been employed by the XYZ voluntary health organization for almost a year now. The job has really gone well. They enjoy the work, like their coworkers, and have been able to use much of what they learned during their health education/promotion professional preparation program. Just recently, the organization received word that it had been awarded a $15,000 grant to conduct a health education/promotion program for a local senior citizens group on living a healthier life. Their supervisor, Ms. Denison, has given Zoyer the responsibility to take the leadership for the project. One restriction on the use of the money is that the program must be planned by a representative group from local voluntary and governmental health education/promotion organizations. Therefore, Zoyer's first task is to invite local groups to send a representative to the initial planning meeting. Zoyer has set the goal of having seven different health voluntary and governmental agencies involved. If you were Zoyer, which organizations would you invite to the initial meeting? Justify why you would select these seven.

Critical Thinking Questions

1. For a number of years, many practicing health education specialists have pushed for a single professional health education/promotion association that would bring together many of the existing associations (i.e., ACHA, ASHA, SOPHE) so that health education/promotion would have a single professional association voice. Would you be in favor of or against combining all the health education/promotion professional associations into a single association? Defend your response. As part of your response, indicate what you think are the strengths and weaknesses of your position.

2. In this chapter, you have read about a number of different professional health education/promotion associations. On graduating from college, few new professionals have enough money to join several different professional groups. Assuming that you have enough money to join one national professional group on graduation, what association/organization would it be? Explain the reasoning you would use to select the one organization to join.

3. One of the major issues facing many professional health education/promotion associations is retaining members from year to year. Some members do not

renew their membership because of cost. Others do not renew because they do not feel that they receive enough benefits. After conducting a membership survey, a professional health association has decided to revamp the benefits provided to members. Assume that you have been appointed as a student member to the executive committee of the professional association and that the president of the association has charged the committee with revamping the membership benefits package. Each member of the executive committee has been asked to create a list of benefits. What would be on your list? Explain why you selected each item.

4. Throughout this book you have been introduced to the work of health education specialists. This chapter focused on the different professional organizations of our profession. We also presented information on the NCHEC. We stated that being a member of a professional organization is different from becoming certified as a health education specialist. Compare and contrast what you see to be the benefits of membership in a professional organization and becoming a CHES® or MCHES®. Aside from the financial costs, do you see any drawbacks of membership and certification?

Activities

1. Closely examine one professional health association/organization and prepare a PowerPoint presentation, poster, or other visual presentation on the history, mission, vision, and other critical information about that association/organization.

2. Interview two health education/promotion faculty members at your school and ask them the following:
   - Do they belong to any professional health education associations/organizations?
   - If they belong, why?
   - What benefits do they see in belonging to them?
   - What association/organization would they recommend that you join?

3. Does your school have a chapter of ESG? If not, make an appointment with the department head/chairperson to inquire about the possibility of starting one on your campus. Be prepared to discuss the benefits of establishing a chapter.

4. Write a one-page paper using the following two sentences to start the paper: "If I could join one professional health association/organization, it would be _____. My reasons for choosing that association/organization are _____."

5. Visit the website of the Coalition of National Health Education Organizations (CNHEO) (http://www.cnheo.org). Once at the site, read the "21st Century" reports: (1) *The Health Education Profession in the Twenty-First Century Progress Report 1995–2001*, (2) *Coalition of National Health Education Organization's 2nd Invitational Conference: Improving the Nation's Health Through Health Education—A Vision for the 21st Century*, and 3) *Profession-wide Strategic Plan*. After reading the reports, create your own list of five activities that you feel the profession should engage in during the next 10 years to move the profession forward. Provide a brief (i.e., a couple of paragraphs) rationale for why you included each activity on your list.

Weblinks

1. **http://www.astho.org**

   The Association for State and Territorial Health Officials (ASTHO)

   This is the website for the ASTHO, which is the national nonprofit organization representing the state and territorial public health agencies of the United States, the U.S. territories, and the District of Columbia. Among other items, this site includes links to each of the state and territorial health departments.

2. **http://www.cancer.org/**

   American Cancer Society (ACS)

   This is the homepage for ACS. The site presents the most up-to-date information on cancer, including treatment and prevention. The site also provides information about the ACS and the resources it can provide for cancer survivors and program planners.

3. **http://www.cnheo.org**

   Coalition of National Health Education Organizations (CNHEO)

   This is the homepage for CNHEO. At the site, you will find information about all of the member organizations, as well as the coalition's mission, goals, *Working Agreement*, the "Code of Ethics for the Health Education Profession," the "21st Century," and the "Profession Wide Strategic Plan" reports.

4. **https://www.heart.org/**

   American Heart Association (AHA)

   This is the home page for the AHA. The AHA provides health education specialists with a wealth of information and materials about many of the cardiovascular diseases and stroke.

5. **https://www.lung.org/**

   American Lung Association (ALA)

   This is the homepage for the ALA. The ALA provides information about various lung diseases, including asthma, chronic obstructive pulmonary disease (COPD), and lung cancer, and stopping smoking resources.

6. **http://www.welcoa.org**

   The Wellness Council of America (WELCOA)

   This is the homepage for the WELCOA. This site provides a variety of resources for those interested in worksite wellness programs.

7. **http://www.cdc.gov/**

   Centers for Disease Control and Prevention (CDC)

   This is the homepage of the CDC. This website includes information for the lay public (e.g., traveler's health and emergency preparedness) as well as information to assist health education specialists (e.g., CDC recommendations, *MMWR*, and special funded initiatives).

8. **http://www.nchec.org**

   National Commission for Health Education Credentialing, Inc.

   This is the homepage for NCHEC. At this site, you can find out more about the CHES® and MCHES® examinations, order publications to help you prepare for the examinations, and get up-to-date on individual credentialing.

   (Note: See Table 8.2 for the URLs of the various professional associations or organizations discussed in this chapter.)

References

American Academy for Health Behavior. (n.d.-a). *Health Behavior Research (HBR) Journal*. Retrieved November 22, 2020, from https://aahb.org/Health-Behavior-Research-HBR-Journal

American Academy for Health Behavior. (n.d.-b). *Mission statement*. Retrieved November 22, 2020, from https://aahb.org/mission_statement

American College Health Association. (n.d.-a). *About ACHA*. Retrieved November 14, 2020, from http://www.acha.org/ACHA/About/

American College Health Association. (n.d.-b). *Journal of American College Health*. Retrieved November 14, 2020, from https://www.acha.org/ACHA/Resources/JACH.aspx

American College Health Association. (n.d.-c). *Membership*. Retrieved November 14, 2020, from http://www.acha.org/ACHA/Membership/

American College Health Association. (n.d.-d). *Regional Affiliates*. Retrieved November 14, 2020, from http://www.acha.org/ACHA/Networks/Regional_Affiliates.aspx

American Public Health Association. (n.d.-a). *About APHA*. Retrieved on November 14, 2020, from https://www.apha.org/about-apha

American Public Health Association. (n.d.-b). *Member Sections*. November 14, 2020, from https://www.apha.org/apha-communities/member-sections

American Public Health Association. (n.d.-c). *Our Work*. Retrieved on November 14, 2020, from https://www.apha.org/About-APHA/Our-Work

American Public Health Association. (n.d.-d). *Publications & Periodicals*. Retrieved November 14, 2020, from https://www.apha.org/publications-and-periodicals

American School Health Association. (n.d.-a). *About*. Retrieved November 17, 2020, from https://www.ashaweb.org/about/

American School Health Association. (n.d.-b). *Journal of School Health*. Retrieved November 17, 2020, from https://www.ashaweb.org/resources/journal-of-school-health/

Capwell, E. M. (2004). Coalition of national health education organizations. *Californian Journal of Health Promotion, 2*(1), 12–15.

Coalition of National Health Education Organizations. (n.d.-a). Coalition of National Health Education Organizations. Retrieved June 28, 2021, from http://www.cnheo.org

Coalition of National Health Education Organizations. (n.d.-b). Member organization and delegates. Retrieved June 28, 2021, from http://www.cnheo.org/organizational-delegates.html

Coalition of National Health Education Organizations. (2003). *The health education profession in the twenty-first century*. http://www.cnheo.org/21stCentury.pdf

Coalition of National Health Education Organizations. (2021). CNHEO working agreement approved document 2.9.2021. Retrieved June 28, 2021, from https://drive.google.com/file/d/1H8xMlCdaS3XOkBc_CcfhMAY64cl02DAs/view

Eta Sigma Gamma. (1991, November). *Eta Sigma Gamma*. Muncie, IN: Author.

Foundation for the Advancement of Health Education. (n.d.). *History of success*. Retrieved January 16, 2021, from https://www.fahefoundation.org/history-of-success/

International Union for Health Promotion and Education. (n.d.-a). Global Health Promotion: *Introduction*. Retrieved November 22, 2020, from https://www.iuhpe.org/index.php/en/global-health-promotion/

International Union for Health Promotion and Education. (n.d.-b). *Mission*. Retrieved November 22, 2020, from http://www.iuhpe.org/index.php/en/iuhpe-at-a-glance/mission

International Union for Health Promotion and Education. (n.d.-c). *Projects*. Retrieved November 22, 2020, from http://www.iuhpe.org/index.php/en/projects

International Union for Health Promotion and Education. (n.d.-d). *Publications*. Retrieved November 22, 2020 from https://www.iuhpe.org/index.php/en/publications

National Commission for Health Education Credentialing, Inc. (NCHEC). (n.d.-a). *Health Education Job Analysis Projects*. Retrieved July 10, 2021 from https://www.nchec.org/HESPA

National Commission for Health Education Credentialing, Inc. (NCHEC). (n.d.-b). *Vision and Mission*. Retrieved November 22, 2020, from https://www.nchec.org/vision-and-mission

National Commission for Health Education Credentialing & Coalition of National Health Education Organizations. (1996). The health education profession in the 21st century: Setting the stage. *Journal of School Health, 66*(8), 291–298.

National Wellness Institute. (n.d.-a). *Join the voices of wellness*. Retrieved December 6, 2020, from https://nationalwellness.org/membership/

National Wellness Institute. (n.d.-b). *Our story*. Retrieved December 6, 2020, from https://nationalwellness.org/about-nwi/

Random House. (2020). Philanthropy. In Dictionary.com *Unabridged*. Retrieved November 11, 2020, from http://https://www.dictionary.com/browse/philanthropy

SHAPE America (Society of Health and Physical Educators). (n.d.-a). *About SHAPE America.* Retrieved November 22, 2020, from http://www.shapeamerica.org/about/

SHAPE America (Society of Health and Physical Educators). (n.d.-b). *Resources and publications.* Retrieved November 22, 2020, from https://www.shapeamerica.org/publications/resources/

Society for Public Health Education. (n.d.-a). *Communities of Practice.* Retrieved June 28, 2021, from https://www.sophe.org/membership/communities-of-practice/

Society for Public Health Education. (n.d.-b). *Journals.* Retrieved June 28, 2021, from https://www.sophe.org/journals

Society for Public Health Education. (n.d.-c). *Our mission.* Retrieved June 28, 2021, from https://www.sophe.org/about/mission

Society for Public Health Education. (n.d.-d). *Publications.* Retrieved June 28, 2021, from https://www.sophe.org/publications

Society for Public Health Education. (n.d.-e). *SOPHE chapters.* Retrieved June 28, 2021, from https://www.sophe.org/membership/sophe-chapters

Society of State Leaders of Health and Physical Education. (n.d.-a). *About the society.* Retrieved November 22, 2020, from https://thesociety.org/about-us

Society of State Leaders of Health and Physical Education. (n.d.-b). *Mission.* Retrieved November 22, 2020, from https://thesociety.org/mission

Werch, C. E. (2000). Editorial: What use, the American Academy of Health Behavior? *American Journal of Health Behavior, 24*(1), 3–5.

Young, K. J., & Boling, W. (2004). Improving the quality of professional life: Benefits of health education and promotion association membership. *Californian Journal of Health Promotion, 2*(1), 39–44.

CHAPTER 9

The Literature of Health Education/Promotion

CHAPTER OBJECTIVES

After reading this chapter and answering the questions at the end, you should be able to:

- Describe the difference between a *primary*, a *secondary*, a *tertiary*, and a *popular press* literature source.
- Write an abstract or a summary of an article from a peer-reviewed journal.
- Critique a journal article using a logical sequence of questions.
- Identify leading journals in the field of health education/promotion.
- Identify the valid online computerized databases for finding health education/promotion information.
- Locate an article related to some aspect of health education/promotion using an online database.
- Conduct an Internet search for information about a health-related topic using one of the website URLs listed in the chapter.
- Critique the validity of the information obtained from searching a site on the Internet.

In her work as a health education special-ist, Georgia administers a federally funded statewide center that distributes prevention information on alcohol, tobacco, and other drugs. Materials in the center include mono-graphs containing the results of research studies on possible treatment protocols and prevention interventions; prevention and education materials from a variety of federal, state, and nonprofit agencies; information on evidence-based practice in both prevention and treatment; and an extensive video library. Almost daily, she and her staff receive requests for information from law enforcement agen-cies, legislators and organizational policymak-ers, community groups, school personnel, counselors, nonprofit organizations, treatment professionals, state agencies, churches, and individual patrons.

Over the past four years, more university health education/promotion students have been visiting to acquire materials for class projects, research studies, or potential thesis topics. These students often request Georgia or her staff to recommend the most up-to-date primary and secondary source materials and the most reputable websites related to sub-stance abuse prevention.

After reading and applying the informa-tion contained in this chapter, you should be able to address questions similar to those received by the staff of the center previously described. Selecting quality health information (Responsibility 6 Communication) is a critical skill that must be acquired by those practicing as health education specialists.

The amount of information about any given topic is growing at an almost exponential rate. Terms such as *information overload* and *information burnout* are being heard more and more. Arguably, the area in which information is growing fastest and in which there is tremendous public interest is health. People today seem obsessed with gathering information about such health topics as diet,

exercise, stress management, vitamins, drugs, sexuality, depression, safety, disease, violence prevention, healthcare policies, health insurance options, and the cost of medical procedures or prescription drugs.

The increasing demand for information, coupled with the fact that data are being produced at an ever greater rate, creates an added need for health education specialists (see Practitioner's Perspective). Two of the major responsibilities of a health education specialist, as discussed in Chapter 6, involve communication (Responsibility 6)

Practitioner's Perspective

Health Education Literature: Ellen Robertson, PhD, MCHES®

CURRENT POSITION: Project Director for Alabama Provider Capacity Project

EMPLOYER: The University of Alabama, School of Social Work VitAL Initiative

DEGREE INFORMATION: PhD in Health Education and Health Promotion (The University of Alabama '09)

MA in Curriculum and Educational Technology (Ball State University '20)

MS in Wellness (University of Mississippi '98)

BS in Exercise Physiology (Mississippi University for Women '94)

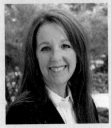

Courtesy of Ellen Robertson.

How I obtained my job: After graduation with my MS degree, I struggled to find my niche in health education. I started teaching part-time and ultimately decided to pursue additional education. At the conclusion of my doctorate, I started teaching full-time. However, I was missing some valuable practical experience in the field. After a few years, an opportunity opened up to work as a Health Promotion Manager at an Air Force base. This position provided me with vast experience using the responsibilities and competencies of a health education specialist. I worked to improve the health of active duty members, families, and retirees. It was a broad audience that provided both great rewards and challenges. After gaining this practical experience, I decided to go back into teaching at the university level. I taught online for seven years; however, I was a casualty of the COVID cutbacks. My position was cut due to funding in July of 2020. I spent many days consulting with peers and contemplating what I wanted to achieve from my next job. I decided to apply for different types of positions within the health education/promotion field. In September of 2020, I was hired to be the project director of the Alabama Provider Capacity Project (APCP) grant within VitAL initiative housed in the School of Social Work at The University of Alabama. VitAL's mission is to improve wellness in Alabama through engagement, collaboration, research, and education. This was a perfect fit for me and utilized the totality of my experience. Through the hard time of COVID cutbacks, I was able to find a position that challenged me, provided me with the opportunity to help change behavior, and educate on health topics.

Describe the duties of your current position: The duties of my position include managing all aspects of a $5 million federal grant. I have daily oversight of Alabama's Demonstration Project to Increase Substance Use Provider Capacity. I work directly with the Substance Use Treatment and

Recovery team to ensure program fidelity as related to the grant guidelines and requirements. A large portion of my duties include maintaining data and reporting requirements and professional documentation. I assist with analyzing data and creating reports of the findings for stakeholders of the project. I also oversee meetings and collaborations between multiple groups who focus on different aspects of the grant. I conduct research to identify gaps and lead the development of implementation activities based on best practices in the field. A main aspect of the job is the development of training and educational materials for providers and substance use disorder treatment professionals. I also play a huge role in the development of a learning management system and online courses to serve the needs of Substance Use Disorder (SUD) professionals to better serve those living in Alabama.

How I utilize health education and the health literature in my job: The most challenging part of my job is thinking creatively about the evolution of initiatives. As a person who is most definitely a "follow the rules" and "inside the box thinker," I rely on research and literature. Others, who are markedly more creative than me, have described tools and ideas that are proven and seen as best practices in the field. One positive outcome of using literature to guide efforts is that executives and funders have confidence in the proven, applied, and best practice efforts. In other words, you can use literature to justify implementation endeavors and provide a logical rationale for initiatives. In my job as a project director, I search the literature for help with almost every aspect of a program. I research the topic area; in this case it is substance use disorders. I research ideas, treatments, prevention, data use, and gaps in services. I also utilize literature to assess the needs of the priority population such as to determine health status, factors that impact health, available resources, and state policies.

What I like most about my job: There are so many things that I like about my job. I love the concrete objective nature of the position. There are so many deadlines and specific objectives; there is no guessing as to what I am supposed to achieve. I love the ever-changing nature of the job; there are so many moving parts; it never gets boring. I love helping people and through this grant, I can see the direct impact on the person, city, and state of Alabama.

What I like least about my job: I really enjoy my job, and there is not much that I do not like. But in choosing one thing I like least, it would be the time constraints of working through a grant. Each grant has a finite amount of time to achieve the goals set forth and a finite employment period. This causes a lot of stress both personally and professionally. However, these are also things I like about the job. I like the ability to set a timeline for accomplishments and the finite employment period allows me to work on different grants, which increases my professional excitement.

Recommendations for those preparing to be health education specialists: My number one recommendation for those entering the health education field is to volunteer to serve the profession. This may be done within a professional organization, the community, or within a particular work setting. My volunteering is through the National Commission for Health Education Credentialing (NCHEC). I have served on a division board, the board of commissioners, and the marketing committee. This has given me a "look behind the curtain" of the profession and helped me to understand where we come from and where we are hoping to go. It is hard to get such a view from professional preparation courses alone, and this view helps with application of the knowledge obtained within the courses. Learn to be proficient in using literature; you will definitely need this skill on the job.

The role of the health education specialist in the future: The role of the health education specialist is evolving. When I was in school, I had this idea that health education specialists can work in a hospital, teach, and teach gym. I was so wrong. As I have been in the field for over 10 years, I have discovered there are many opportunities for us to work in the workplace, colleges, private sector, grantsmanship, nursing homes, and so many more. There is not a one-size-fits-all area for health education specialists. We will have a huge role in the community in the coming years. COVID has enlightened many on the benefits of maintaining health and creating policy, both of which have the potential to reduce healthcare costs. Health education specialists will have an essential role in the future; we need to continuing expanding our reach and "thinking outside the box."

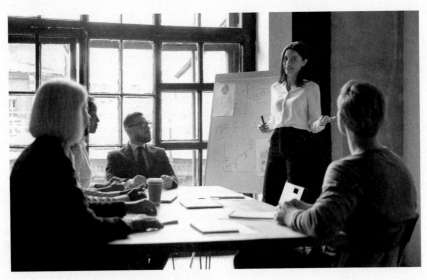

Figure 9.1 Health education specialists often make presentations to community groups.
© fizkes/Shutterstock.

and advocating to others about health education needs, concerns, and resources (Responsibility 5) (see **Figure 9.1**). When seeking out current and accurate information, the health education specialist must be able to find and evaluate its credibility. Then the facts and ideas are disseminated to consumers through appropriate channels and explained in a manner that is meaningful to the intended audience. This chapter introduces prospective health education students to the most common sources of health-related information used by health education specialists. It also describes how to access the subject matter from these sources. When searching for valid and reliable materials, it is always wise to seek the assistance of a reference librarian if questions arise.

Types of Information Sources

When accessing information, it is important to note whether the source is primary, secondary, or tertiary. **Primary sources** of data or information are published studies or

eyewitness accounts written by the people who actually conducted the experiments or observed the events in question. A journal that publishes original manuscripts only after they have been read by a panel of experts in the field (peer-reviewers) and recommended for publication is termed a **peer-reviewed journal or refereed**. Examples of primary sources are research articles written by the researcher(s); personal records (autobiographies); podcasts or video/audio recordings of actual lectures (which may also be secondary sources depending on whether the information presented is the speakers' own work [primary] or a compilation of the works of self and others [secondary]); speeches, debates, or events; official records of legislative sessions or minutes of community meetings; newspaper eyewitness accounts; and annual reports.

Of note is the fact that some peer-reviewed journals now are published only in electronic format. Some of these electronic journals follow the subscription-only format of their print counterparts. Other electronic journals are **open-access journals** that come in a variety of reader-access levels. Some articles are immediately available to individual subscribers or subscribing institutions; others allow delayed access to articles for anyone with an Internet connection; and some of the publishing sites have a mixture of the two availability types. The "open access" designation means that the article is copyrighted but generally can be used more liberally than articles with more traditional copyrights. Databases such as BioMed Central (biomedcentral.com) are repositories of these types of journals, many of which are new and most of which use scientists who have been editorial board members on highly prestigious paper-based journals for their editorial review boards. The increased cost of paper-based journals and publishing company charges will undoubtedly expand the number of electronic-only primary sources of information in the future.

Secondary sources are usually written by someone who was not present at the event or did not participate as part of the study team. The value of these sources is that they often provide a summary of several related studies or chronicle a history or sequence of events. The writers of secondary sources may also provide editorial comments or alternative interpretations of the study or event. Secondary sources often provide a bibliography of primary sources. Examples of secondary sources are journal review articles, editorials, and non-eyewitness accounts of events occurring in the community, region, or nation.

Although peer-reviewed journals usually publish primary source articles, they occasionally contain secondary source articles. The types of secondary source articles most likely to be found in a peer-reviewed journal are articles summarizing the results of several studies, editorials, or positions deemed important enough (by a panel of expert reviewers) to be interesting and useful to those who read the journal.

Tertiary sources contain information that has been distilled and collected from primary and secondary sources. Examples include handbooks, informational pamphlets or brochures from governmental organizations

(or hospitals, or national nongovernmental agencies such as the American Cancer Society or March of Dimes), newsletters such as the Nutrition Action Letter, almanacs, encyclopedias, fact books, dictionaries, abstracts, and other reference tools. At this stage, information from such sources is accepted as fact by the scientific community. The operative word in the preceding sentence is *fact*. Information that has no documentation and is laced with opinion or intended for marketing a service or product is not considered a tertiary source; publications of that type are classified as popular press sources.

A fourth source of health information, **popular press publications**, is probably the most difficult to check for credibility. Popular press publications range from weekly summary-type magazines (e.g., *Time, Newsweek,* and *U.S. News & World Report*), regular articles in newspapers (e.g., Dr. Oz's column), and newspaper supplements (e.g., *Parade*) to monthly magazines (e.g., *Shape, Prevention,* and *Men's Health*) and tabloids (e.g., *The Star, People,* and *Us* Weekly). At times, any of these may contain a primary source of information (as in an interview). Most often; however, they are secondary sources at best. Often, articles in the popular press include opinions or editorials that express the bias of the author or the editor of the publication. Popular press articles should be heavily scrutinized as to the source of the information before being cited as authentic and accurate.

Before concluding this discussion, it is important to note that, with the exception of open access journals, no website references were included in the literature types described. This is because websites are generally not peer reviewed. Just about anyone can publish an article on the Internet without an impartial reader or group of readers reviewing it beforehand. To be sure, websites are often wonderful sources of information, but they can just as often be replete with bad information. A discussion of methods to determine the accuracy of material on the Internet is included later in this chapter. Sorting through the maze of health information can be a daunting task, even for the most skilled health education specialist. To equip the health education specialist to assume the responsibilities of providing and disseminating information, several tasks need to be mastered. The next several sections of this chapter are designed to provide background for the student in (1) identifying the components of a research article; (2) critically reading a research article; (3) ascertaining the accuracy of the information in non–research-based articles or are from secondary or popular press sources; (4) writing an abstract or a summary of a journal article; (5) identifying and locating primary and secondary sources most commonly used by health education specialists using indexes, abstracts, and computerized databases; and (6) retrieving health-related information on the Internet.

Identifying the Components of a Research Article

A research article usually begins with an abstract, which is a brief description of the study's results. The abstract describes the research questions that were tested, outlines the study design, and lists one or two major findings from the study. The abstract is meant to communicate essential information, so that readers will know whether the study has information related to the topic they are interested in. An example of an abstract (Hibbard & Greene, 2013) follows:

Patient engagement is an increasingly important component of strategies to reform health care. In this article, we review the available evidence of the contribution that patient activation—the skills and confidence that equip patients to become actively engaged in their health care—makes to health outcomes, costs, and patient experience. There is a growing body of evidence showing that patients who are more activated have better health outcomes and care experiences, but there is limited evidence to date about the impact on costs. Emerging evidence indicates that interventions that tailor support to the individual's level of activation, and that build skills and confidence, are effective in increasing patient activation. Furthermore, patients who start at the lowest activation levels tend to increase the most. We conclude that policies and interventions aimed at strengthening patients' roles in managing their health care can contribute to improved outcomes and that patient activation can—and should—be measured as an intermediate outcome of care that is linked to improved outcomes. (p. 207)

The paper's Introduction, which sometimes is divided into subsections, follows the abstract. Its purpose is usually threefold: (1) to give readers a more detailed description of the research question(s) or hypotheses being tested, (2) to review related literature, and (3) to explain the need for or the significance of the study. This section communicates the rationale behind the researchers' decision to conduct the study.

The methodology section comes directly after the introductory material. In this section, there is usually a description of (1) the research design used, (2) the subjects who took part in the research, (3) the instruments used to gather the data necessary to answer the research questions, and (4) any administrative procedures involved in conducting the research, such as methods used to select the subject(s), gather the data, or protect the rights of the subject(s).

Following the methodology section are the results and discussion sections. The results section gives the research findings by describing the results of the statistical procedures used in analyzing the data (in the case of studies involving quantitative methods—methods involving the analyses of numerical data) and provides an overall answer to the research questions or hypotheses that were described in the introductory section. The discussion section provides a forum for the researcher to interpret the conclusions and meanings and to comment on the implications of the data analyses. In addition, the researcher often includes a narrative about the limitations of the study and makes recommendations for further research on the topic.

Critically Reading a Research Article

The volume of articles on any single health topic continues to escalate. It is important to be able to evaluate the information for accuracy and significance from sources of all types. Research articles serve as primary sources of valuable information for health education specialists. Beginning students in the field of health education/promotion are not expected to be able to immediately understand every nuance in a research article. It is essential, however, to begin to frequently read scientific reports and journal articles to become familiar with their style. Often, preformulating generic questions suitable for critiquing any study can help when evaluating study results. The following is a sequence of questions found to be of help when such an evaluation is necessary. The list is adapted from (Subramanyam, 2013)

1. What were the aims and objectives of the research study?
2. What was the research/study hypothesis?
3. Who were the subjects, how were they recruited and how was the sampling done
4. Were the design and location of the study described clearly?
5. Were the data collection instruments described and appropriate?
6. Were reliability and validity reported for the instruments?
7. Did the results answer the research questions or hypotheses?
8. Were the tables and figures understandable and help explain the results?
9. Were the conclusions reasonable and based on the data and analyses performed?
10. Were the conclusions reasonable, logical and useful to other researchers/practitioners?
11. Were the study implications meaningful to the population you serve?

The final test comes when students can read an article and begin to view themselves in the position of a reporter who has the task of describing the study, its findings, and its limitations to an audience in no more than five minutes. People who can restate study findings and limitations in their own words have accomplished much in becoming critical consumers of scientific and nonscientific literature as well as better resources for others.

Evaluating the Accuracy of Non–Research-Based Sources

As with journal articles that are research based, it is important to be able to evaluate whether the information presented is reliable, regardless of the source. Cottrell (1997) conducted a search for instruments that could assist him in teaching his students to assess the accuracy of information found in almost any type of journal or magazine. The six questions are still relevant today:

1. What are the author's qualifications? Does the person have an academic degree in the field being written about? (A note of caution—a degree does not make someone absolutely qualified, but it provides evidence that *suggests* that the person is qualified.)

2. What is the style of presentation? Look for health information written in a scientific style of writing, not a style that uses generalities or testimonials.

3. Are references included? A well-written article provides references to the primary sources used. Be aware when someone is writing about another person's research because that individual may be interpreting the results in a different way than the author did.

4. What is the purpose of the publication? Be aware of publications, news or otherwise, that contain advertisements designed to sell items discussed in the articles.

5. What is the reputation of the publication? Is it peer reviewed? Professional journals are good sources of information. Popular press publications can sometimes have poor information related to health issues.

6. Is the information new? When reading for the first time, be skeptical. Information must be validated over time. New information is newsworthy but may not be valid.

It is important to realize that becoming a skeptical, critical consumer of printed and web-based health information is an important first step in being seen by others as credible. For the public to use the expertise and training of health education specialists to a greater degree, the health education specialist must develop a reputation for providing accurate and current information.

Writing an Abstract or a Summary

Another valuable skill when reading and interpreting health-related literature of any kind (primary, secondary, tertiary, or popular press) involves learning to write an abstract or a summary of an article. Although abstracts and summaries are both short forms of describing a research study, the major differences lie in the extent of the content. Abstracts are short (usually 150–250 words). They are written to identify the purpose of the research, the study questions, the methods used by the researcher, and one or two major findings. Summaries, on the other hand, may be two to three pages in length and include all of the elements of the abstract. In addition, summaries are meant to reveal any secondary findings, to describe study limitations, and to provide a more detailed review of the researcher's conclusions and recommendations from the viewpoint of the summary's author.

It is recommended that beginning health education specialists practice writing both abstracts and summaries of the articles they read. Using this technique sharpens the ability of the health education specialist to discriminate between health-related articles that are reliable and credible for health education/promotion and those that contain erroneous or misleading claims or information.

Locating Health-Related Information

Health education specialists serve as major health information resource persons for many constituencies. It does not matter if they are employed in the school, the clinic, the worksite, or the community setting. In all cases, inquiries from a variety of people wanting to know about a health topic or wanting interpretation of the latest research findings are directed to health education specialists. Therefore, it is essential that the latter be knowledgeable about how to find the information requested. The next section identifies resources that health education specialists can use to locate information on health education/promotion and explains how to access it.

Journals

As has been previously mentioned, much of the evidence that health education specialists use to make decisions when planning, implementing, and evaluating health promotion programs can be found in journals that publish primary research articles and position papers about health topics and health programs. The following are examples of journals commonly used by health professionals. The list by no means includes all journals of benefit to the health education specialist.

1. ***AIDS Education and Prevention.*** An international journal designed to support the efforts of professionals working to prevent HIV and AIDS, *AIDS Education and Prevention* includes scientific articles by leading authorities from many disciplines, research reports on the effectiveness of new strategies and programs, debates about key issues, and reviews of books and video resources. The journal also covers a wide range of public health, psychosocial, ethical, and public policy concerns related to HIV and AIDS.

2. ***American Journal of Health Behavior*** (formerly ***Health Values***). Articles feature research about the impact of personal behavior patterns and practices on health promotion. The journal emphasizes efforts at fostering a better understanding of the multidisciplinary interface of systems and individuals as they impact behavior. Examples of successful multidisciplinary approaches to improving health at the community level are featured. Only available online after 2009.

3. ***American Journal of Health Education.*** Includes research findings, community health intervention and learning strategies, and health promotion strategies. Some articles are designed as self-study courses.

4. ***American Journal of Health Promotion.*** This journal features original research articles, the testing of health behavioral theory on selected populations, and program evaluation. It is an excellent source of worksite health promotion articles.

5. ***American Journal of Public Health.*** Published by the American Public Health Association, this journal features reports related to health research, program evaluations, and health policy analysis, as well as articles on special topics on the health of selected groups and communities.

6. ***Evaluation and the Health Professions.*** Articles generally focus on practitioner-friendly research related to the development, implementation, and evaluation of community-based health programs. Healthcare researchers and evaluators can find examples of state-of-the-art tools and methods for conducting meaningful evaluations.

7. ***Family and Community Health.*** Presents creative, multidisciplinary perspectives and approaches for effective public and community health programs. Issues focus on a single topic and addresses problems of concern to a wide variety of population groups with diverse ethnic backgrounds, including children and the elderly, men and women, and rural and urban communities.

8. ***Health Affairs.*** This journal is published bimonthly and features health policy-related articles of national concern or interest. The journal serves as a major source of primary research concerning healthcare coverage, health economics, health reform, and the impact of policy on the health of the populace.

9. ***The Health Educator: The Journal of Eta Sigma Gamma.*** Published by Eta Sigma Gamma, the health education honor society, this journal includes articles related to most health education/promotion topics in a variety of settings. Many of the studies and commentaries are submitted by students in health education/promotion and/or public health programs.

10. ***The Hastings Center Report.*** This journal focuses on the ethical, social, legal, and economic factors in health policy, medicine, healthcare delivery, and public health.

11. ***Health Education & Behavior*** (formerly ***Health Education Quarterly***). The official publication of the Society for Public Health

Education, Inc. (SOPHE), its articles center on health behavior and education, case studies in health, program evaluation, and strategies to improve social and behavioral health. Each submission includes a commentary on the application of findings to the practice setting.

12. **Health Education Research.** Official publication of the International Union for Health Promotion and Education and features articles concerning health promotion program planning, implementation, and evaluation. Articles focus on application of results in the practice of health promotion.

13. **Health Promotion International.** The majority of research studies and commentaries are on issues related to health promotion in schools, clinics, worksites, and communities located outside of the United States. Unique to this journal is the fact that submissions describing spontaneous activities, organizational change interventions, and social and environmental development are featured too.

14. **Health Promotion Practice.** Publishes articles devoted to the practical application of health promotion and education in a variety of settings including community, health care, educational, worksite, and international. Articles focus on best practices and their application to health policies that promote health and disease prevention.

15. **Global Journal for Health Education and Promotion (GJHEP)** (formerly **The International Electronic Journal of Health Education**). Features articles on nearly every aspect of health education, including school health, community health, worksite health promotion, the ethical implications of health education, and the philosophy of health education. Published by Sagamore Publishing.

16. **The Journal of American College Health.** Published by the American College Health Association in cooperation with Heldref Publications, its articles are limited to those that relate to health promotion or health service provision in the college or university environment. This is the *only* journal written by college health professionals for college health professionals.

17. **Journal of Community Health.** This journal features articles relating to the practice, teaching, and research of community health; preventive medicine; and analysis of delivery of healthcare services.

18. **Journal of Health Communication.** This journal is published eight times a year. It presents the latest developments in the field of health communication, including research in risk communication, health literacy, social marketing, communication (from interpersonal to mass media), psychology, government, policymaking, and health education around the world.

19. **Journal of Nutrition Education and Behavior.** The official publication of the Society of Nutrition Education and Behavior, this journal publishes articles that are germane to the interface between nutrition education and behavior as practiced worldwide. It serves as a resource for anyone interested in nutrition education or diet and physical behavior.

20. **Journal of School Health.** Published for the American School Health Association, articles in this journal are related to the public or private school setting from pre-K through grade 12. Articles generally focus on children's health issues but may include information related to other aspects of coordinated school health programs.

21. **Global Health Promotion.** This is an official publication of the International Union for Health Promotion and Education (IUHPE), published by Sage Publications. Most issues are topical in nature (e.g., environmental health, population health, and infectious disease prevention) and feature articles related to the application of public health and health promotion in countries around the globe. Articles are published in several languages.

22. **National *Journal of Rural Health.*** Published by Wiley-Blackwell Publishing, Inc. for the Rural Health Association, this journal's articles focus on professional practice, research, theory development, and policy issues related to health in the rural setting.

23. ***Pedagogy in Health Promotion: The Scholarship of Teaching and Learning.*** A quarterly journal first published in 2016. Curriculum and course design, assessment, and administration relevant to teaching and learning are topics that provide focal points for articles in this publication.

24. ***Public Health Reports.*** Published by the Association of Schools of Public Health, this journal reports findings from many avenues of research related to health services acquisition, health policy development, and health promotion at the community level.

25. ***Health Behavior and Policy Review.*** A bi-monthly journal that was first published in January of 2014. The journal features articles on policy development impacting health behaviors that are population rather than individual focused. Research guiding policy development and prioritizing health policy choices is also a focus.

Indexes and Abstracts

Indexes and **abstracts** provide links to articles from many peer-reviewed journals, books, and research reports. An index references articles from journals, books, and reports pertaining to topics that fall under the subject headings for which the index was created (e.g., health behavior, physical activity, methamphetamine treatment, or corporate health education/promotion programs). An abstract provides somewhat similar information but also includes short summaries of the article's content to help the researcher determine whether the article contains the information they are seeking.

Although some indexes and abstracts can still be found in hard copy, many are online or electronic formats. The cost of publishing paper versions plus the ease of user access to online materials is reducing the number of paper-version editions of either indexes or abstracts. *Index Medicus*, an abstract that has been printed for more than a century, is an example of a publication that is no longer available in paper copy because of the high cost of printing the volumes. In its place, the National Library of Medicine and the National Institutes of Health have created a site (http://www.ncbi.nlm.nih.gov/pubmed/) that combines the information formerly available in *Index Medicus* with many other sources to create a database that is accessible to anyone with a computer.

Government Documents

The U.S. Government Printing Office (GPO) publishes volumes of materials of use to health education specialists. This section (adapted from the University of Akron library website [University of Akron, n.d.]) is meant to provide a generic description of the types of documents that can be accessed in the government documents section of an academic library. Because each library has slightly different procedures for finding these documents, students are encouraged to communicate with the government documents librarian at their university for the specifics on locating documents. It should be noted that the U.S. government is shifting away from issuing paper copies and is increasing the number of documents available online.

Government publications range from official documents including laws, court decisions, and records of congressional actions to the results of government-sponsored technical and scientific studies. Information on topics such as obesity, water treatment, or exercise can also be found in a government documents section.

Government documents are not organized under the same classification scheme as a traditional general collection. Instead, they are organized and shelved according to Superintendent of Documents (SuDocs) numbers. The SuDocs number is unique in that it has a colon. For example, A1:1 is an annual report from the Agriculture Department. Numbers of the documents are arranged alphabetically by agency, and the numbers are whole numbers, not decimals (e.g., HE 1.6 comes before HE 1.9). The letter that begins the SuDocs number signifies the publishing agency, as noted:

A	Agriculture Department
C	Census Bureau
ED	Department of Education
HE	Health and Human Services
NA	National Academy of Science
X–Y	Congress

Government documents contain a storehouse of valuable and current information and should not be overlooked when seeking information on a health topic of interest. Most libraries have online search capabilities for government documents, so as with many traditional sources of information, accessing them has become much less labor intensive.

Electronic Databases

Electronic databases often provide a preferred alternative to manually searching indexes or abstracts (see **Figure 9.2**). As mentioned previously, most, if not all, of the publishers of the hardcopy abstracts and indexes either have converted or are converting their documents to an online format. Much like an index or abstract, each database has a general subject area (e.g., medicine, education, psychology, and community health). The electronic database provides access via the Internet. Computer searches using databases are significantly faster than manual searches, and they have the advantage of enabling the user to link several concepts together to provide focus for a search.

For example, if a person wanted to search for articles about "health behavior" and the influence of "health communication" on behavior, an electronic database would allow the user to enter both terms into the computer and connect them by placing the word *and* between them. The result will be to eliminate any articles that do not have both *health behavior* and *health communication* as key terms. Other terms can be used to further narrow a search to be as specific as desired. The main concern the computer database user faces is to accurately specify the key terms associated with the information desired, so the resulting list of references that is generated will be of use. Computerized searches require little computer knowledge; however, it is always advisable to seek the assistance of a librarian when beginning to seek information. Users should also know that just because the information is readily available online, it is not necessarily free. Academic libraries spend hundreds of thousands of dollars per year to ensure that students and faculty have access to the free or low-cost materials they need. The databases most used by health education specialists are

1. **ERIC (Education Resource Information Center).** It includes the *Current Index to Journals in Education (CIJE)* and *Resources in Education (RIE)*. ERIC is sponsored by the U.S. Department of Education. It is an online resource that indexes journal articles, books, and grey literature pertaining to educational research.

2. **MEDLINE.** This is the premier biomedicine database indexing more than 3,000 journals. It covers the fields of medicine, nursing, dentistry, veterinary medicine, and preclinical sciences. MEDLINE is also the commercial version of PubMed. The major differences between the two versions are that PubMed goes back before 1966, uses a different search platform, indexes books available on the NCBI bookshelf, and indexes prepublication journal articles.

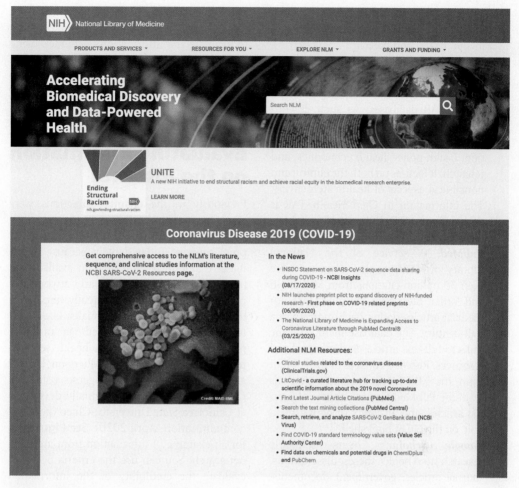

Figure 9.2 Electronic databases such as the National Library of Medicine (NLM) provide ready access to information on a particular topic.

Courtesy of the U.S. National Library of Medicine.

3. ***ScienceDirect.*** This is one of the largest full-text scientific databases in the world covering physical sciences, life sciences, health sciences, and engineering material. It indexes more than 2,500 peer-reviewed journals and over 42,000 e-books, books, major reference books and book series.

4. **CINAHL Database.** CINAHL indexes nursing and allied health from 1983 to the present. It indexes over 5,000 journals. The database also provides access to books,

book chapters, nursing dissertations, selected conference proceedings, some audiovisuals, and standards of practice.

5. ***ETHXWeb.*** This database covers the years 1974–2009 and is no longer being updated. Topics include ethical, legal, and public policy issues surrounding health care and biomedical research. Citations are derived from the literature of law, religion, ethics, social sciences, philosophy, the popular media, and the health sciences.

6. **PsycINFO.** This is the largest database of peer-reviewed literature in the areas of mental health and behavior sciences.

7. **Ovid Healthstar.** Ovid Healthstar includes data from the National Library of Medicine's (NLM) MEDLINE and former HealthSTAR databases. As such, it contains citations of the published literature in health services, technology, administration, health policy, health economics, and research. It focuses on both the clinical and nonclinical aspects of healthcare delivery. The information in Ovid HealthSTAR is derived from MEDLINE, the Hospital Literature Index, and selected journals.

8. **PubMed.** A service of the National Library of Medicine that contains more than 30 million citations from MEDLINE and other lifescience journals for biomedical articles dating back more than a half-century. The database includes some links to full-text articles and other related resources. PubMed consists of the content from the MEDLINE database, citations from the PubMed Central archive of journal articles, and an index of books available on the NCBI bookshelf.

9. **Google Scholar.** Covers scholarly research from books, theses, dissertations, journal articles, government documents, etc. It indexes professional societies, online repositories, university sites, government websites, etc. If you use settings, you can customize it to link to your university library's resources.

Application Scenario

Assume you are a newly employed health education specialist in a hospital outpatient clinic. One of your jobs is to provide information to patients after they have seen the physician. A skeptical Ms. X has just been diagnosed with coronary artery disease, and the physician has sent her to you to discuss the impact of lifestyle on her condition. Search for several sources of information that you could give her to read that might assist you with the education process. Make certain to evaluate the information's accuracy using the criteria in the section that follows because it is highly likely Ms. X will need some assurance that the information you are providing her is accurate.

Evaluating Information on the Internet

Previously in the chapter, directions were given for evaluating the accuracy and validity of information from journal and popular press sources. Today, largely because of the massive amount of information available on the Internet and because nearly anyone can publish on the Web, it is equally imperative that the health education specialist know how to evaluate material obtained via an Internet search. T. J. Madden, a health sciences reference specialist in the Albertson Library at Boise State University, suggests using the CRAAP test, which was originally developed at California State University, Chico (personal communication, April 2020). See **Figure 9.3** for an example of information from an Internet search. You can use the criteria below to evaluate the credibility of the information shown on the website.

Evaluation Criteria

Currency: *The timeliness of the information.*

- When was the information published or posted?
- Has the information been revised or updated?
- Does your topic require current information or will older sources work as well?
- Are the links functional?

Relevance: *The importance of the information for your needs.*

- Does the information relate to your topic or answer your question?

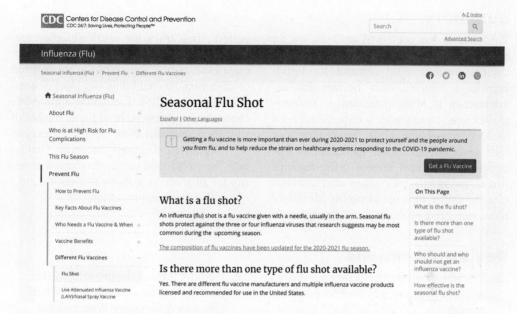

Figure 9.3 Centers for Disease Control and Prevention website with information about the flu vaccine.

Reproduced from Centers for Disease Control and Prevention. (n.d.). *Seasonal flu shot.* Retrieved April 8, 2021, from https://www.cdc.gov/flu/prevent/flushot.htm

- Who is the intended audience?
- Is the information at an appropriate level (i.e., not too elementary or advanced for your needs)? Have you looked at a variety of sources before determining this is one you will use?
- Would you be comfortable citing this source in your research paper?

Authority: *The source of the information.*

- Who is the author, publisher, source, or sponsor?
- What are the author's credentials or organizational affiliations?
- Is the author qualified to write on the topic?
- Is there contact information, such as a publisher or email address?
- Does the URL reveal anything about the author or source? (examples: .com, .edu, .gov, .org, or .net)

Accuracy: *The reliability, truthfulness, and correctness of the content.*

- Where does the information come from?
- Is the information supported by evidence?

- Has the information been peer reviewed?
- Can you verify any of the information in another source or from personal knowledge?
- Does the language or tone seem unbiased and free of emotion?
- Are there spelling, grammar, or typographical errors?

Purpose: *The reason the information exists.*

- What is the purpose of the information?
- Is it to inform, teach, sell, entertain, or persuade?
- Do the authors or sponsors make their intentions or purpose clear?
- Is the information fact, opinion, or propaganda?
- Does the point of view appear objective and impartial?

SIFT is another great resource to help you spot online misinformation. SIFT was created by Mike Caulfield, a digital literacy expert at Washington State University in Vancouver (Caulfield, 2019).

Summary

This chapter has presented an overview on accessing and evaluating health-related information. An increasing demand for health knowledge, coupled with the fact that the information is being produced at an ever-greater rate, creates added responsibility for health education specialists. Two of the major roles of health education specialists as discussed in Chapter 6 involve being resource people for health information and communicating with others about health education/promotion needs, concerns, and resources. To perform these tasks, the health education specialist must have the skills to find information, must evaluate the source of the information to determine its credibility, and must disseminate the information through the appropriate channels to consumers. In addition, the health education specialist must be able to explain the information effectively. Becoming familiar with the tools found in this chapter is a necessity for all students wanting to enter the field of health education/promotion.

Review Questions

1. Describe the difference between primary, secondary, tertiary, and popular press sources.
2. How do an article abstract and an article summary differ in content?
3. What are the questions you should ask yourself when critiquing a journal article? What are the differences between the questions asked when evaluating a primary research article and those asked when evaluating a secondary source or popular press article?
4. Pick any three of the previously listed journals that focus on the field of health education/promotion. What types of information would you expect to find in each of the journals you named?
5. What advantage might the information from a government document have over another source on the same topic?
6. How does one go about evaluating information retrieved from the Internet?

Case Study

As a health education/promotion major, you have just finished studying about the Responsibilities and Competencies for Entry-Level Health Education Specialists (found in Appendix B of this text). During this unit, the instructor invited a group of practicing health education specialists to the class to participate in a panel discussion on the validity of the various roles in the real-life practice of health education/promotion.

Following the presentation, each of the panelists offered to host two to three students from the class for four hours per week for three weeks at their place of work. This opportunity resulted from student questions to the panelists concerning their desire to transfer the classroom learning to the work setting. Several of the students expressed frustration at what they perceived to be the emphasis on theory and the lack of application in their courses and coursework. The panelists readily conceded that the 12-hour block of time each student would spend at the worksite with them would not totally solve theory-practical application problems, but they hoped it might help the students to see that, at least in the case of the majority of the responsibilities and competencies, what they studied about in class was what the health education specialist was doing.

After a quick meeting between the instructor and the panel members, placement assignments were made for the students. Because of your interest in becoming a health education specialist in a clinical setting, you were assigned to a community health clinic to shadow a physician to see what kind of health education is given to patients.

On your first day, the physician to whom you are assigned requests that you accompany her into the examination room as she sees patients. During the first two hours, she sees three patients for colds or influenza, two patients for hypertension, one patient for emphysema, one patient for diabetes, one for a broken hand, and two teenage patients for sports physicals. After these appointments, she takes some time to visit with you and discuss your initial perceptions. During the conversation, she asks if you are aware of any good health education/promotion information sites for teens on the Internet. You promise to do some research on this question and bring the information on your next visit. What information do you think would be of benefit to teens? Which two or three sites would you recommend and why?

Critical Thinking Questions

1. Assume that all information about any topic is available on the Internet. If that were true, would there be any need for health education specialists? Defend your answer.
2. Make a list of two advantages and two disadvantages of the Internet from your perspective. Assuming that your answers reflect universal truths about the Internet, how might you persuade someone who is not computer literate to use a computer to search for health information?
3. Given that so much information is available online, under what circumstances does it make sense to use the library?
4. If the Internet had been developed in the early 1900s, how might the U.S. healthcare system and the role of health education specialists differ from what they are today?

Activities

1. You are employed as a health education specialist in a district health department and have just received a call from a member of a local coalition wanting to know where to find some peer-reviewed studies that summarize the content and effectiveness of available school-based sexuality education curricula. Use an index to find a reference to an article that meets those criteria.
2. Was the article you located in Activity 1 a primary or secondary source of information? Provide a rationale for your answer.
3. Using a database (CINAHL, MEDLINE, PsycINFO, or ERIC), find a primary research article relating to motorcycle safety (e.g., the use of a helmet, wearing protective gear, or road surfaces). Critique the article by applying the questions found in the "Critically Reading a Research Article" section of this chapter.
4. Use your choice of a browser and look up the term *endometriosis*. Then evaluate at least two of the sites that appear using the CRAAP methodology.
5. Perform an Internet search on the topic of breast cancer. Compare the results of your findings from a primary source, a government publication, and a popular press publication.

Weblinks

Epidemiological and Statistical Information

1. **https://wonder.cdc.gov/**

   CDC WONDER

   Wide-ranging online data for epidemiological research—an easy-to-use, menu-driven system that makes the information resources of the CDC available to public health professionals and the public at large. It provides access to a wide array of public health information.

2. **https://www.cdc.gov/nchs/index.htm**

   National Center for Health Statistics (NCHS)

   NCHS is the nation's principal health statistics agency. Their website offers access to an extensive collection of health statistics intended to guide those working to improve public health.

3. **https://www.cdc.gov/mmwr/index .html**

   Morbidity and Mortality Weekly Report (MMWR)

   MMWR is a weekly report prepared by the CDC. State health departments report their findings to MMWR. The site offers access to studies and reports and also provides useful information on a wide range of diseases.

4. **https://www.census.gov/**

   U.S. Bureau of the Census

   The website of the U.S. Census Bureau allows the user to access specific data for their state, county, or city. View results from Census 2000 and Census 2010 and access analytical reports on population change, race, age, family structure, and more.

Infectious Diseases

5. **https://www.cdc.gov/datastatistics /index.html**

   Centers for Disease Control and Prevention—Data & Statistics

   With the mission of preventing illness, disability, and death, the CDC conducts epidemic investigations, laboratory research, and public education programs to attempt to prevent and control diseases and disorders of all types.

Chronic Diseases

6. **https://www.cdc.gov/chronicdisease /index.htm**

   National Center for Chronic Disease Prevention and Health Promotion (NCCDPHP)

   This section of the CDC is dedicated to chronic diseases and provides links to a variety of helpful sites, including a diabetes public health resource and sites discussing heart disease, nutrition, and physical activity.

7. **https://www.cancer.gov/**

   National Cancer Institute (NCI)

   The NCI's website covers information on a variety of cancer topics, discussing treatment, prevention, research, and much more. The NCI supports prevention and treatment of cancer, rehabilitation, and continued care of cancer patients and their families.

8. **https://www.diabetes.org/**

   American Diabetes Association (ADA)

   The ADA provides diabetes research, scientific findings, information, and advocacy. The site contains helpful information for people with diabetes, their families, health professionals, and the public.

Disease Control and Prevention

9. **https://www.samhsa.gov/**

    SAMHSA: Substance Abuse and Mental Health Services Administration

    This site has links to ordering government materials online that focus on professional and research topics; issues in the field of treatment, prevention, and recovery; and information on conditions and disorders.

10. **https://www.samhsa.gov/about-us /who-we-are/offices-centers/csap**

    Center for Substance Abuse Prevention (CSAP)

    CSAP is funded by the Substance Abuse and Mental Health Services Administration (SAMHSA) and is responsible for improving the access to and quality of substance abuse prevention services to the public. CSAP provides national leadership in the development of policies, programs, and services to prevent the onset of illegal drug use and underage alcohol and tobacco use, and to reduce the negative consequences of using substances.

11. **https://www.whitehouse.gov/ondcp**

    Office of National Drug Control Policy (ONDCP)

    With the goal of reducing illicit drug use, substance abuse-related crimes, drug trafficking, and drug-related health problems, the ONDCP is working to establish a national strategy to fight these dilemmas. The site contains national priorities, annual reports, and a tremendous amount of drug information.

12. **https://www.cdc.gov/nchhstp/eis /DHAP.html**

    Division of HIV/AIDS Prevention (EIS 2021)/CDC

    With a mission to prevent HIV infection and reduce the incidence of HIV-related illness, the CDC's Division of HIV/AIDS Prevention Website provides useful information for those working in the health field. The site includes such topics as prevention tools, research, brochures, and fact sheets.

13. **https://www.childrenssafetynetwork .org/**

    Children's Safety Network

    The Children's Safety Network, funded by the Maternal & Child Health Bureau (MCH) and the U.S. Department of Health and Human Services, provides technical assistance, training, and resources to MCH and other injury prevention professionals in an extensive effort to reduce the burden of injury and violence to our nation's children.

14. **https://www.fda.gov/home**

    Food and Drug Administration (FDA)

    This site not only outlines national programs intended to increase food safety awareness but it also contains information concerning the laws enforced by the FDA and provides helpful tips on preventing food-related illness.

15. **https://www.oncolink.org/**

    OncoLink

    OncoLink, provided by the Abramson Cancer Center of the University of Pennsylvania, is the Web's first cancer resource. The site provides up-to-date cancer news and research. Locate information on the causes of cancer, screening and prevention, clinical trials, and other resources on cancer.

16. **https://wwwnc.cdc.gov/**

    Travelers' Health

    Locate health information for specific destinations, stay up to date on outbreaks throughout the world, and learn how to avoid illness from food and water.

17. **https://www.cdc.gov/nchhstp/eis /DTBE.html**

CDC's Division of Tuberculosis Elimination

With the mission of "preventing, controlling and eventually eliminating tuberculosis from the United States," the website of the CDC's Division of Tuberculosis Elimination contains useful information to aid that mission. Learn all there is to know about tuberculosis, locate statistics on its occurrence, and obtain education and training materials on it.

18. **https://www.healthywomen.org/**

Healthy Women

Their mission is to educate women between 35 and 64 to make informed health choices.

19. **https://www.menshealthnetwork.org/**

Men's Health Network

The Men's Health Network is an informational and educational organization recognizing men's health as a specific social concern.

20. **https://kidshealth.org/Nemours**

KidsHealth

Nemours KidsHealth is the largest and most visited site on the Web, providing doctor-approved health information about children from before birth through adolescence. Created by the Nemours Foundation's Center for Children's Health Media, the award-winning KidsHealth provides families with accurate, up-to-date, and jargon-free health information they can use.

21. **https://www.nsc.org/**

National Safety Council

The National Safety Council is focused on providing safety and health information to reduce the number of injuries and deaths from preventable accidents. Their website contains information on new policies and laws

enacted to prevent unintentional injuries. It also provides statistics and helpful tips regarding this health topic.

22. **https://ctb.ku.edu/en**

Community Tool Box

The goal of the Community Tool Box is to support work in community health promotion and development. The Tool Box provides multiple pages of practical skill-building information on more than 250 different topics related to community development. Topic sections include step-by-step instruction, examples, checklists, and related resources.

National Agencies

23. **https://www.cdc.gov**

CDC—Centers for Disease Control and Prevention

The CDC is recognized as the leading federal agency for protecting the health and safety of the public, providing credible information to enhance health decisions and promote health. The website of the CDC includes a variety of helpful health and safety topics. The information covers everything from health promotion to vaccines to traveler's health. Data, statistics, publications, and products are also available.

24. **https://www.hhs.gov**

USDHHS—Department of Health and Human Services

The Department of Health and Human Services is the U.S. government's principal agency for health protection and the provision of human services. Its site is divided into health topics such as Safety & Wellness, Diseases & Conditions, and Families & Children. Readers can also use the Resource Locator and Reference Collections to find such things as healthcare facilities and publications.

25. **https://www.epa.gov/**

    U. S. EPA—Environmental Protection Agency

    The EPA is focused on protecting human health and the environment by working for a cleaner, healthier environment. The site provides air quality reports, current environmental news stories, and tips on how the public can make the environment healthier. The QuickFinder allows fast and easy access to a variety of environmental topics.

26. **https://www.ihs.gov/**

    IHS—Indian Health Service

    Indian Health Service is the Federal Health Program for American Indians and Alaska Natives. IHS is focused on improving the health of these groups while attempting to ensure that they have access to culturally acceptable health services.

27. **https://www.ama-assn.org/**

    American Medical Association

    This website is divided into a section for physicians and medical students and a section for patients. The patient section allows the user to search for a doctor and obtain health information and resources. The physician section provides information on such topics as medical education, legal issues, and advocacy.

28. **https://www.nih.gov/**

    National Institutes of Health (NIH)

    The NIH site has a wide variety of great health information. It contains an A–Z index of health resources, a wealth of grant information, and a section dedicated to scientific resources.

29. **https://www.govinfo.gov/**

    Govinfo/Government Publications Office (GPO)

    Offers free online access to official publications from all three branches of the Federal Government.

International Agencies

30. **https://www.who.int/home**

    WHO—World Health Organization

    The website of WHO is an incredible resource with many health and development topics linked to WHO projects, initiatives, activities, information products, and contacts.

31. **https://www.paho.org/en**

    PAHO—Pan American Health Organization

    PAHO, affiliated with WHO, focuses on a multitude of public health topics, with the mission of promoting health in the Americas.

32. **https://library.un.org/**

    The Dag Hammarskjold Library/United Nations

    Includes health-related information on diseases, policies, legislation, and the health status of countries around the globe.

INTERNET-Based MEDLINE Search Systems

33. **https://pubmed.ncbi.nlm.nih.gov/**

    PubMed

    PubMed is a service of the NLM. It includes literally millions of citations for biomedical articles going back to the 1950s. The citations are from MEDLINE and additional lifescience journals. PubMed includes links to many sites providing full-text articles and other related resources.

34. **https://www.medscape.com/**

    Medscape

    Medical news, drug and disease information

35. **https://www.nlm.nih.gov/**

    National Library of Medicine (NLM)

    The NLM, on the campus of the NIH in Bethesda, Maryland, is the world's largest medical library. Excellent central source of current information on results of health research for the lay person, the practicing health professional, the health researcher, and health librarians. Updated daily.

36. **https://medlineplus.gov/**

    MedlinePlus

    Health professionals and the general public alike can easily access information on MedlinePlus that is accurate and up to date. MedlinePlus has extensive information from the National Institutes of Health and other trusted sources on numerous diseases and conditions.

Public Health Practice

37. **https://www.cdc.gov/publichealth gateway/about-cstlts/index.html**

    Center for State, Tribal, Local, and Territorial Support (CSTLTS)

    The priority of the CSTLTS is to improve the capacity and performance of the public health system at all levels. The office works both within the CDC and in the field to identify gaps, opportunities for collaboration, and the strategies needed to support growth and enhancement of public health work.

38. **https://www.apha.org**

    American Public Health Association (APHA)

    The APHA is the world's largest and oldest organization of public health professionals. Useful sections include Continuing Education, Newsroom, and Science and Programs.

State and Local Public Health Departments

39. **https://www.astho.org/**

    Association of State and Territorial Health Officials (ASTHO)

    ASTHO is the national nonprofit organization representing the public health agencies of the United States, the U.S. Territories, and the District of Columbia, as well as the 120,000 public health professionals these agencies employ. ASTHO members, the chief health officials of these jurisdictions, are dedicated to formulating and influencing sound public health policy and to ensuring excellence in state-based public health practice.

40. **https://www.healthguideusa.com /index.htm**

    Health Resource Guide USA

    Health Guide USA provides quick reference to healthcare-related resources throughout the United States. It provides locations of state and local health departments, as well as medical schools and medical licenses.

General Health Information

41. **https://www.google.com**

    Google

    Google is a great tool for finding anything on the Web. Google has several specialized search features such as Blog Search and Alerts. Blog Search can help find health related blogs. You can set up an Alert and receive regular email updates.

42. **https://www.optum.com/business /solutions/population-health /prevention/center-wellbeing -research.html**

    OPTUM Center for Wellbeing Research

    Provides MD-reviewed information on a variety of health topics. The information is easy to understand and can be used by a health education specialist to research background information related to all aspects of health.

43. **https://www.webmd.com**

    WebMD

    Site devoted to providing current and relevant consumer health information on a variety of topics. Medical facts are reviewed by physicians prior to posting.

44. **https://www.yahoo.com/lifestyle /well-being**

Yahoo!Life—Wellbeing

Get in-depth coverage on a variety of health issues, including a directory of the most popular websites related to a particular health topic.

45. **https://www.mayoclinic.com**

Mayo Clinic

The Mayo Clinic offers a wealth of health information developed and reviewed by more than 2,000 physicians and scientists. The site also allows access to healthy living tools, such as a personal health card and a first-aid and self-care guide.

46. **https://www.berkeleywellness.com**
47. **https://www.healthfinder.gov**

Healthfinder®

Healthfinder, developed by the Department of Health and Human Services, directs the user to various health resources depending on their needs. Resources include such things as online publications, clearinghouses, support groups, government agencies, and websites.

48. **https://www.usa.gov/health**

USA.gov-Health

The Health and Nutrition section of the U.S. Government's Official web portal is filled with great health information. The Healthfinder link enables access to the Personal Health Tools link, which features tools for calculating body mass index (BMI) and taking an online checkup. The site also features health topics for population groups and helps the user locate health services in their area.

49. **https://candid.org/**

Candid (formerly Foundation Center and GuideStar)

Candid collects information on non-profits, foundations, and grants.

50. **https://www.goaskalice.columbia.edu/**

Go Ask Alice!

Go Ask Alice's Q&A database houses numerous health-related questions and answers. It is produced by Columbia University's Health Education Program.

51. **https://health.gov/our-work/health -literacy/resources/national-health -information-center**

National Health Information Center (NHIC)

The NHIC is a health information referral service that puts health professionals and consumers who have health questions in touch with organizations that are best able to provide answers.

News Stories

52. **https://www.reuters.com/news/health**

Reuters Healthcare and Pharmaceuticals

Reuters is the premier supplier of health and medical news on the Internet. The Healthcare and Pharmaceuticals section is written for the general public.

53. **https://amp.usatoday.com/news /health/**

USA Today Health

This section of *USA Today* provides current health news stories

Health Education/Health Promotion Jobs

54. **https://sph.emory.edu/careers/index .html**

Rollins School of Public Health at Emory—Careers

Includes a section titled Public Health Employment

Health Policy

55. **https://www.nashp.org**

    National Academy for State Health Policy

    The National Academy for State Health Policy conducts policy analysis; provides training and technical assistance to states; produces informational resources; and convenes state, regional, and national forums. This site enables the user to access these services and the results of policy studies that have been completed.

56. **https://www.heritage.org**

    The Heritage Foundation

    This site provides access to well-written and well-documented health policy research and analysis papers that reflect a more conservative perspective.

57. **https://rwjf.org/**

    The Robert Wood Johnson Foundation

    The Robert Wood Johnson Foundation has a goal of funding projects that improve the health and health care of all Americans. This site features many of the foundation's policy papers, current and future studies, and projects that the foundation is or will consider funding. The organization is considered nonpartisan.

58. **https://kff.org/**

    The Kaiser Family Foundation

    The Kaiser Family Foundation is a nonprofit, privately operating foundation focusing on the major healthcare issues facing the nation. The foundation is an independent voice and source of facts and analysis for policymakers, the media, the healthcare community, and the general public.

59. **https://www.commonwealthfund.org/**

    The Commonwealth Fund

    This site contains policy briefs and full-text health policy papers that are well written and well documented and are often from a more liberal perspective.

60. **https://www.statecoverage.org/**

    State Coverage Initiatives (SCI)

    The SCI program is a national initiative of The Robert Wood Johnson Foundation that works with states to plan, execute, and maintain health insurance expansions, as well as to improve the availability and affordability of healthcare coverage. The site includes the results of many states' initiatives to increase health insurance coverage for their residents.

General

61. **http://findarticles.com/p/articles /tn_health**

    Find articles

    Provides free access to millions of articles from many top publications.

62. **https://scholar.google.com/**

    Google Scholar

    This site provides another alternative to search through scholarly literature across many disciplines and sources, including theses, books, abstracts, and articles. Use the "More" link, choose "Settings", then click on Library links to link to electronic materials at libraries where you have borrowing rights.

References

California State University Chico. (2020). Evaluating information applying the CRAAP test. Retrieved May 5, 2021, from https://library.csuchico.edu/sites/default/files/craap-test.pdf. Licensed under a Creative Commons Attribution 4.0 International License.

Caulfield, M. (2019). Web literacy for student fact-checkers. Retrieved January 17, 2021, from https://webliteracy.pressbooks.com/. Licensed under a Creative Commons Attribution 4.0 International License.

Cottrell, R. R. (1997). *A guide to evaluating a journal article.* Unpublished manuscript.

Hibbard, J. H., & Greene, J. (2013). What the evidence shows about patient activation: Better health outcomes and care experiences; fewer data on costs. *Health Affairs, 32*(2), 207–214.

Subramanyam R. (2013). Art of reading a journal article: Methodically and effectively. *Journal of Oral and Maxillofacial Pathology, 17*(1), 65–70. https://doi.org/10.4103/0973-029X.110733

University of Akron. (n.d.). *Government documents.* Retrieved May 27, 2013, from http://www.uakron.edu/libraries/services/services-detail.dot?inode=360659&title=Government%20Documents

CHAPTER 10

Future Trends in Health Education/Promotion

CHAPTER OBJECTIVES

After reading this chapter and answering the questions at the end, you should be able to:

- Identify a setting in which health education specialists will practice in the next five years to a greater degree than they do today.
- Describe four major societal changes that will influence the practice of health education/promotion in the next 10 years.
- Explain at least one major implication of credentialing for future health education specialists.
- Compare and contrast the roles of health education specialists in the four practice settings.
- Identify several reasons that health education specialists should be optimistic about future employment opportunities.

It is said that one of the few constants in life is change. Societal trends impact the health education/promotion profession too. People are interested in a wide variety of health topics and can look up all kinds of information. There have been and continue to be changes to the Affordable Care Act, demographic patterns, and health care. Healthcare costs are spiraling, we rely evermore on technology, and there is a heightened skepticism of the medical establishment and health insurance companies. The work environment for a health education specialist in 2040 will significantly differ from 2010. These changes present the health education specialist with enormous opportunities. This chapter will explore future

developments in the discipline of health education/promotion, and we hope, to create a sense of excitement and anticipation about the challenges that lie ahead.

Go to YouTube and look up a news show from 2000 based solely on that program and the commercial messages during the station breaks, how would you describe the lives of people 20 years ago? Look at current shows; how has life changed? Although it is not the purpose of this chapter to dwell on comparative history, it is noteworthy that, in a brief span of 30-plus years, the communication methods and patterns in the United States and the world have changed dramatically. For example, in the early 1990s, there was effectively no online access to information of any sort. In 2016, 80% of all U.S. adults using the Internet reported that they used it to find health information (LaValley, Kiviniemi & Gage-Bouchard, 2017). Societal changes will also impact the work of health education/promotion specialists.

First, we will discuss changing demographic patterns, then societal trends, and then issues related to credentialing and preparation. Using this information as a foundation, the chapter concludes by postulating about the impact of these changes for the health education specialist in the school, public health, worksite, and medical care settings. Obviously, no one knows exactly what the future will hold. The information presented is meant to stimulate your thinking about the role health education specialists will play going forward within the next 15 years.

Demographic Changes

Over the past 30 years, the population growth rate in the United States has increased at about 1% per year but the pace of growth is slowing (Pollard et al., 2020). A more in-depth study of the **demographic profile**—the breakdown of the U.S. population by age group, sex, race, and ethnicity—shows a dramatically altered picture from that of just 10 years ago. This consistently changing demographic profile—specifically, a greater percentage of minority residents and an ever-aging population—has important implications for the future practice of health education specialists (see **Figure 10.1**). The Census Bureau anticipates that starting in 2030, immigration will be the primary source of population growth in the United States. (Vespa et al., 2020).

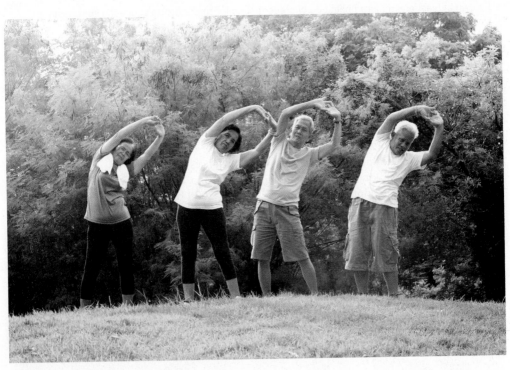

Figure 10.1 The demand for older-adult focused, health-promotion programs will continue to grow.
© SUPERMAO/Shutterstock.

Population Changes

Clark's (2014) comments, written midway through the last decade of the 20th century, remain cogent today. She states, "We are undergoing a massive change in culture in our society. We are literally looking different as a nation and the conventional majority values and norms are being challenged as we become a more diverse, more ethnic, more integrated culture. Health educators have long prided themselves with working across cultures....The cultural changes are...greater than we have experienced previously" (p. 137).

It seems that the increased racial and ethnic diversity in the United States has several major causes. In the 1800s and early to mid-1900s, the bulk of immigrants to the United States came from Western Europe. Hale (2000) mentions that worsening economic conditions in Mexico and Central America over the decade from 2000 to 2010 are largely responsible for the large number of immigrants from those areas. According to Khullar and Chokshi (2019) about a fifth of the world's immigrants, 46 million, live in the United States. Immigration status, citizenship, ethnicity and location all greatly impact the health and access to health care of each person. Changing federal and state policies present new challenges (and opportunities) for the public health community. California, Florida, and Texas all have high percentages of immigrants. These three states have almost 30% of the US population but from 2014–2015 accounted for 48% of U.S. population growth (Mather, 2015). Immigrants have higher rates of fertility than native-born peoples, which means that the shifts in culture and the challenges to majority norms alluded to by Clark are likely here to stay.

The 2010 census found that the U.S. minority population was composed of 12.4% African American, 16.3% Hispanic, 5.0% Asian or Pacific Islander, and 0.9% Native American. **Table 10.1** shows the projected percentage figures for each of these population groups by the year 2060 (U.S. Census Bureau, 2012).

From Table 10.1, it is readily apparent that the greatest percentage increase over the next 40 years will come from the Hispanic and Asian/Pacific Islander groups. The projected percentage increase of Hispanics and Asians from 2015 until 2060 is 115% and 143%, respectively. While the percentage of non-Hispanic Whites will fall from 62.2%, 2015 to about 43.6% in the year 2060, a decrease of about 8.2% of the overall 2060 U.S. all-races population.

At least one ramification of these changes, increasing numbers of ethnic minority students in public school, is already being felt in the classrooms of our nation. In 2020, approximately 56% of the children in public schools in the United States were minorities as

Table 10.1 Projected U.S. Population Percentages of African Americans, Hispanics, Native Americans, and Asians or Pacific Islanders: 2010 and 2060

Race	2010 (%)	2060 (%)
African American	12.4	14.3
Hispanic	16.3	28.6
Native American	0.9	0.7
Asian/Pacific Islander	5.0	11.7

Data from U.S. Census Bureau. (2012). *Most children younger than age 1 are minorities.* http://www.census.gov/newsroom/releases/archives/population /cb12-90.html reported by the National Center for Education Statistics (2020). According to the U.S. Census Bureau, in 2012, the majority (50.4) of children under one year of age in the United States are minority children (U.S. Census Bureau, 2012). From schools in Caldwell, Idaho, with a student population of nearly 65% Hispanic, to Chicago, Illinois, with a Hispanic and other minority race student population of more than 80%, the escalating minority population makes an already diverse nation even more so. This trend presents health education specialists with an ever-widening array of opportunities and challenges as the 21st century continues to unfold.

Aging

Another demographic factor that will impact the practice of health education/promotion in the future is the aging population. More Americans are living longer than ever before. According to the United States Census Bureau, all baby boomers will be at least age 65 by 2030 and by 2060, nearly 1 in 4 Americans will be over 65 (Vespa et al., 2020). Other causative factors accentuating changes in age demographics are that married couples in the United States are having fewer children, and the baby boomers (those born between 1946 and 1964) are retiring. In 2020, more people retired than in 2019 (Pew Research, 2020). To further illustrate this trend, the median age of the U.S. population in 2010 was 37.2. In the year 2020, it is estimated to be 38.3; and in 2050, it will be 41.

Societal Trends

There probably has not been a time when societal change was as rapid as in the latter decades of the 20th century. For example, since 1960, there have been changes in societal mores and practices, such as more openness to cohabitation, a greater tolerance for premarital sex, more vocal and open gay relationships including the legalization of gay marriage, a greater number of single-parent households, an increase in child abuse, more violence, an increase in the amount and availability of pornographic materials, massive changes in the number of ethical issues related to medicine, alterations in the way the medical establishment is organized and medical care is delivered, a decreasing respect for authority of any kind, declining state and federal support for K–12 public schools and higher education institutions, an infusion of and a reliance on technology, and a distrust of the political establishment in general. All of these factors play a big role in shaping the structure of society in the future. This section discusses several of the major societal trends that experts agree will impact health education/promotion in the new millennium.

Technology

Certainly, the boom in **technology** has affected, if not transformed, the lives of many people around the globe. Many of the advances in communication, transportation, medicine, engineering, and ease of access to information have created an enhanced quality of life for people worldwide. The increased availability and use of technology also creates many opportunities for the prospective health education specialist in the planning, design, implementation, and evaluation of programs and materials.

Today, it is impossible to find a campus without numerous student computer labs and secure WiFi everywhere. In 2021, many courses and even entire degree programs are online, enabling the student to participate in class sessions in "real time," their time, and from anywhere. The constantly expanding technological capabilities in the education field have created a learning environment in which information is readily available and lessons can be easily structured to require a greater degree of critical thinking and be more interactive than was the case only a few years ago. An increasing number of journals are published only in electronic form; no printed hard copy is available (Prabha, 2006). Google, Amazon, and Internet Archive have digitized millions of books and monographs, making the information contained in those publications not only more readily accessible but the content is also more searchable (Kahle, 2017). There is no doubt that ready availability of information and technology will continue to impact our profession.

The COVID-19 pandemic highlights the importance of helping people find valid sources of information and the deadly impact of misinformation (Adams, & Gonzales, 2020). As technological developments accelerate, it is imperative to keep current on the modalities and develop innovative communication mechanisms in multiple languages and different literacy levels (Guest et al., 2020). The focus of the 2018 Digital Health Promotion Executive Leadership Summit, included

- The role of digital technology in addressing current public health issues such as mental health, opioids, suicide and the impact of social media on children and teens.
- Examples of success public health interventions on social media.
- Privacy issues, digital health and confidentiality, data sharing, patient protection.
- Future trends in the use of digital technology to improve individual and population health.

The expanding number and use of social media sites and messaging over the past 10 years have clearly shown the need for people to have access to credible sources that are culturally relevant. Providers should use evidence-based health communication interventions that are rigorously evaluated. The creators of digital health interventions should anticipate unintended consequences the campaign may have on vulnerable populations (Abroms, et al., 2018).

Researchers, Guistini, Ali, Fraser, Boulos (2018) and Korda and Itani (2013) found that social media can work to not only inform and

change attitudes but also to alter behavior. As with most "in person" interventions; however, crafting the messages using behavioral theory and making certain that the message is designed in such a manner that two-way communication is achieved greatly increase the chances of success. In the Health Education Specialist Practice Analysis (HESPA II, 2020), Eight Areas of Responsibility for Health Education, Area IV focuses on communication and subcompetency 6.1.3 specifically identifies social as a means of communicating with different populations (NCHEC, 2020).

Clearly, technology will continue to shape the delivery of health education/promotion into the future. SOPHE Digital Health Promotion Executive Leadership Summit focuses on new ways to explore technology so that it can be used to enhance health and health education. SOPHE also recognizes individuals or groups that apply innovative, noncommercial technology in health education that can impact our practice and be broadly disseminated with the Digital Technology & Communications Award (SOPHE, 2020). Students of health education/promotion must become familiar with the various media methods available to gather and deliver information including the creation of messages usable across multiple devices and in multiple languages. Social media such as Twitter, Facebook, Pinterest, Instagram, Reddit, and YouTube are all ways to communicate around specific health conditions. New platforms are being created all the time and in 2017, the health-related mobile applications available to consumers surpassed 400,000—nearly double the number available in 2015—with approximately 200 new apps added to the market each day (IQVIA). People use digital devices to track activity, stress, sleep, calories, and water. While mobile health (mHealth) apps can send alerts to move more, take medications, provide health information updates, and find support groups only a small number are regulated by the FDA(Larson, 2018). Healthcare apps are being used to help diabetic patients track their blood sugar, provide personalized online mental health therapy, connect new moms to individualized infant information, and educate patients about a myriad of health conditions. These are examples of new opportunities for health education specialists to provide personalized client messages (Morgan, 2018).

Due to the increasing popularity of social media, many health education professionals are now utilizing these platforms in health education/promotion and behavior change (Alber et al., 2016).

Family Structure

The U.S. family structure has changed dramatically since the 1960s (see **Figure 10.2**). The **traditional family** (two parents and their children) is becoming less and less common because of factors such as high rates of divorce, smaller families, postponed marriage and childbearing, teenage and nonmarital

childbearing, stepfamilies, homosexual couples, and dual-earner marriages (Acock & Demo, 1994). According to Cilluffo & Cohn (2019), one in four parents were married in 2017 and only one in five parents stayed home. Only 61% of households fit the definition of a family having both a married male and female at home, and one fourth of those homes are in a remarriage situation. Thirty-two percent of families have children younger than 18 living with them. More 18–29 year olds are living with their parents, which is higher than during the Great Depression (Fry et al., 2020).

Divorce rates have dropped from 3.6 per 1,000 to 2.9 per 1,000 (National Center for Health Statistics (2020).

In addition, about 33% of Americans live alone or in nonfamily combinations, such as housemates, friends, or partnerships outside of legal marriage.

From 1968 to 2020, the percentage of children younger than 18 who lived with both

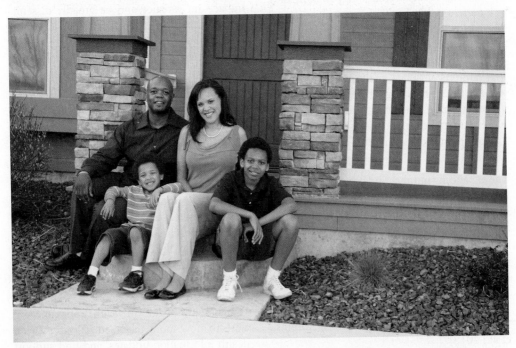

Figure 10.2 Keep in mind the different family structures, such as extended families or single parents, when planning programs and policies.

© Daniel Hurst/iStock/Thinkstock.

parents declined from 85 to 69%. The percentage of children living with only a mother increased from 10 to 20%. Almost 10.5% of children under 18 lived with grandparents or other relatives. (Census, 2020; AARP, 2017).

The impact caused by these new structures is being felt throughout our society. Children are the most affected. The Pew Research Center (2015) reported that 31% of children under 6 today have experienced a major change in their family structure including parental divorce, separation, marriage, cohabitation, or death (p. 17).

With the high cost of goods and services in the United States, the number of mothers in the workforce with children under 18 has changed dramatically. According to Christnacht & Sullivan (2020), working mothers account for nearly one-third of all working women. A 2019 Pew Research Center study found that 72% of mothers are now in the workforce—an increase of nearly 80% since 1980. This even places a strain on nuclear families with two parents; affordable daycare services for the children must be obtained. For many low-income and single-parent families, the choice is no care or supervision at all—a situation that puts children at risk. Under the Affordable Care Act (ACA), more people have health insurance through the state health exchanges, Medicaid expansion, and employers. In 2014, the first year people were required to purchase insurance under the ACA, 89.6% of people had health insurance coverage for part or all of the year (Smith & Medalia, 2015) and that increased to 92% in 2019 (Keisler-Starkey, & Bunch, 2019). Currently, there are 12 states that have chosen not to expand Medicaid so there are still millions of people without health insurance who typically work in service-oriented positions that often pay minimum wage and are a major source of employment for many low-skilled workers (Kaiser Family Foundation, 2020). As a result, nearly 32% of children under 18 in the United States are living in poverty. This is the highest rate in the industrialized world

and most poor children are Latino, Black, and American Indian (Yang, Ekono, and Skinner, 2016). The linkage between these factors may be a predisposing condition leading to an increased rate of child abuse (McKenzie et al., 2008). Finally, it is no secret that the economic downturn since 2008 has contributed significantly to increasing the number of families and children under economic stress as a result of job loss or underemployment. COVID has severely impacted the job market and in December of 2020, the unemployment rate was 6.7%, up from 4% in December 2018 (Bureau of Labor Statistics, 2021) The U.S. Census Bureau noted in 2019 that overall poverty levels in the United States were the lowest they had been since 2007 at 10.5%.

The changes previously noted have significant implications for health education specialists. Family structures will likely remain diverse in the coming years and will probably operate on a new set of norms. In other words, new methods of reaching individuals, families, and communities will need to be created to improve the health of all family members in accordance with their needs.

Political Climate

As was mentioned previously, there remains little doubt that today there is an increasing frustration with politics and politicians in general. Whether a person is a **conservative**, one who generally distrusts governmental regulations and tax-supported programs for addressing social or economic problems; a **moderate**, one who usually acts in a more situationally specific manner with regard to using tax-supported programs to solve societal problems; or a **liberal**, one who generally supports government programs to attack social and economic problems; there seems to be no end to the bickering and infighting among and between members of various political parties. Many of the political issues considered in Congress relate to health. For example, the landmark agreement between the tobacco industry and the states over the sale and marketing of tobacco products to minors; the addition of prescription drug benefits to Medicare; determination of Medicaid eligibility and Medicaid expansion; the repeal of a motorcycle helmet law in Texas; the passage of physician-assisted suicide laws in California, Oregon, Washington, Montana, and Vermont; the escalating cost of prescription drugs; debates as to whether to allow health insurance companies to offer coverage across state lines; immigration reform and whether to offer healthcare coverage for those undocumented immigrants currently in the United States; climate change; pornography as a public health issue; minimum wage; timely physical and mental health care for veterans returning from wars in Iraq and Afghanistan; passage of and stages of implementation of the Affordable Care Act; community health center legislation; gun control; and the debate as to whether to increase spending on school lunches at the expense of Supplemental Nutrition Assistance Program (SNAP), aka, food stamp allotments, are examples of political issues that directly impact the health of the populace.

Politics and health seem to be inextricably linked. Some governmental officials and legislators worry that public health professionals infringe on personal autonomy by advocating for seat belt laws, wearing masks to help prevent COVID, tobacco laws, worksite wellness programs, helmet laws, air bags, environmental protection, healthier options in fast foods and public schools, gun control laws, and health insurance for all. Others believe that legislation fostering a social climate that enhances the health of the population as a whole is worth the sacrifice of some personal choice and autonomy.

As citizens and professionals, the involvement of health education specialists in the political process is important. O'Rourke (2006) states, "Health education not only seeks to change lifestyles, but to create public understanding of the political issues involved in public health programs" (p. 9). He goes on to challenge all health education specialists to assume a **macrolevel** view of health problems. Using this approach, health education specialists move from a position of assisting behavior change, one person at a time, to community-based interventions. In implementing the community-based programs, success often depends on the health education specialist's having a working knowledge of the political process and how it impacts every decision. Hunter (2008) supports the fact that public health professionals can no longer be bystanders but must become passionate advocates for healthy change in individuals and communities. He believes that the collective advocacy of all public health practitioners is vital in moving governmental bodies to support and improve health.

There is little doubt that health education specialists must become participants in the political process. O'Rourke (2006) eloquently makes a case for enhancing the effectiveness of health education/promotion through an approach that encompasses collective responsibility and community involvement through participation in the political process and service on county health boards, city councils, and school boards. In these capacities, health educators can influence the health of entire communities and not rely on the 'one person at a time' model of improving health through individual responsibility. (p. 8)

To that end, a method for health education specialists to increase their visibility and political clout is advanced by McDermott (2000) when he challenges present and future health education specialists to consider the importance of research in the practice of health education/promotion. For interventions to be effective, health education specialists must use evidence-based practices when these practices are known. Future gains in the effectiveness and scope of prevention programs probably will be made only when health education specialists insist on pushing the research envelope to determine the factors that affect health and cause health disparities in populations, are components of effective intervention programs, and allow for dissemination of these programs across a variety of settings. Including community partners, community-based participatory research, and legislators in these research efforts are a strategy proven to gain trust and allies more welcoming to the benefit of macrolevel initiatives.

Advocacy is such an important part of our professional competencies that it is now a new standalone responsibility for health education specialists (HESPA II 2020) Area V: Advocacy includes these major competencies 5.1 Identify a current or emerging health issue requiring policy, systems, or environmental change, 5.2 Engage coalitions and stakeholders in addressing the health issue and planning advocacy efforts, 5.3 Engage in advocacy, and 5.4 Evaluate advocacy. Learning how to effectively use our voices and engage with others to advocate for changes at the policy and systems level is essential for improving health outcomes.

Medical Care Establishment and the Affordable Care Act

The healthcare system in the United States continues to be in need of an overhaul. Passage of the Affordable Care Act in early 2010 was a start in the right direction, but the exact impact of that legislation is far from certain (see Chapter 1). Meanwhile, the cost of care continues to escalate, and the system seems stuck in an unsustainable model of reimbursement for procedures (fee-for-service) instead of a capitated reimbursement structure for helping people stay well. Citizens increasingly desire to be participants in their own care and to be provided with options. Enhancing the quality of life as opposed to simply increasing longevity is becoming a prevalent goal of U.S. healthcare consumers.

There are several reasons for this trend. Although few would deny that our medical care system has been responsible for saving countless lives, clearly, health is largely a reflection of the nature of the environments in which a person resides, personal lifestyle choices, and standards of living, and not the medical care system. In the United States, medical care tends to concentrate on secondary and tertiary care and to ignore the value of primary prevention. In the United States, only three cents of every healthcare dollar are spent on prevention, and well more than 75% of healthcare costs are attributable to preventable disease conditions (Forsberg & Fichtenberg, 2012).

These points are substantiated by Williams et al., (2010) and Goodarz and colleagues (2010) when they state that healthier lives are best fostered in a climate of a culture of health. What seems to be most important in creating and maintaining health are the actions taken by individuals and communities to select and support habits like choosing what food we eat, having healthy relationships, staying physically active, and investing in safe and environmentally friendly neighborhoods. Much of health is not only tied to medical intervention but also to primary prevention.

The ACA has increased the opportunities for health education specialists. Koh and Sebelius (2010) document that this law "promotes wellness in the workplace, providing new health promotion opportunities for employers and employees" (p. 4). In addition, the act strengthens the community role in promoting prevention and serves to enhance partnerships between state and local government and community groups and nonprofits.

While COVID-19 has brought to light the strains, underfunded local and state health departments face, it has also demonstrated the incredible work of public health professionals. Undergraduate programs are growing and 2020 saw a 20% increase in applications to Masters in Public Health (MPH) programs (Association of Schools and Programs of Public Health, 2021).

The Boise, Idaho–based nonprofit corporation, Healthwise, the provider of the web-based health information found in WebMD and responsible for much of the health education/promotion content disseminated by major insurance companies and hospitals around the country, offers an example of the value of health education/promotion in a clinical arena. Healthwise, professionals have developed a health information and education prescription format tailored to consumers so that they can obtain the information they need to make choices about their own care. In addition, the information equips them to ask for the care that they need and facilitates their saying no to care that they do not need. Thus, patient autonomy is enhanced.

This approach bodes well for enhanced opportunities for health education specialists who desire to practice in a healthcare setting in large part because of the myriad set of situations, policies, and approaches that seem to have no solution: high pharmaceutical costs, nearly 29 million Americans currently without health insurance (Tolbert et al., 2020), continuous federal tinkering with both the Medicare and Medicaid systems, lack of oversight for universal quality-of-care standards, high-cost care with limited emphasis on quality, lack of affordability of private pay insurance, inconsistent chronic disease management protocols, and frustration with a lack of emphasis on prevention. Given these circumstances, health education specialists can facilitate patient choice by helping patients understand their options regarding physician choice, healthcare insurance plan, type of care, and intensity of services. In addition, they can assist medical organizations by increasing patient satisfaction through contributing to more one-on-one contact, improving patterns of communication between patient and provider, evaluating outcomes, and enhancing patient compliance with treatment regimens (T. Epperly, personal communication, Family Medicine Residency of Idaho, Boise, May 2015).

Some key trends in healthcare now and beyond show that the healthcare industry is moving toward wellness as part of a value-based system of care. "Virtual care and the use of technology will allow a continued focus on population health, which is an increasing challenge for states when balancing their urban vs. rural areas. Similarly, challenges remain with balancing the economics of healthcare delivery with state financial obligations (e.g., pensions, Medicaid, infrastructure services) and the politics of running a state government" Vogenberg, & Santilli (2019).

Healthy People 2030 uses 355 data-driven national objectives as the backbone of all efforts to improve health and well-being for the next 10 years. These objectives are organized by health conditions, health behaviors, populations, settings and systems, and the Social Determinants of Health (SDH). Economic stability, education access and quality, healthcare access and quality, neighborhood and built environment, and social and community context all impact health, functioning and quality-of-life outcomes (Healthy People 2030). Health education specialists can work on the "upstream" factors to reduce health disparities and improve health. Where we live, zip code, has a bigger impact on health outcomes than genetic code (Belsky et al., 2019).

Professional Preparation and Credentialing

Although the issues of professional preparation and credentialing were extensively covered in Chapter 6, both have implications for the future practice of health education/promotion. Thus, the reasons why health education/promotion practice might be affected by these issues are of some importance.

Professional Preparation

In this discussion, it is not our intent to provide a list of courses that must be taken to become a "better" health education specialist. Coursework is by nature specific to the institution you are attending. Course titles and descriptions vary widely from one program to another. As you are aware, the coursework you will take in your degree program is interdisciplinary. We attempt to provide some ideas, concepts, and objectives for you to consider as you enter your preparation program.

The social changes previously discussed in this chapter are the challenges driving health education specialists of the future to be proactive in meeting the demands placed on them. What tasks will a health education specialist need to be able to perform effectively in the decades ahead? Clark (2014) described the skills health education/promotion professionals would need and they are still relevant:

1. The mission will be less about providing factual information and more about helping people become better analytical thinkers...
2. There will be...stronger partnerships with the medical establishment....
3. Health education specialists will need... Long-term, not short-term, thinking...
4. ...Education at the community level will be the focus of most health interventions.
5. There will be an enhanced need for quality research...
6. Health education specialists must...use technology to help people learn.
7. ...The gap between school and community services will close.
8. Environmental activism will continue to emerge...
9. ...people will judge the success of health education/promotion by whether or not their quality of life has improved.

In our work, there is an ever-growing need to facilitate health education/promotion interventions at the community level (as opposed to the individual level, or **microlevel**). Inherent in this charge is that those who reside in the community where the intervention occurs will be totally involved in the planning from the outset.

Three additional documents that provide information about the competencies health education specialists must possess into the future are described next. The first two can be found using the Weblinks at the end of this chapter. The first document features the deliberations by members of the Committee on Educating Public Health Professionals for the 21st Century (Institute of Medicine of the National Academies, 2003). The workshop participants who wrote the article "Who Will Keep the Public Healthy? Workshop Summary" (Weblinks #3) identify eight new content areas that should be added to the curricula of individuals studying to practice public health: informatics, genomics, communication, community-based participatory research, global health, health policy, health law, and public health ethics. Although the report is largely directed at universities offering graduate programs, even a cursory glance finds several suggested content areas that are relevant to the practice of health education/promotion. The list also shows the rapidly expanding knowledge base the future health education specialist will need to have to successfully interact with health professionals from a variety of other fields. The more understanding a health education specialist has about the vocabulary and nature of the work of other health providers, the more likely they are to be an accepted and valued member of the healthcare community.

The second document is the website for the National Commission for Health Education Credentialing (NCHEC) (2020), which features the results of a study titled, "2020 Health Education Specialist Practice Analysis (HESPA)II" commissioned by the Society for Public Health Education (SOPHE) and the National Commission for Health Education Credentialing (NCHEC). The findings report on changes in health education practice since the 2015 Health Education Specialist Practice Analysis (HESPA) study.

The third document, a cogent paper written by McKenzie (2004), cautions that those in charge of health education preparation programs must not assume that it is possible or even advisable to prepare "generic" health education specialists. The four practice settings to which he refers in the quote that follows are discussed later in this chapter. McKenzie states, "...even though the responsibilities and competencies of health educators are similar regardless of the settings, the work is indeed different and the preparation cannot be the same..." (p. 48).

In June of 2014, the Council on Education for Public Health (CEPH) released updated accreditation standards for Standalone Baccalaureate Programs (SBP). This allows for health education programs not associated with schools of public health to go through a nationally recognized accreditation process. The curriculum must cover 11 domains and required competencies if preparing students to sit for CHES (King, 2018).

It is apparent that tomorrow's health education specialists must be able to respond rapidly to changes in all avenues of society. When planning, implementing, and evaluating programs and working in multidimensional settings, they must enter into collaborative relationships with healthcare professionals from other disciplines in the spirit of cooperation. They understand how the Social Determinants of Health impact every aspect of one's health. Health education specialists who are not afraid to be innovative, who respect but do not fear change, who are not just purveyors of information but community builders, who are politically active and facilitators of learning, who continue to be curious and learn themselves, who have a sense of adventure, and who seek the truth through thoughtful research, study, and dialogue are the individuals who will lead our profession into the next several decades.

Credentialing

The history of and reasons for credentialing were thoroughly covered in Chapter 6. There are, however, several facets of credentialing that need reemphasis because they have profound implications for the future practice of health education/promotion.

The credentialing process as it now stands begins with the candidate's submitting a transcript of coursework in health education to the NCHEC. On verification by NCHEC that the candidate has completed coursework leading to a degree and the coursework has focused on the responsibilities and competencies of an entry-level health education specialist, the applicant is permitted to sit for the certification exam. Exam questions are based on the eight responsibilities and competencies for entry-level health education specialists. Individuals who pass the exam are awarded a Certified Health Education Specialist (CHES) credential. Those individuals must then complete continuing education units on a regular basis to maintain their credential.

All health education specialists, regardless of setting, have certain generic skills that they perform: assessing, planning, implementing and evaluating. Depending on the setting, we may need to refine or expand on the skills needed to perform in a particular work environment.

Health education specialists practice in a variety of settings (e.g., school, worksite, community, and health care), they may work with different populations (e.g., adults, the aged, children, and minorities), they may be process specialists (e.g., program planners, program implementers, and program evaluators), or they may be content specialists (e.g., HIV/AIDS, cancer prevention, injury or violence prevention, and nutrition). A potentially important consequence of having a CHES credential is that of eligibility for reimbursement for services rendered. As different care models are advanced with prevention as a focus (thanks to the ACA), insurers are limiting the types of providers eligible for reimbursement. Without some external credential or license, it is highly unlikely that any health education services rendered in a medical care setting will be reimbursed (Idaho Blue Shield Human Resources Department, personal communication, April 2015).

The credentialing process is here to stay. The bottom line is that this certification program does establish a national standard for individual health education specialists. In the past, certifications could differ by state, and some states or regions had local certifications and registries. Having a national certification better ensures that health education specialists in every state or setting have the same training and academic requirements. The CHES process works well and is endorsed by prevention specialists and organizations nationwide. Potential changes to the credentialing process and necessary competencies that emanate from the 2020 Health Education Specialist Practice Analysis (HESPA) II referenced in the previous section of this chapter will most likely occur. Students should stay abreast of developments in credentialing by visiting the NCHEC and SOPHE websites on a regular basis.

As the profession of health education/ promotion continues to evolve and health education specialists become more visible partners in the delivery of health services, students considering careers in this field should seriously consider obtaining CHES certification. The CHES credential assists employers in identifying practitioners who have met national standards, and it assures the consumers of health education/promotion services that the health educators with whom they work are competent professionals.

It is important to note that the Affordable Care Act focuses on prevention and several states now include health education specialists in the list of approved providers in Medicaid reimbursed programs such as nutrition classes (Auld, 2017). Each health education specialist needs to check with their state to see if this action applies in their locale.

Implications for Practice Settings

Chapter 7 detailed the variety of settings in which health education specialists can practice: the worksite, school, clinical/health care, and public health. Each setting has unique characteristics, and the practice set of skills or competencies may vary from one setting to another. However, the settings also are similar in that the goal of health education/promotion is to create a climate that facilitates the improvement of health status for every member of the population served by each entity. The first part of this chapter described various influences destined to impact the health of the populace into the next century. This section briefly summarizes the future role of the health education specialist in each setting.

School Setting

"It is important to note that there is clear evidence that the level of an individual's education is related to health outcomes in adulthood, and clear evidence that healthier children learn better and are more likely to be academically successful than those with health issues" (Birch, 2017). In 2015, Congress passed the Every Student Succeeds Act (ESSA), and for the first time, health education has been included as a "core subject" (United States 114th Congress, 2015–16). Providing high-quality health education in schools means more students will learn how to increase positive health behaviors and reduce negative ones. These statements characterize the goal and importance of school health education and provide direction for school health education specialists.

If children's well-being is to be maintained or enhanced, a coordinated approach to providing health education is needed (Allensworth & Kolbe, 1987). The Centers for Disease Control and Prevention (CDC) uses the Whole School, Whole Community, Whole Child (WSCC) model to address health in schools. This model uses a unified and collaborative approach to improve learning and health in our schools (CDC, 2020) Model components include (1) health education, (2) nutrition environment and services, (3) employee wellness, (4) social and emotional school climate, (5) physical environment, (6) health services, (7) counseling, psychological, and social services, (8) community involvement, (9) family engagement, and (10) physical education and physical activity.

Should you choose to practice health education/promotion in a school setting, what skills and abilities must you possess if schools are to incorporate a coordinated health education/promotion program to address the health needs of children and adolescents, both now and in the future? In light of the information on influences on health in this chapter and that on settings for health education/promotion from Chapter 7, we think that the following skills are imperative. You must be able to

1. Create a logical scope and sequence to health content units that incorporate age-appropriate information.
2. Prepare and deliver lessons that are participatory in nature, stress skill development, and foster attitudes necessary for problem solving and informed decision making.
3. Use technology and social media to assist in both updating your own skills and delivering health education/promotion messages to your school and community. Teach students how to be critical users of social media.
4. Acquire sound oral and written communication techniques.
5. Apply behavior-change strategies and what is known about environmental influences on behavior to the classroom setting.
6. Teach and promote the enhancement of strategies to increase health literacy among the population served to reduce health disparities (Hasnain-Wynia & Wolf, 2010).
7. Use both qualitative and quantitative strategies to evaluate your lessons, your units, and the district health education/ promotion program.
8. Assess the health needs of the students, faculty, and staff.
9. Ensure that health and counseling services are provided for students.
10. Read and interpret the findings of health research on effective health programs and practices.
11. Learn about the influence of culture on health, cultivate sensitivity toward it, and instill an awareness of it in your teaching.
12. Assist teachers at all grade levels in obtaining age-appropriate health education materials and help coordinate a classroom scope and sequence for all grade levels in your district.
13. Work both independently and as a member of a team.
14. Collaborate with health education specialists practicing in the community, worksite, or healthcare setting to coordinate the delivery of disease prevention and health promotion messages and programs.
15. Create or coordinate a parent/community health education/promotion advisory council.
16. Actively participate in local, state, regional, and national professional organizations.
17. Serve as resource person and liaison between the school health setting and other settings in which health education might occur.

Each of the above skills are included within the responsibilities, competencies, and subcompetencies of a health education specialist. School health educators who possess these skills will be well prepared to lead programs that enhance the health of the students, teachers, and staff in their schools.

Work-Site Setting

The workplace of today bears little resemblance to that of only 20 years ago. Because many employers want to attract the best employees and realize that employee satisfaction is key in productivity and retention, worksites have introduced programs for employees and their families that provide continuing education, recreational opportunities, health promotion, and financial planning. In particular, worksites have become an increasingly important setting for health education/ promotion programs. Examples of programs offered include stress management, worksite safety, drug and alcohol abuse prevention, and tobacco cessation. As noted previously in this chapter, the ACA also signals the advent of a renewed emphasis on worksite health promotion (Chait & Glied, 2018).

The influence of changing demographic patterns on health education/promotion in general was discussed previously. However, another factor must be taken into account when specifically anticipating the future direction of worksite health promotion. The greatest percentage of persons joining the workforce in the decades between 2015 and 2050 will be women and minorities.

The expansion of worksite health promotion programs bodes well for the future of health education/promotion and the concurrent need for an increasing number of trained health education specialists. This truth has broad implications for the future practice of work-site health education/promotion. Together with the information presented both earlier in this chapter and in Chapter 7, the following competencies represent a baseline for the future practice of health education/promotion in worksite settings:

1. Become familiar with the culture inherent in a business setting.
2. Use up-to-date technology to market programs to worksite supervisors, employees, and their families through newsletters, brochures, Internet chat groups, and social media.
3. Plan and manage a budget.
4. Acquire grant writing skills.
5. Implement programs in a manner consistent with management philosophy.
6. Coordinate needs assessments of worksite populace, keeping in mind how social determinants of health impact different populations. Conduct evaluations of program components.
7. Design and employ evaluation strategies that are outcome-based to assess program effectiveness.
8. Conduct fitness assessments and participate in health screenings.

9. Function as a resource person for health information for employees and their families.
10. Identify and work with aspects of the corporate organizational climate that facilitate or impede participation.
11. Recognize the importance of cultural and demographic influences on individual and group health behavioral choices.
12. Attain a working knowledge of epidemiological and statistical principles and applications.
13. Acquire sound oral and written communication techniques.
14. Gain a thorough understanding of current, relevant literature and well-designed research studies that influence health promotion practice in the worksite setting.
15. Work both independently and as a member of a team.
16. Teach and promote the enhancement of strategies to increase health literacy among the population served to reduce health disparities (Hasnain-Wynia & Wolf, 2010).
17. Prepare and conduct prevention presentations to worksite subgroups.
18. Coordinate employee coalitions and steering committees to maximize employee input into program components.
19. Be able to apply behavior-change strategies and what is known about environmental influences on behavior to the worksite setting.

Incorporating competencies such as those listed previously into the professional preparation program will help ensure that you are ready to begin practice as a worksite health education specialist.

Public Health Setting

The community setting (called the *public health setting* in this text) has a myriad of options for the practice of health education/promotion. For example, health education specialists are employed in many local, city, state, and federal health departments; in many federal agencies; in county extension agencies; in nonprofit and volunteer health organizations (e.g., American Cancer Society, American Heart Association, American Red Cross); in churches; in homeless shelters; in grassroots community organizations; and in prisons. One reason for the diversity of opportunities is that the mission, goals, and objectives of one community agency may differ dramatically from those of another. Some agencies might have a health education specialist serving as a coordinator of services or as a fundraiser, whereas in another agency, the educator might plan, conduct, and evaluate programs. Another, more obvious, reason for increased employment opportunities is that almost every locale in the United States has one of the aforementioned groups.

The purpose of community health organizations is to both monitor and improve the health of the public they serve. Goodman (2000) mentions that when health education specialists combine forces with people from other professional disciplines (e.g., ecologists, economists, anthropologists, communication specialists), the probability of reducing the health risks of populations is heightened. Consequently, collaboration with community organizations and with other professionals to address population health is a skill that all health education specialists must develop. In this era of using health education/promotion to help reduce healthcare costs while improving the quality of care, and with an increasing need for community-level programs, public health education specialists are well positioned to participate in improving the health of citizens from all regions of the United States.

With employment opportunities for health education specialists in the public setting on the rise (Bureau of Labor Statistics, 2020), what skills will the public health education specialists of the future need to function effectively? The following is a list of basic competencies or attributes that will be critical to the effective practice of public health education. They are not listed in any specific order of importance.

1. Recognize the importance of social determinants of health and how cultural and demographic influences on individual and group health behavioral choices. More focus on discriminatory systems related to race, ethnicity, LGBTQ+, immigration status and disability, more inclusive programming to meet diverse health needs.

2. Maintain competence in the use of technology and social media to access and deliver health-related information.

3. Learn to be flexible because the job will probably change and the responsibilities will be varied. Telecommuting and flexible schedules vs. 8–5.

4. Learn another language.

5. Learn and use strategies to seek information, guidance, and support from community members regarding their health needs. Intentionally involve the people being served at the earliest stages of programming.

6. Assess strengths of communities in building a plan to assist them in meeting their health needs.

7. Design and employ evaluation strategies that are outcomes based to assess program effectiveness.

8. Gain a thorough understanding of current, relevant literature and well-designed research studies that influence practice in the community setting (i.e., community-based participatory research). Gain an understanding of data visualization.

9. Apply behavior-change strategies and what is known about environmental influences on behavior to the public health setting.

10. Learn and practice research-based, coalition-building strategies, more shift to strategic planning, including being the backbone agency for community coalitions/initiatives.

11. Actively participate in local, state, regional, and national professional organizations.

12. Work independently and as a member of a team.
13. Advocate policies that enhance the role of prevention and provide for universal access to health services when needed. Health care is seeing the value of prevention and self-care practices as part of the comprehensive healthcare model.
14. Foster the ability to work in a multidisciplinary and a multicultural environment.
15. Teach and promote the enhancement of strategies to increase health literacy among the population served to reduce health disparities (Hasnain-Wynia & Wolf, 2010).
16. Study and apply the fundamentals of obtaining extramural funding. It is important to leverage partners to maximize fluctuating funding. More and more programs from similar topic areas are increasingly working together to maximize their resources and effectiveness.
17. Use a variety of marketing strategies and branding to reach diverse community constituencies.
18. Attain a working knowledge of epidemiological and statistical principles and applications.
19. Acquire excellent oral and written communication techniques.
20. The silos of public health are dissolving and programs from similar topic areas are increasingly working together to maximize their resources and effectiveness.

A well-trained community health education specialist will undoubtedly make an increased contribution to the health of diverse populations. With the increasing health awareness of U.S. citizens and the multitude of cultural changes in society, community health education specialists have a bright and exciting future.

Clinical or Healthcare Setting

Healthcare settings employ health education specialists in a variety of institutions and a multitude of ways. Health education specialists can be employed in for-profit and public hospitals, health maintenance organizations (HMOs), health insurance corporations, medical care clinics, and home health agencies. They might be involved in conducting one-on-one patient education; planning and implementing education programs for enrollees or other medical providers; coordinating community education programs on a variety of health topics; conducting program evaluations; marketing the health services available through the hospital, clinic, or HMO; conducting health education/promotion activities for the employees; or serving as a member of a community health promotion team.

Epperly (personal communication, May 2013) feels that healthcare providers, insurance companies, and the public in general are becoming more receptive to the notion that accurate and timely health information is an important part of any treatment regimen. Lack of adequate health education/promotion can negate potential positive contributions in the prevention and management of disease. With no end in sight to the skyrocketing costs of health care, the word *prevention* is being incorporated into more care plans than ever before.

Yarnall and colleagues (2003) note that the evidence of preventive services is well established but the rate of the delivery of preventive services by medical providers is severely lacking. Their study of time burdens required to deliver preventive care concluded that the major reason for the lack of delivery is that, to fulfill the U.S. Preventive Health Services Task Force recommendations, a primary care physician with a "normal" practice would have to dedicate nearly 7.5 hours per day solely to the delivery of preventive services. Obviously, this time allocation is impossible because physicians need to spend most of their time diagnosing and treating disease. Yarnall's study concludes with the following statement: "Our current system of preventive care delivery—provided by physicians…no longer meets national needs. New methods of preventive care delivery are required, as well as a clearer focus on which services can be best provided, and by whom" (p. 640).

The shift in practice norms by most clinical healthcare professionals requires trained personnel to ensure that education in the healthcare setting meets the needs of both the patient and the provider and motivates the patient to adopt a healthier lifestyle and to comply with any treatment regimen.

Given the medical community's acceptance of the value of health education/promotion in patient care, the outlook is positive for more employment opportunities for health education specialists in healthcare settings. Employment opportunities have increased for the health education specialist at Federally Qualified Community Health Clinics (FQHC's), serving the underserved. They are working in patient education, quality, informatics, and compliance. (Blanco, T personal communication, January 14, 2021) What skills, competencies, and attributes will be absolutely necessary for the health education specialist of the future who seeks employment in a healthcare setting? The following is a list of suggested competencies in no particular order:

1. Learn to perform basic health-screening techniques like blood pressure monitoring and pulse and respiration measurements.
2. Obtain a working knowledge of epidemiological and statistical principles and applications.
3. Maintain competence in the use of technology to access and deliver health-related information.
4. Acquire sound oral and written communication techniques.
5. Become familiar with the clinical disease process.
6. Learn a second language.
7. Obtain a working knowledge of the role of informatics in assisting in prevention at all vulnerable points in the causal chains leading to disease, injury, or disability (Davies et al., 2001).

8. Recognize the importance of cultural and demographic influences on individual and group health behavioral choices. Health education specialists should be culturally competent. Learn how to develop awareness of health equity and how to deliver tools necessary to reduce barriers to care.
9. Be able to apply behavior-change strategies and what is known about environmental influences on behavior to the healthcare setting.
10. Coordinate interdisciplinary teams or steering committees to maximize input into program components. Increased focus on policy, system and environmental change to address social influencers of health that impact health outcomes and costs.
11. Teach and promote the enhancement of strategies to increase health literacy among the population served to reduce health disparities (Hasnain-Wynia & Wolf, 2010).
12. Provide training in health education/promotion theory to other members of the healthcare team.
13. Become familiar with technological innovations to provide better outreach to patients, employees, and their families through using electronic and print media that meet the client's needs.
14. Advocate policies that enhance the role of prevention and provide for universal access to health services when needed. Stay current with the continued evolution of coverage models.
15. Work independently and as a member of a team.
16. Prepare and deliver lessons that are participatory in nature and research-based, that stress skill development, and foster attitudes necessary for problem solving and informed decision making.
17. Learn to be flexible, as the job probably will involve changing and varied responsibilities.

18. Serve as a liaison between the healthcare setting and other settings in which health education might occur.
19. Learn about public health emergency response and preparedness because fires, floods, hurricanes, and pandemics are constant and you can help lead efforts.
20. Function as a resource person for health information for patients and their families.

With rapid changes occurring in medical care delivery today, there is much reason for health education specialists to be optimistic about employment opportunities. As the public demands health education/promotion and disease prevention as a part of their medical care treatment plan, health education specialists will increasingly be identified as the best prepared to assist individuals in adopting healthy lifestyles.

Alternative Settings

Besides the four traditional practice settings previously discussed, there are several other viable alternatives for the practice of health education/promotion into the next century. In this section, we briefly introduce these choices so that individuals who are interested can research them further.

The first alternative is to teach health education/promotion in a **postsecondary institution**, usually defined as community college, college, or university. There will continue to be a need for qualified instructors. Minimum standards for obtaining one of these positions is usually a master's degree in health education and two to five years of experience for a community college or vocational school position, and a doctorate and two to five years of experience for a college or university position.

Students who are interested in combining the fields of health education/promotion and journalism can find positions in both the print (traditional print media as well as using blogging, Twitter, and reporting for online sources) and TV media as health reporters for newspapers, magazines, and TV stations. A broad-based knowledge of health issues and a passion for writing or speaking are necessary qualifications.

Because of the increasing interdependence among nations and because there are many areas of the world in which health assistance is badly needed, health education specialist positions will continue to be available in foreign countries. Examples include positions with organizations such as the Peace Corps, Project Hope, the United Nations, the Pan American Health Organization, and the World Health Organization. Many national church organizations also send interdisciplinary health teams to international locations to improve the health of the populace. Often, the health education specialist must have a college degree, some experience, and the ability to speak a foreign language.

Medical supply companies, pharmaceutical companies, sports equipment manufacturers, health topical curriculum developers or companies, health food stores, and textbook publishers often employ health education specialists in sales positions. A college degree is required. In addition, a willingness to travel, excellent oral and written communication skills, critical thinking, an ability to analyze research information (what is "real" and what is "hype"), and an ability to work with all types of people are necessary prerequisites.

Because of the aging of the U.S. population, demand for health education specialists in long-term care institutions and retirement communities is escalating. Elders are living longer and want to be active in their retirement years; thus, employment opportunities continue to grow. Usually, a college degree is required. Excellent oral and written communication skills are essential, as is a desire to listen and learn from older adults.

The diversity of our country and continued problems people have in accessing care has increased the demand for individuals who can work with a health education specialist to enhance outreach and impact within specific communities. **Community Health Workers** are these lay members of the community who volunteer or work with health education specialists in public health departments, local health care entities situated in both rural and urban environments. They live within the community they serve and have the unique ability to communicate with residents in multiple ways. They serve as a bridge between community members, health care, and public health departments (Berthold, 2016).

There continues to be an increasing number of opportunities for health education specialists in entrepreneurial and consultant roles. As self-employed persons, these individuals are free to set up their own practice, hiring out as consultants to organizations that temporarily need someone with expertise in grant writing, program planning and evaluation, software development, professional speaking, or technical writing. Other possibilities include contracting with several small businesses to conduct worksite health promotion; freelancing with HMOs and other insurance providers to offer health education/promotion services (reimbursement will be an issue); serving as a content specialist (e.g., stress management, eating disorders, substance abuse) to businesses and corporations; becoming a certified personal trainer; and teaching part-time in colleges, community colleges, or evening community education/promotion programs.

Now that we have explored the differences in the various practice settings, we reemphasize the fact that there are common tasks for health education specialists that transcend the individual practice settings. Dr. John Seffrin, former director of the American Cancer Society, eloquently reminds us of the direction health education/promotion must take, no matter what the practice setting, if it is to realize its potential. His scholar's address (Seffrin, 1997), given to members of the former American Association for Health Education AAHE, describes four actions for present and future health education specialists that still ring true today:

1. Look at ourselves as major players in keeping Americans healthy; to that end, work with policymakers to affect legislation that truly promotes health.
2. Collaborate with other health professionals in both the for-profit and the not-for-profit sectors.
3. Strive to exhibit greater professional solidarity; be an advocate for health education/promotion and the role that trained health education specialists can play as part of the healthcare team.
4. Advocate for those who do not have a voice; be a spokesperson in the political arena and work to ensure that health services and health education/promotion are available for all.

Summary

This chapter began with the notion of change as a constant. Although no one can actually "see" into the future, it is obvious that flexibility is imperative to adapt to ongoing change. This is an exciting time to become a health education specialist. Opportunities have never been greater, and the future has never looked brighter. The job outlook for health education specialists is anticipated to increase by 13% over the next 10 years (Bureau of Labor Statistics, 2020). There is little doubt that health education/promotion will continue to expand in all of the more traditional as well as some of the nontraditional settings. Health education specialists have the training and expertise to make a positive difference in enhancing the quality of life for all people. We wish you success as you begin your journey.

Review Questions

1. Identify three worksite settings in which health education specialists will practice to a greater degree than they currently do.
2. How will each of the societal changes discussed in the chapter impact the practice of health education/promotion in the worksite setting? The clinical/medical care setting? The school setting? The public health setting?
3. What are the implications for health education/promotion graduates who choose not to become credentialed (CHES)?
4. Using the list of basic competencies listed under the section on practicing in the clinical care setting, which of the items in the list fit into the following categories: assessment, instruction, and collaboration? Which are the most difficult to classify?
5. What is meant by the statement "Health education specialists need to become enhanced advocates for the profession"?
6. How has the passage of the Affordable Care Act impacted the practice of health education/promotion?

Case Study

One day, you see on the department website that the health education/promotion program in which you are enrolled is seeking national accreditation. The announcement includes information from the department chair on the reasons for accreditation along with a request for student assistance in working with faculty to prepare the necessary self-study documentation before the visit from an outside review team. Because you are entering the second semester of your junior year, you decide that a great way to learn more about the health education/promotion program and the field of health education/promotion in general would be to volunteer.

You notify the department chair of your willingness to help, and she appoints you to one of the program study committees, specifically the committee dealing with the use of the online health education/promotion curriculum.

You are excited about that committee because the campus has a strictly online program and a more traditional in-person program with some online offerings. Some of your classmates are not fans of online classes and say they are as rigorous as in-person classes, and they do not allow for as much interaction among students as traditionally delivered courses.

At the first meeting of the study committee, the committee chair outlines tasks that will need to be accomplished and suggests a timeline for completion. One of the major tasks is to determine whether the online program is meeting the accreditation goals for which they are designed. What key questions would you need to ask to obtain that information? What methods would you use to collect the data? How might the findings be used by health education/promotion programs in planning for the future?

Critical Thinking Questions

1. After reading the chapter and in your opinion, what major demographic trend will most impact the delivery of health education/promotion in the next several decades? Given your answer, describe the health education specialist in the year 2025.
2. Compare and contrast the lists of competencies noted in the chapter for the four major practice settings in

which a health education specialist might practice. Based on your findings, should professional preparation programs include coursework specific to the settings in which graduates will practice? Why or why not?

3. Read the 2020 HESPA II report commissioned by SOPHE and NCHEC that was referred to in the chapter. Using the information from that report, what duties might you assign to health education specialists desiring to practice in the clinical setting? How might your choices influence the Centers for Disease Control and Prevention goal of **Nurturing public health**—to have strong, well-resourced public health leaders and capabilities at national, state, and local levels to protect Americans from health threats? Look up the Centers for Disease Control and Prevention: Mission, Role and Pledge.

4. Assume that it is the year 2050 and you are retiring after many years as a practicing health education specialist. At your retirement banquet, you have been asked to spend five minutes summarizing the accomplishments of your profession. What will you say?

5. What are two ways in which the health education/health promotion community can make the message of prevention more appealing to the public? What are the major barriers you must address? How might you implement your ideas?

Activities

1. Make a list of your five strongest attributes. Make a second list of the five tasks you most like to do. Using these lists and what you know about health education/promotion, write a paragraph describing the "perfect" health education/promotion job for you.

2. Construct and administer a short survey to the health education/promotion faculty at your institution to determine their thoughts on the major factors influencing the current and future practice of health education/promotion. Compile your results.

3. Conduct an informational interview with a graduate from your school's health education/promotion program who is now practicing in the field as a certified health education specialist. Ask their feelings about their career path, current position, what their daily responsibilities are, and future trends in their field.

4. Write a job description that will be used to advertise for a new public health education specialist position in a worksite setting. In the document, be sure to include necessary applicant qualifications and expected duties.

Weblinks

1. **https://health.gov/healthypeople**

   Healthy People 2030

   Website of the national *Healthy People 2030* documents that describe U.S. goals and objectives for creating a healthier population by 2030.

2. **https://www.kingcounty.gov/depts /health.aspx**

   Public Health—Seattle and King County

   This outstanding website was launched by the Seattle King County Health

Department to help health education specialists and the public obtain current information on a variety of pertinent public health topics such as bioterrorism preparedness, family planning and reproductive health, diabetes, COVID-19, and others.

3. **https://www.ncbi.nlm.nih.gov/books /NBK221182/**

   "Who Will Keep the Public Healthy?"

   This 2003 report from the Institute of Medicine of the National Academies suggests specific ways to improve public health professionals' capabilities to address new and complex challenges. The report emphasizes that public health professionals in government health departments, other health services, community agencies, and universities have a shared responsibility to prevent illness and injury and keep communities healthy.

4. **http://www.nchec.org/**

   National Commission for Health Education Credentialing

   Provides information on the competencies to be a health education specialist including updated competencies as

a result of the 2020 HESPA II Study referenced earlier in the chapter.

5. **https://www.kff.org/**

   The Henry J. Kaiser Family Foundation

   The Kaiser Family Foundation website highlights health policy issues and enables the user to access background information on several current health policy topics. Modules and slide tutorials explaining that the policy issues are also included.

6. **https://www.rwjf.org/**

   The Robert Wood Johnson Foundation

   The Robert Wood Johnson Foundation features papers on health policy, health issue analyses, grant opportunities, and research and commentaries on healthcare reform.

7. **https://www.cdc.gov/health communication/index.html/**

   The CDC's website on health communications and marketing strategies for health promotion programs. Features examples of programs that have been successful. Also has a portal to the *Health Communication Science Digest* journal.

References

The American Association of Retired Persons. (2017). *GrandFacts.* https://www.aarp.org/content/dam/aarp /relationships/friends-family/grandfacts/grandfacts -national.pdf

Abroms, L., Allegrante, J., Auld, E., Gold, R., Riley, W., Smyser. J. (2019). Toward a common agenda for the public and private sectors to advance digital health communication. *American Journal of Public Health. 109*(2), 221–222. https://doi.org/10.2105/AJPH.2018 .304806

Acock, A. C., & Demo, D. H. (1994). *Family diversity and well-being.* Sage.

Adams, P., & Gonzales, S. (2020). Practicing information hygiene, Corona virus misinformation and COVID-19 journalism, News Literacy Project. https://newslit.org /educators/sift/the-sift-practicing-information-hygiene -coronavirus-misinformation-covid-19-journalism/

Alber, J. M., Paige, S., Stellefson, M., & Bernhardt, J. M. (2016). Social media self-efficacy of health education specialists: Training and organizational development implications. *Health Promotion Practice, 17*(6), 915–921. https://doi.org/10.1177%2F1524839916652389

Allensworth, D. D., & Kolbe, L. J. (1987). The comprehensive school health program: Exploring an expanded concept. *Journal of School Health, 57*(10), 409–412.

Association of Schools and Programs of Public Health. (2021, January 22). Media mentions: Florida trend— coronavirus spurs students to seek public health degrees. https://www.aspph.org/media-mentions/

Auld, E. (2017). Health education careers in a post-health reform era. *Health Promotion Practice, 18*(5), 629–635. https://doi.org/10.117/1524839917726495

Belsky, D. W., Caspi, A., Arseneault, L., Corcoran, D. L., Domingue, B. W., Harris, K. M., Houts, R. M., Mill, J. S., Moffitt, T. E., Prinz, J., Sugden, K., Wertz, J., Williams, B., & Odgers, C. L. (2019). Genetics and the geography of health, behaviour and attainment. *Nature Human Behaviour, 3,* 576–586. https://doi.org/10.1038/s41562-019-0562-1

Berthold, T. (Ed.) (2016). *Foundations for community health workers* (2nd ed.). Jossey-Bass.

Birch, D. A. (2017). Improving schools, improving school health education, improving public health: The role of SOPHE members. *Health Education & Behavior, 44*(6), 839–844. https://doi.org/10.1177%2F1090198117736353

Bureau of Labor Statistics, U.S. Department of Labor. (2020). *Occupational Outlook Handbook.* https://www.bls.gov/ooh/community-and-social-service/health-educators.htm

Bureau of Labor Statistics (2021). *The employment situation.* https://www.bls.gov/news.release/pdf/empsit.pdf

Centers for Disease Control and Prevention. (2019). *Community health worker (CHW) toolkit.* https://www.cdc.gov/dhdsp/pubs/toolkits/chw-toolkit.htm

Centers for Disease Control and Prevention. (2020). *Whole School, Whole Community, Whole Child (WSCC).* https://www.cdc.gov/healthyschools/wscc/index.htm

Chait, N., & Glied, S. (2018). Promoting prevention under the Affordable Care Act. *Annual Review of Public Health 39,* 507–524. https://doi.org/10.1146/annurev-publhealth-040617-013534

Christnacht, C., & Sullivan, B. (2020). *About two-thirds of the 23.5 million working women with children under 18 worked full-time in 2018.* https://www.census.gov/library/stories/2020/05/the-choices-working-mothers-make.html

Cilluffo, A., & Cohn, D. (2019). *6 demographic trends shaping the U.S. and the world in 2019.* https://www.pewresearch.org/fact-tank/2019/04/11/6-demographic-trends-shaping-the-u-s-and-the-world-in-2019/

Clark, N. M. (2014). Health educators and the future: Lead, follow, or get out of the way. *Journal of Health Education, 41*(3), 492–498. https://doi.org/10.1177/1090198114547509

Davies, J., Smith, G., & Gustafson, D. (2001). Public health informatics transforms the notifiable condition system. *Northwest Public Health, Spring/Summer,* 14–17.

English, G. M., & Videto, D. M. (1997). The future of health education: The knowledge to practice paradox. *Journal of Health Education, 28*(1), 4–12.

Forsberg, V., & Fichtenberg, C. (2012). *The prevention and public health fund: A critical investment in our nation's physical and fiscal health.* American Public Health Association, Center for Public Health Policy Issue Brief. https://www.apha.org/-/media/files/pdf/topics/aca/apha_prevfundbrief_june2012.ashx

Fry, R., Passel, J. S., & Cohn, D. (2020). A majority of young adults in the U.S. live with their parents for the first time since the Great Depression. *Pew Research Center.* https://www.pewresearch.org/fact-tank/2020/09/04/a-majority-of-young-adults-in-the-u-s-live-with-their-parents-for-the-first-time-since-the-great-depression/

Danaei, G., Rimm, E. B., Oza, S., Kulkarni, S. C., Murray, C. J. L., & Ezzati, M. (2010). The promise of prevention: The effects of four preventable risk factors on national life expectancy and life expectancy disparities by race and county in the United States. *PLOS Medicine, 7*(3), 1–13.

Goodman, R. M. (2000). On contemplation at 50: SOPHE Presidential Address, November 1999. *Health Education & Behavior, 27*(4), 423–429.

Giustini, D. M., Ali, S. M., Fraser, M., & Kamel Boulos, M. N. (2018). Effective uses of social media in public health and medicine: A systematic review of systematic reviews. *Online Journal of Public Health Informatics, 10*(2), e215. https://doi.org/10.5210/ojphi.v10i2.8270

Guest, J. L., del Rio, C., & Sanchez, T. (2020). The three steps needed to end the COVID-19 pandemic: Bold public health leadership, rapid innovations, and courageous political will. *JMIR Public Health Surveillance, 6*(2), e19043. https://doi.org/10.2196/19043

Hale, C. (2000). Demographic trends influencing public health practice. *Washington Public Health, Fall,* University of Washington, 1–3.

Hasnain-Wynia, R., & Wolf, M. S. (2010). Promoting health care equity: Is health literacy a missing link? *Health Services Research, 45*(4), 897–903.

Hunter, D. J. (2008). Health needs more than health care: The need for the new paradigm. *European Journal of Public Health, 18*(3), 217–219.

IQVIA. (2017). *IQVIA Institute for Human Data Science Study: Impact of digital health grows as innovation, evidence and adoption of mobile health apps accelerate.* https://www.iqvia.com/newsroom/2017/11/impact-of-digital-health-grows-as-innovation-evidence-and-adoption-of-mobile-health-apps-accelerate#:~:text=The%20use%20of%20Digital%20Health,estimated%20%247%20billion%20per%20year

Kaiser Family Foundation. (2020). Status of state Medicaid expansion decisions: Interactive map. https://www.kff.org/medicaid/issue-brief/status-of-state-medicaid-expansion-decisions-interactive-map/

Kahle, B. (2017). Transforming our libraries from analog to digital: A 2020 vision, *EDUCAUSE Review, 52*(2). https://er.educause.edu/articles/2017/3/transforming-our-libraries-from-analog-to-digital-a-2020-vision

Keisler-Starkey, K., & Bunch, L. N. (2020). Health insurance coverage in the United States: 2019.

U.S Census Bureau. https://www.census.gov/library/publications/2020/demo/p60-271.html

King, L. (2018). *Accreditation criteria: Standalone baccalareate programs*. https://media.ceph.org/wp_assets/2018.SBPcriteria.pdf

Korda, H., & Itani, Z. (2013). Harnessing social media for health promotion and behavior change. *Health Promotion Practice, 14*(1), 15–23.

Khullar, D., & Chokshi,D. (2019). Challenges for immigrant health in the USA—the road to crisis. *The Lancet, 393*(10186), 2168–2174. https://doi.org/10.1016/S0140-6736(19)30035-2

Larson, R. (2018). A path to better-quality mHealth apps. *JMIR Mhealth UHealth, 6*(7), e10414. https://doi.org/10.2196/10414

LaValley S. A., Kiviniemi M.T., & Gage-Bouchard E. A. (2017). Where people look for online health information. *Health Information and Libraries Journal, 34*(2), 146–155. https://doi.org/10.1111/hir.12143

Levine, S., Malone, E., Lekiachvili, A., Briss, P. (2019). Health care industry insights: Why the use of preventive services is still low. *Preventing Chronic Disease, 16*, E30. https://doi.org/10.5888/pcd16.180625

Mather, M. (2015) *Three States Account for Nearly Half of U.S. Population Growth*. https://www.prb.org/us-3-states-account/

McDermott, R. J. (2000). Health education research: Evolution or revolution (or maybe both)? *Journal of Health Education, 31*(5), 264–271.

McKenzie, J. F. (2004). Professional preparation: Is a generic health educator really possible? *American Journal of Health Education, 35*(1), 46–48.

McKenzie, J. F., Kotecki, J. E., & Pinger, R. R. (2008). *An introduction to community health.* Jones and Bartlett.

Morgan, B. (2018). *10 Examples of personalization in healthcare.* https://www.forbes.com/sites/blakemorgan/2018/10/22/10-examples-of-personalization-in-healthcare/?sh=139eb7a224e0

National Center for Education Statistics. (2020). Racial and ethnic enrollment in public schools. Retrieved January 17, 2021, from https://nces.ed.gov/programs/coe/indicator_cge.asp

National Center for Health Statistics (2020, May 5) Marriage and divorce. https://www.cdc.gov/nchs/fastats/marriage-divorce.htm

National Commission for Health Education Credentialing. (2020). HESPA II 202. Areas of responsibility, competencies and sub-competencies for health education specialist practice analysis II 2020 (HESPA II 2020). https://www.nchec.org/assets/2251/hespa_competencies_and_sub-competencies_052020.pdf

National Heart, Lung, and Blood Institute. (2014). Role of community health workers. https://www.nhlbi.nih.gov/health/educational/healthdisp/role-of-community-health-workers.htm

Neiger, B. L., Thackery, R., Van Wagenen, S. A., Hanson, C. L., West, J. H., Barnes, M. D., & Fagen, M. C. (2012). Use of social media in health promotion: Purposes, key performance indicators, and evaluation metrics. *Health Promotion Practice, 13*(2), 159–164.

O'Rourke, T. (2006). Philosophical reflections on health education and health promotion: Shifting sands and ebbing tides. *The Health Education Monograph Series, 23*(1), 7–10.

Pew Research Center. (2019). *A majority of mothers are now employed full time*. https://www.pewresearch.org/fact-tank/2019/09/12/despite-challenges-at-home-and-work-most-working-moms-and-dads-say-being-employed-is-whats-best-for-them/ft_19-09-11_workingparents_majority-mothers-employed-full-time/

Pew Research (2020). *The pace of boomer retirements has accelerated in the past year*. https://www.pewresearch.org/fact-tank/2020/11/09/the-pace-of-boomer-retirements-has-accelerated-in-the-past-year/

Pollard, K. M., Jacobsen, L. A., & Mather, M. (2020) *The U.S. population is growing at the slowest rate since the 1930s.* https://www.prb.org/the-u-s-population-is-growing-at-the-slowest-rate-since-the-1930s/

Prabha, C. (2007). Shifting from print to electronic journals in ARL university libraries. *Serials Review, 33*(1), 4–13. https://doi.org/10.1016/j.serrev.2006.12.001

Seffrin, J. R. (1997). *AAHE scholar's address.* American Alliance for Health, Physical Education, Recreation, and Dance Convention.

Smith, J. C., & Medalia, C. (2015). *Health insurance coverage in the United States: 2014. U.S. Census Bureau.* https://www.census.gov/content/dam/Census/library/publications/2015/demo/p60-253.pdf

Society for Public Health Education. (2020). *Digital health technology & communications award.* https://www.sophe.org/about/awards-fellowships-scholarships/technology-award/

Thackery, R., Neiger, B. L., Hanson, C. L., & McKenzie, J. F. (2008). Enhancing promotional strategies within social marketing programs: Use of web 2.0 social media. *Health Promotion Practice, 9*(4), 338–343.

Tolbert, J., Orgera, K. & Damico, A. (2020). *Key facts about the uninsured population.* https://www.kff.org/uninsured/issue-brief/key-facts-about-the-uninsured-population/

United States 114th Congress. (2015–16). *Every Student Succeeds Act (ESSA).* https://www.congress.gov/bill/114th-congress/senate-bill/1177/text

U.S. Census Bureau. (2012). *Most children younger than 1 are minorities.* http://www.census.gov/newsroom/releases/archives/population/cb12-90.html

U.S. Census Bureau. (2020). *Measuring the nation's social and economic well-being.* https://www.census.gov/library/visualizations/2020/comm/measuring-nations-well-being.html

Census. (2020). *Historical living arrangements of children.* https://www.census.gov/data/tables/time-series/demo/families/children.html

Vespa, J., Medina, L., & Armstrong, D. M. (2020). Demographic turning points for the United States: Population projections for 2020 to 2060. Population estimates and projections. *Current Population Reports.* https://www.census.gov/content/dam/Census/library/publications/2020/demo/p25-1144.pdf

Vogenberg, F. R., & Santilli, J. (2019). Key trends in healthcare for 2020 and beyond. *American Health & Drug Benefits, 12*(7), 348–350.

Williams, D. R., McClellan, M. B., & Rivlin, A. M. (2010). Beyond the Affordable Care Act: Achieving real improvements in Americans' health. *Health Affairs, 29*(8), 1481–1488.

Jiang, Y., Ekono, M., & Skinner, C. (2016). *Basic facts about low-income children: Children under 18 years, 2014. National Center for Children in Poverty.* http://www.nccp.org/publications/pub_1145.html

Appendix A

Code of Ethics for the Health Education Profession

CODE OF ETHICS FOR THE HEALTH EDUCATION PROFESSION
PREAMBLE

The Code of Ethics provides a framework of shared values within Health Education professions. The Code of Ethics is grounded in fundamental ethical principles, including: value of life, promoting justice, ensuring beneficence, and avoiding harm. A Health Education Specialist's responsibility is to aspire to the highest possible standards of conduct and to encourage the ethical behavior of all those with whom they work.

Health Education professionals are dedicated to excellence in the practice of promoting individual, family, group, organizational, school, community, public, and population health. Guided by common goals to improve the human condition, Health Education Specialists are responsible for upholding the integrity and ethics of the profession as they perform their work and face the daily challenges of making ethical decisions. Health Education Specialists value equity in society and embrace a multiplicity of approaches in their work to support the worth, dignity, potential, quality of life, and uniqueness of all people.

Health Education Specialists promote and abide by these guidelines when making professional decisions, regardless of job title, professional affiliation, work setting, or populations served.

Article I: Core Ethical Expectations

1. Health Education Specialists display personal behaviors that represent the ethical conduct principles of honesty, autonomy, beneficence, respect, and justice. The Health Education Specialist should, under no circumstances, engage in derogatory language, violence, bigotry, racism, harassment, inappropriate sexual activities or communications in person or through the use of technology and other means.

2. Health Education Specialists respect and support the rights of individuals and communities to make informed decisions about their health, as long as such decisions pose no risk to the health of others.

3. Health Education Specialists are truthful about their qualifications and the qualifications of others whom they recommend. Health Education Specialists know their scope of practice and the limitations of their education, expertise, and experience in providing services consistent with their respective levels of professional competence, including certifications and licensures.

4. Health Education Specialists are ethically bound to respect the privacy, confidentiality, and dignity of individuals and organizations. They respect the rights of others to hold diverse values, attitudes, and opinions. Health Education Specialists have a responsibility to engage in supportive relationships that are free of exploitation in all professional settings (e.g.: with clients, patients, community members, students, supervisees, employees, and research participants.)

5. Health Education Specialists openly communicate to colleagues, employers, and professional organizations when they suspect unethical practices that violate the profession's Code of Ethics.

6. Health Education Specialists are conscious of and responsive to social, racial, faith-based, and cultural diversity when assessing needs and assets, planning, and implementing programs, conducting evaluations, and engaging in research to protect individuals, groups, society, and the environment from harm.

7. Health Education Specialists should disclose conflicts of interest in professional practice, research, evaluation, and the dissemination process.

Article II: Ethical Practice Expectations

Section 1: Responsibility to the Public
Health Education Specialists are responsible for educating, promoting, maintaining, and improving the health of individuals, families, groups, and communities. When a conflict or issue arises among individuals, groups, organizations, agencies, or institutions, Health Education Specialists must consider all issues and give priority to those that promote the health and well-being of individuals and the public, while respecting both the principles of individual autonomy, human rights, and equity as long as such decisions pose no risk to the health of others.

A: Health Education Specialists advocate and encourage actions and social policies that promote maximal health benefits and the elimination or minimization of preventable risks and health inequities for all affected parties.

B: Health Education Specialists contribute to the profession by redefining existing practices, developing new practices, and by sharing the outcomes of their work.

C: Health Education Specialists actively involve individuals, groups, stakeholders, and communities in the entire educational process to maximize the understanding and personal responsibilities of those who may be affected.

Section 2: Responsibility to the Profession
Health Education Specialists are responsible for their professional behavior, the reputation of their profession, promotion of certification for those in the profession, and promotion of ethical conduct among their colleagues.

A: Health Education Specialists recognize the boundaries of their professional competence and are accountable for their professional activities and actions.

B: Health Education Specialists maintain, improve, and expand their professional competence through continued education, research, scholarship, membership, participation, leadership in professional organizations, and engagement in professional development.

C: Health Education Specialists contribute to the profession by refining existing professional health-related practices, developing new practices, and by sharing the outcomes of their work.

D: Health Education Specialists give recognition to others for their professional contributions and achievements.

Section 3: Responsibility to Employers
Health Education Specialists are responsible for their professional behavior in the workplace and for promoting ethical conduct among their colleagues and employers.

A: Health Education Specialists apply current, evidence informed standards and theories when fulfilling their professional responsibilities.

B: Health Education Specialists accurately represent and report service and program outcomes to employers.

C: Health Education Specialists maintain competence in their areas of professional practice through continuing education on a regular basis to maintain their competence.

Section 4: Responsibility in the Delivery of Health Education/Promotion

Health Education Specialists deliver evidence informed practices with integrity. They respect the rights, dignity, confidentiality, inclusivity, and worth of all people by using strategies and methods tailored to the needs of diverse populations and communities.

A: Health Education Specialists remain informed of the latest scientific information and advances in health education theory, research, and practice.

B: Health Education Specialists support the development of professional standards grounded in theory, best-practice guidelines, and data.

C: Health Education Specialists adhere to a rigorous and ethical evaluation of health education/promotion initiatives.

D: Health Education Specialists promote healthy behaviors through informed choice and advocacy, and do not use coercion or intimidation.

E: Health Education Specialists disclose potential benefits and harms of proposed services, strategies, and actions that affect individuals, organizations, and communities.

F: Health Education Specialists actively collaborate with a variety of individuals and organizations, and demonstrate respect for the unique contributions provided by others.

G: Health Education Specialists do not plagiarize.

Section 5: Responsibility in Research and Evaluation

Through research and evaluation activities, Health Education Specialists contribute to the health of populations and the profession. When planning and conducting research or evaluation, Health Education Specialists abide by federal, state, and tribal laws and regulations, organizational and institutional policies, and professional standards and ethics.

A: Health Education Specialists ensure that participation in research is voluntary and based upon the informed consent of participants. They follow research designs and protocols approved by relevant institutional review committees and/or boards.

B: Health Education Specialists respect and protect the privacy, rights, and dignity of research participants and honor commitments made to those participants.

C: Health Education Specialists treat all information obtained from participants as confidential, unless otherwise required by law, and inform research participants of the disclosure requirements and procedures.

D: Health Education Specialists take credit, including authorship, only for work they have performed and give appropriate authorship, co-authorship, credit, or acknowledgment for the contributions of others.

E: Health Education Specialists report the results of their research and evaluation objectively, accurately, and in a timely manner.

F. Health Education Specialists promote and disseminate the results of their research through appropriate formats while fostering the translation of research into practice.

Section 6: Responsibility in Professional Preparation and Continuing Education

Those involved in the professional preparation and training of Health Education students and continuing education for Health Education Specialists, are obligated to provide a quality education that meets professional standards and benefits the individual, the profession, and the public.

A: Health Education Specialists foster an inclusive educational environment free from all forms of discrimination, coercion, and harassment.

B: Health Education Specialists engaged in the delivery of professional preparation and continuing education demonstrate careful planning; state clear and realistic expectations; present material that is scientifically accurate, developmentally appropriate, and inclusive; conduct fair assessments; and provide reasonable and prompt feedback to learners.

C: Health Education Specialists provide learners with objective and comprehensive guidance about professional development and career advancement.

D: Health Education Specialists facilitate meaningful opportunities for the professional development and advancement of learners.

Code of Ethics Taskforce Members:

Christopher Ledingham, MPH, PhD (Co-Chair)
Keely Rees, PhD, MCHES® (Co-Chair)
Andrea L. Lowe, MPH, CPH
Elisa "Beth" McNeill, Ph.D., CHES®
Fran Anthony Meyer, PhD, CHES®
Holly Turner Moses, PhD, MCHES®, FESG
Larry Olsen, MAT, MPH, Dr. P.H., MCHES®
Lori Paisley, B.S., MA.
Kerry J. Redican, MPH, PhD, CHES ®
Jody Vogelzang, PhD, RDN, CHES®, FAND
Gayle Walter, PhD, CHES®

Suggested Citation:

Code of Ethics for the Health Education Profession®. (2020). Coalition for National Health Education Organizations (CNHEO). [Document]. http://cnheo.org/ethics-of-the-profession.html

The Code of Ethics for the Health Education Profession® update by the CNHEO Task Force: Christopher Ledingham, MPH, PhD (Co-Chair) Keely Rees, PhD, MCHES® (Co-Chair) Andrea L. Lowe, MPH, CPH Elisa "Beth" McNeill, Ph.D., CHES® Fran Anthony Meyer, PhD, CHES® Holly Turner Moses, PhD, MCHES®, FESG Larry Olsen, MAT, MPH, Dr. P.H., MCHES®, Lori Paisley, BS, MA, Kerry J. Redican, MPH, PhD, CHES ® Jody Vogelzang, PhD, RDN, CHES®, FAND, Gayle Walter, PhD, CHES®. *The Task Force was organized by the CNHEO Committee in 2019. Significant contributions to the Code were also made by the broader CNHEO members and full memberships. This Code was updated from a Task Force in 2011 and adopted by the CNHEO in February 2020.*

Appendix B

Areas of Responsibility, Competencies, and Subcompetencies for Health Education Specialist Practice Analysis II 2020 (HESPA II 2020)

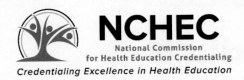

NCHEC
National Commission
for Health Education Credentialing
Credentialing Excellence in Health Education

AREAS OF RESPONSIBILITY, COMPETENCIES AND SUB-COMPETENCIES FOR HEALTH EDUCATION SPECIALIST PRACTICE ANALYSIS II 2020 (HESPA II 2020)

The Eight Areas of Responsibility contain a comprehensive set of Competencies and Sub-competencies defining the role of the health education specialist. These Responsibilities were verified by the 2020 Health Education Specialist Practice Analysis II (HESPA II 2020) project and serve as the basis of the CHES® and MCHES® exam beginning 2022.

The Eight Areas of Responsibility for Health Education Specialists are:
Area I: Assessment of Needs and Capacity
Area II: Planning
Area III: Implementation
Area IV: Evaluation and Research
Area V: Advocacy
Area VI: Communication
Area VII: Leadership and Management
Area VIII: Ethics and Professionalism

Color Key:

Advanced – 1
Advanced – 2

The Sub-competencies shaded yellow and blue in the table below are advanced-level only and will not be included in the entry-level, CHES® examination. However, the advanced-level Sub-competencies will be included in the MCHES® examination.

HEALTH EDUCATION SPECIALIST PRACTICE ANALYSIS II 2020 (HESPA II 2020)
Competencies and Sub-Competencies

	Area I: Assessment of Needs and Capacity
1.1	**Plan assessment.**
1.1.1	Define the purpose and scope of the assessment.
1.1.2	Identify priority population(s).
1.1.3	Identify existing and available resources, policies, programs, practices, and interventions.
1.1.4	Examine the factors and determinants that influence the assessment process.
1.1.5	Recruit and/or engage priority population(s), partners, and stakeholders to participate throughout all steps in the assessment, planning, implementation, and evaluation processes.
1.2	**Obtain primary data, secondary data, and other evidence-informed sources.**
1.2.1	Identify primary data, secondary data, and evidence-informed resources.
1.2.2	Establish collaborative relationships and agreements that facilitate access to data.
1.2.3	Conduct a literature review.
1.2.4	Procure secondary data.
1.2.5	Determine the validity and reliability of the secondary data.
1.2.6	Identify data gaps.
1.2.7	Determine primary data collection needs, instruments, methods, and procedures.
1.2.8	Adhere to established procedures to collect data.
1.2.9	Develop a data analysis plan.
1.3	**Analyze the data to determine the health of the priority population(s) and the factors that influence health.**
1.3.1	Determine the health status of the priority population(s).
1.3.2	Determine the knowledge, attitudes, beliefs, skills, and behaviors that impact the health and health literacy of the priority population(s).
1.3.3	Identify the social, cultural, economic, political, and environmental factors that impact the health and/or learning processes of the priority population(s).
1.3.4	Assess existing and available resources, policies, programs, practices, and interventions.
1.3.5	Determine the capacity (available resources, policies, programs, practices, and interventions) to improve and/or maintain health.
1.3.6	List the needs of the priority population(s).
1.4	**Synthesize assessment findings to inform the planning process.**
1.4.1	Compare findings to norms, existing data, and other information.

1.4.2	Prioritize health education and promotion needs.
1.43	Summarize the capacity of priority population(s) to meet the needs of the priority population(s).
1.4.4	Develop recommendations based on findings.
1.4.5	Report assessment findings.

	Area II: Planning
2.1	**Engage priority populations, partners, and stakeholders for participation in the planning process.**
2.1.1	Convene priority populations, partners, and stakeholders.
2.1.2	Facilitate collaborative efforts among priority populations, partners, and stakeholders.
2.1.3	Establish the rationale for the intervention.
2.2	**Define desired outcomes.**
2.2.1	Identify desired outcomes using the needs and capacity assessment.
2.2.2	Elicit input from priority populations, partners, and stakeholders regarding desired outcomes.
2.2.3	Develop vision, mission, and goal statements for the intervention(s).
2.2.4	Develop specific, measurable, achievable, realistic, and time-bound (SMART) objectives.
2.3	**Determine health education and promotion interventions.**
2.3.1	Select planning model(s) for health education and promotion.
2.3.2	Create a logic model.
2.3.3	Assess the effectiveness and alignment of existing interventions to desired outcomes.
2.3.4	Adopt, adapt, and/or develop tailored intervention(s) for priority population(s) to achieve desired outcomes.
2.3.5	Plan for acquisition of required tools and resources.
2.3.6	Conduct a pilot test of intervention(s).
2.3.7	Revise intervention(s) based on pilot feedback.
2.4	**Develop plans and materials for implementation and evaluations.**
2.4.1	Develop an implementation plan inclusive of logic model, work plan, responsible parties, timeline, marketing, and communication.
2.4.2	Develop materials needed for implementation.
2.4.3	Address factors that influence implementation.

| 2.4.4 | Plan for evaluation and dissemination of results. |
| 2.4.5 | Plan for sustainability. |

Area III: Implementation

3.1	**Coordinate the delivery of intervention(s) consistent with the implementation plan.**
3.1.1	Secure implementation resources.
3.1.2	Arrange for implementation services.
3.1.3	Comply with contractual obligations.
3.1.4	Establish training protocol.
3.1.5	Train staff and volunteers to ensure fidelity.
3.2	**Deliver health education and promotion interventions.**
3.2.1	Create an environment conducive to learning.
3.2.2	Collect baseline data.
3.2.3	Implement a marketing plan.
3.2.4	Deliver health education and promotion as designed.
3.2.5	Employ an appropriate variety of instructional methodologies.
3.3	**Monitor implementation.**
3.3.1	Monitor progress in accordance with the timeline.
3.3.2	Assess progress in achieving objectives.
3.3.3	Modify interventions as needed to meet individual needs.
3.3.4	Ensure plan is implemented with fidelity.
3.3.5	Monitor use of resources.
3.3.6	Evaluate the sustainability of implementation.

Area IV: Evaluation and Research

4.1	**Design process, impact, and outcome evaluation of the intervention.**
4.1.1	Align the evaluation plan with the intervention goals and objectives.
4.1.2	Comply with institutional requirements for evaluation.
4.1.3	Use a logic model and/or theory for evaluations.
4.1.4	Assess capacity to conduct evaluation.

4.1.5	Select an evaluation design model and the types of data to be collected.
4.1.6	Develop a sampling plan and procedures for data collection, management, and security.
4.1.7	Select quantitative and qualitative tools consistent with assumptions and data requirements.
4.1.8	Adopt or modify existing instruments for collecting data.
4.1.9	Develop instruments for collecting data.
4.1.10	Implement a pilot test to refine data collection instruments and procedures.
4.2	**Design research studies.**
4.2.1	Determine purpose, hypotheses, and questions.
4.2.2	Comply with institutional and/or IRB requirements for research.
4.2.3	Use a logic model and/or theory for research.
4.2.4	Assess capacity to conduct research.
4.2.5	Select a research design model and the types of data to be collected.
4.2.6	Develop a sampling plan and procedures for data collection, management, and security.
4.2.7	Select quantitative and qualitative tools consistent with assumptions and data requirements.
4.2.8	Adopt, adapt, and/or develop instruments for collecting data.
4.2.9	Implement a pilot test to refine and validate data collection instruments and procedures.
4.3	**Manage the collection and analysis of evaluation and/or research data using appropriate technology.**
4.3.1	Train data collectors.
4.3.2	Implement data collection procedures.
4.3.3	Use appropriate modalities to collect and manage data.
4.3.4	Monitor data collection procedures.
4.3.5	Prepare data for analysis.
4.3.6	Analyze data.
4.4	**Interpret data.**
4.4.1	Explain how findings address the questions and/or hypotheses.
4.4.2	Compare findings to other evaluations or studies.
4.4.3	Identify limitations and delimitations of findings.
4.4.4	Draw conclusions based on findings.
4.4.5	Identify implications for practice.

4.4.6	Synthesize findings.
4.4.7	Develop recommendations based on findings.
4.4.8	Evaluate feasibility of implementing recommendations.
4.5	**Use findings.**
4.5.1	Communicate findings by preparing reports, and presentations, and by other means.
4.5.2	Disseminate findings.
4.5.3	Identify recommendations for quality improvement.
4.5.4	Translate findings into practice and interventions.

Area V: Advocacy

5.1	**Identify a current or emerging health issue requiring policy, systems, or environmental change.**
5.1.1	Examine the determinants of health and their underlying causes (e.g., poverty, trauma, and population-based discrimination) related to identified health issues.
5.1.2	Examine evidence-informed findings related to identified health issues and desired changes.
5.1.3	Identify factors that facilitate and/or hinder advocacy efforts (e.g., amount of evidence to prove the issue, potential for partnerships, political readiness, organizational experience or risk, and feasibility of success).
5.1.4	Write specific, measurable, achievable, realistic, and time-bound (SMART) advocacy objective(s).
5.1.5	Identify existing coalition(s) or stakeholders that can be engaged in advocacy efforts.
5.2	**Engage coalitions and stakeholders in addressing the health issue and planning advocacy efforts.**
5.2.1	Identify existing coalitions and stakeholders that favor and oppose the proposed policy, system, or environmental change and their reasons.
5.2.2	Identify factors that influence decision-makers (e.g., societal and cultural norms, financial considerations, upcoming elections, and voting record).
5.2.3	Create formal and/or informal alliances, task forces, and coalitions to address the proposed change.
5.2.4	Educate stakeholders on the health issue and the proposed policy, system, or environmental change.
5.2.5	Identify available resources and gaps (e.g., financial, personnel, information, and data).
5.2.6	Identify organizational policies and procedures and federal, state, and local laws that pertain to the advocacy efforts.
5.2.7	Develop persuasive messages and materials (e.g., briefs, resolutions, and fact sheets) to communicate the policy, system, or environmental change.

5.2.8	Specify strategies, a timeline, and roles and responsibilities to address the proposed policy, system, or environmental change (e.g., develop ongoing relationships with decision makers and stakeholders, use social media, register others to vote, and seek political appointment).
5.3	**Engage in advocacy.**
5.3.1	Use media to conduct advocacy (e.g., social media, press releases, public service announcements, and op-eds).
5.3.2	Use traditional, social, and emerging technologies and methods to mobilize support for policy, system, or environmental change.
5.3.3	Sustain coalitions and stakeholder relationships to achieve and maintain policy, system, or environmental change.
5.4	**Evaluate advocacy.**
5.4.1	Conduct process, impact, and outcome evaluation of advocacy efforts.
5.4.2	Use the results of the evaluation to inform next steps.
	Area VI: Communications
6.1	**Determine factors that affect communication with the identified audience(s).**
6.1.1	Segment the audience(s) to be addressed, as needed.
6.1.2	Identify the assets, needs, and characteristics of the audience(s) that affect communication and message design (e.g., literacy levels, language, culture, and cognitive and perceptual abilities).
6.1.3	Identify communication channels (e.g., social media and mass media) available to and used by the audience(s).
6.1.4	Identify environmental and other factors that affect communication (e.g., resources and the availability of Internet access).
6.2	**Determine communication objective(s) for audience(s).**
6.2.1	Describe the intended outcome of the communication (e.g., raise awareness, advocacy, behavioral change, and risk communication).
6.2.2	Write specific, measurable, achievable, realistic, and time-bound (SMART) communication objective(s).
6.2.3	Identify factors that facilitate and/or hinder the intended outcome of the communication.
6.3	**Develop message(s) using communication theories and/or models.**
6.3.1	Use communications theory to develop or select communication message(s).
6.3.2	Develop persuasive communications (e.g., storytelling and program rationale).
6.3.3	Tailor message(s) for the audience(s).

6.3.4	Employ media literacy skills (e.g., identifying credible sources and balancing multiple viewpoints).
6.4	**Select methods and technologies used to deliver message(s).**
6.4.1	Differentiate the strengths and weaknesses of various communication channels and technologies (e.g., mass media, community mobilization, counseling, peer communication, information/digital technology, and apps).
6.4.2	Select communication channels and current and emerging technologies that are most appropriate for the audience(s) and message(s).
6.4.3	Develop communication aids, materials, or tools using appropriate multimedia (e.g., infographics, presentation software, brochures, and posters).
6.4.4	Assess the suitability of new and/or existing communication aids, materials, or tools for audience(s) (e.g., the CDC Clear Communication Index and the Suitability Assessment Materials (SAM).
6.4.5	Pilot test message(s) and communication aids, materials, or tools.
6.4.6	Revise communication aids, materials, or tools based on pilot results.
6.5	**Deliver the message(s) effectively using the identified media and strategies.**
6.5.1	Deliver presentation(s) tailored to the audience(s).
6.5.2	Use public speaking skills.
6.5.3	Use facilitation skills with large and/or small groups.
6.5.4	Use current and emerging communication tools and trends (e.g., social media).
6.5.5	Deliver oral and written communication that aligns with professional standards of grammar, punctuation, and style.
6.5.6	Use digital media to engage audience(s) (e.g., social media management tools and platforms).
6.6	**Evaluate communication.**
6.6.1	Conduct process and impact evaluations of communications.
6.6.2	Conduct outcome evaluations of communications.
6.6.3	Assess reach and dose of communication using tools (e.g., data mining software, social media analytics and website analytics).

	Area VII: Leadership and Management
7.1	**Coordinate relationships with partners and stakeholders (e.g., individuals, teams, coalitions, and committees).**
7.1.1	Identify potential partners and stakeholders.
7.1.2	Assess the capacity of potential partners and stakeholders.
7.1.3	Involve partners and stakeholders throughout the health education and promotion process in meaningful and sustainable ways.
7.1.4	Execute formal and informal agreements with partners and stakeholders.
7.1.5	Evaluate relationships with partners and stakeholders on an ongoing basis to make appropriate modifications.
7.2	**Prepare others to provide health education and promotion.**
7.2.1	Develop culturally responsive content.
7.2.2	Recruit individuals needed in implementation.
7.2.3	Assess training needs.
7.2.4	Plan training, including technical assistance and support.
7.2.5	Implement training.
7.2.6	Evaluate training as appropriate throughout the process.
7.3	**Manage human resources.**
7.3.1	Facilitate understanding and sensitivity for various cultures, values, and traditions.
7.3.2	Facilitate positive organizational culture and climate.
7.3.3	Develop job descriptions to meet staffing needs.
7.3.4	Recruit qualified staff (including paraprofessionals) and volunteers.
7.3.5	Evaluate performance of staff and volunteers formally and informally.
7.3.6	Provide professional development and training for staff and volunteers.
7.3.7	Facilitate the engagement and retention of staff and volunteers.
7.3.8	Apply team building and conflict resolution techniques as appropriate.
7.4	**Manage fiduciary and material resources.**
7.4.1	Evaluate internal and external financial needs and funding sources.
7.4.2	Develop financial budgets and plans.
7.4.3	Monitor budget performance.

7.4.4	Justify value of health education and promotion using economic (e.g., cost-benefit, return-on-investment, and value-on-investment) and/or other analyses.
7.4.5	Write grants and funding proposals.
7.4.6	Conduct reviews of funding and grant proposals.
7.4.7	Monitor performance and/or compliance of funding recipients.
7.4.8	Maintain up-to-date technology infrastructure.
7.4.9	Manage current and future facilities and resources (e.g., space and equipment).
7.5	**Conduct strategic planning with appropriate stakeholders.**
7.5.1	Facilitate the development of strategic and/or improvement plans using systems thinking to promote the mission, vision, and goal statements for health education and promotion.
7.5.2	Gain organizational acceptance for strategic and/or improvement plans.
7.5.3	Implement the strategic plan, incorporating status updates and making refinements as appropriate.
	Area VIII: Ethics and Professionalism
8.1	**Practice in accordance with established ethical principles.**
8.1.1	Apply professional codes of ethics and ethical principles throughout assessment, planning, implementation, evaluation and research, communication, consulting, and advocacy processes.
8.1.2	Demonstrate ethical leadership, management, and behavior.
8.1.3	Comply with legal standards and regulatory guidelines in assessment, planning, implementation, evaluation and research, advocacy, management, communication, and reporting processes.
8.1.4	Promote health equity.
8.1.5	Use evidence-informed theories, models, and strategies.
8.1.6	Apply principles of cultural humility, inclusion, and diversity in all aspects of practice (e.g., Culturally and Linguistically Appropriate Services (CLAS) standards and culturally responsive pedagogy).
8.2	**Serve as an authoritative resource on health education and promotion.**
8.2.1	Evaluate personal and organizational capacity to provide consultation.
8.2.2	Provide expert consultation, assistance, and guidance to individuals, groups, and organizations.
8.2.3	Conduct peer reviews (e.g., manuscripts, abstracts, proposals, and tenure folios).
8.3	**Engage in professional development to maintain and/or enhance proficiency.**

8.3.1	Participate in professional associations, coalitions, and networks (e.g., serving on committees, attending conferences, and providing leadership).
8.3.2	Participate in continuing education opportunities to maintain or enhance continuing competence.
8.3.3	Develop a career advancement plan.
8.3.4	Build relationships with other professionals within and outside the profession.
8.3.5	Serve as a mentor.
8.4	**Promote the health education profession to stakeholders, the public, and others.**
8.4.1	Explain the major responsibilities, contributions, and value of the health education specialist.
8.4.2	Explain the role of professional organizations and the benefits of participating in them.
8.4.3	Advocate for professional development for health education specialists.
8.4.4	Educate others about the history of the profession, its current status, and its implications for professional practice.
8.4.5	Explain the role and benefits of credentialing (e.g., individual and program).
8.4.6	Develop presentations and publications that contribute to the profession.
8.4.7	Engage in service to advance the profession.

Updated: 10/31/19

Glossary

A

A New Perspective on the Health of Canadians The Canadian publication that presented the epidemiological evidence supporting the importance of lifestyle and environmental factors on health and sickness and called for numerous national health promotion strategies to encourage Canadians to become more responsible for their own health.

Abstract Provides short summaries of an article's content to help the researcher determine whether the article contains the information they are seeking.

Accreditation The process by which an agency or organization evaluates and recognizes an institution as meeting certain predetermined standards.

Action stage The stage in which people have made specific overt modifications in their lifestyles within the past six months. Because action is observable, the overall process of behavior change often has been equated with action.

Actual behavioral control The extent to which a person has the skills, resources, and other prerequisites needed to perform the behavior in question.

Adjusted rate Expressed for a total population but is statistically adjusted for a certain characteristic, such as age.

Advocacy Any attempt to influence procedures, policy, public opinion, and/or attitudes that directly affect people's lives.

American Academy of Health Behavior (AAHB) It is a society of researchers and scholars in the areas of health behavior, health education, and health promotion.

American College Health Association (ACHA) Founded originally as the American Student Health Association in 1920. In 1948, the name of the association was changed to its current name. ACHA's mission is to "serve as the principal leadership organization for advancing the health of college students and campus communities through advocacy, education, and research."

American Public Health Association (APHA) Champions the health of all people and all communities.

American Red Cross (ARC) ARC has several "official" responsibilities given to it by the federal government such as providing relief to victims of natural disasters (Disaster Services) and serving as the liaison between members of the active armed forces and their families during family emergencies (Services to the Armed Forces and Veterans). ARC also provides many nongovernmental services such as its blood drives and safety services classes such as water safety, first aid, and CPR.

American School Health Association (ASHA) The mission of ASHA "is to transform all schools into places where every student learns and thrives."

Anonymity When no one, including those conducting the program, can relate a participant's identity to any information pertaining to the program.

Asclepiads A brotherhood of men present at the Greek temples who initially claimed descent from Asclepius.

Asclepius A Thessalian chief who had received instruction in the use of drugs. By the beginning of the eighth century BCE, tradition had enshrined him as the god of medicine.

Attitude toward the behavior The degree to which performance of the behavior is positively or negatively valued.

B

Bacteriological period of public health Tremendous advancement in bacteriology made during the second half of the 19th century.

Behavior change philosophy Involves a health education specialist using behavioral contracts, goal setting, and self-monitoring to try to foster a modification of an unhealthy habit in an individual with whom they are working.

Beneficence Describes the principle of doing good, demonstrating kindness, showing compassion, and helping others.

Benevolence Compassion to do good.

C

Caduceus The staff and serpent of the physician symbol.

Capacity Refers to both individual and collective resources that can be brought to bear for health enhancement.

Certification A process by which a profession grants recognition to an individual who, upon completion of a competency-based curriculum, can demonstrate a predetermined standard of performance.

Certified Health Education Specialist One who has passed the certification exam and met all the certification requirements of the National Commission for Health Education Credentialing.

Chain of infection A model used to explain the spread of a communicable disease from one host to another.

CHES Certified Health Education Specialist.

Coalition of National Health Education Organizations, USA (CNHEO) A nonprofit federation of organizations dedicated to advancing the health education/promotion profession.

Code of ethics Document that maps the dimensions of the profession's collective social responsibility and acknowledges the obligations individual practitioners share in meeting the profession's responsibilities.

Code of Hammurabi Named after the king of Babylon. It contained laws pertaining to health practices and physicians, including the first known fee schedule.

Cognitive-based philosophy Focuses on the acquisition of content and factual information. The goal is to increase the knowledge of the individuals or groups so that they are better armed to make decisions about their health.

Communicable disease model The minimal requirements for the presence and spread of a communicable disease in a population.

Communicable diseases Also referred to as infectious diseases; illnesses caused by infectious agents or its toxins that are transmissible from one individual to another.

Community empowerment Refers to the process of enabling communities to increase control over their lives.

Community health "The health status of a defined group of people and the actions and conditions to promote, protect and preserve their health" (Joint Committee, 2021).

Community Health Workers Lay members of the community who volunteer or work with health education specialists in public health departments, local health care entities situated in both rural and urban environments.

Competencies Skills or abilities necessary for successful performance as a health education specialist.

Competencies Update Project The first initiative to update the competencies of a health education specialist which was completed in 2004.

Comprehensive school health education The health curriculum component of the Whole School Whole Community, Whole Child (WSCC) model.

Concepts The primary elements of theories.

Confidentiality Confidentiality exists when only those responsible for conducting a program can link information about a participant with the individual and do not reveal such information to others.

Conservative One who generally distrusts governmental regulations and tax-supported programs for addressing social or economic problems.

Construct A concept that has been developed, created, or adopted for use with a specific theory.

Contemplation stage People are intending to start the healthy behavior in the foreseeable future (defined as within the next 6 months).

Continuum theory Variables that influence actions (i.e., beliefs, attitudes), quantify the variables, and combine those variables into a single equation that predicts the likelihood of action.

Coordinated school health program Consists of eight interactive components that work together to enhance the health and well-being of the students, faculty, staff, and community.

Coordinated school health An integrated set of planned, sequential, school-affiliated strategies, activities, and services designed to promote the optimal physical, emotional, social, and educational development of students.

Credentialing The "planned and systematic activities" used to increase confidence that the product or service—in this case, health education specialists—is meeting the requirements of the profession.

Crude rate The rate expressed for a total population.

Cue to action The stimulus needed to trigger the decision-making process to accept a recommended health action.

Cultural competence A developmental process defined as a set of values, principles, behaviors, attitudes, and policies that enable health professionals to work effectively across racial, ethnic, and linguistically diverse populations.

Culturally responsive Positive, strengths-based approach to health education that is rooted in respect and appreciation for the role of culture in learning and development.

D

Death rates (The number of deaths per 100,000 resident population), sometimes referred to as *mortality* or *fatality rates*, are probably the most frequently used means of quantifying the seriousness of injury or disease.

Decision-making philosophy A health education approach that presents simulated problems, case studies, or scenarios to students or clients. Each problem, case, or scenario requires decisions to be made in seeking a "best approach or answer."

Demographic profile The breakdown of the U.S. population by age group, sex, race, and ethnicity.

Deontological theories The belief that certain actions are good or bad, regardless of the consequences of those actions.

Determinants of health (1) Genetics (e.g., sex, age, and individual characteristics), (2) individual behavior (e.g., diet, physical activity, and alcohol use), (3) social circumstances (e.g., education, socioeconomic status, housing, and crime), (4) environmental and physical influences (e.g., safe water, where a person lives, and crowding conditions), and (5) health services (e.g., access to quality health care, cost, and lack of insurance coverage).

Diffusion Theory (DIF)   How new products, ideas, techniques, behaviors, or services (known as innovations) are adopted within populations.

Dimension of health and wellness   "The many aspects of a person's life, including the emotional, physical, occupational, intellectual, financial, social, environmental, and spiritual areas. These dimensions are considered interconnected as one area builds upon another" (Joint Committee, 2021).

Disability-adjusted life years (DALYs)   One lost year of "healthy" life as a result of being in states of poor health or disability.

Disease prevention   "The process of reducing risks and alleviating disease to promote, preserve, and restore health and minimize suffering and distress" (Joint Committee, 2001, p. 99).

Distributive justice   The idea that one has indeed acted justly toward a person when that person has been given what is due or owed.

E

Early adopters   People who are very interested in innovation, but they do not want to be the first involved. Early adopters are respected by others in the social system and considered opinion leaders.

Early majority   People who may be interested in the innovation but need some external motivation to get involved.

Eclectic health education/promotion philosophy   Any health education/promotion approach that seems appropriate to the situation.

Ecological assessment   A systematic assessment of factors in the social and physical environment that interact with behavior to produce health effects or quality-of-life outcomes.

Elaboration Likelihood Model of Persuasion (ELM)   Designed to help explain how persuasion messages (communication), aimed at changing attitudes, are received and processed by people.

Elaboration   The amount of cognitive processing (i.e., thought) that a person puts into receiving messages.

Electronic databases   Provide a preferred alternative to manually searching indexes or abstracts. The electronic database provides access via the Internet. Computer searches using databases are significantly faster than manual searches, and they have the advantage of enabling the user to link several concepts together to provide focus for a search.

Empowerment   Social action process for people to gain mastery over their lives and the lives of their communities.

Endemic   Occurs regularly in a population as a matter of course, such as heart disease in the United States.

Environment   Includes all those matters related to health that are external to the human body and over which the individual has little or no control.

Epidemic   An unexpectedly large number of cases of an illness, specific health-related behavior, or other health-related event in a population, like the opioid overdose epidemic in the United States.

Epidemiological data   Data gathered at the local, state, and national levels to assist with the prevention of disease outbreaks or control those in progress and to plan and assess health education/promotion programs.

Epidemiology   The study of the distribution and determinants of health-related states or events (including disease), and the application of this study to the control of diseases and other health problems.

Epistemology   The study of knowledge.

Eta Sigma Gamma (ESG)   The national health education honorary.

Ethical   Refers to how choices are made related to acceptable and unacceptable behavior within the norms of a particular group.

Ethical dilemma A situation that forces a decision that involves breaking some ethical norm or contradicting some ethical value.

Ethics The study of morality.

Evidence Data that can be used to make decisions about planning.

Evidence-informed practices When health education specialists practice in such a way that they systematically find, appraise, and use evidence as the basis for decision making when planning health education/promotion programs.

F

Formalism The primary means by which ethical theories have been categorized has been to place them in the category of deontology.

Freeing or functioning philosophy A reaction to traditional approaches of health education/promotion that ran the risk of blaming victims for practicing health behaviors that were often either out of their control or not considered in their best interests.

G

Generalized model A model that contains the following five tasks assessing needs, setting goals and objectives, developing interventions, implementing interventions, and evaluating results.

Global health promotion "Placing priority on improving health and achieving equity for all people worldwide. Work is directed to help all people reach the 'highest attainable standard of health' goal set by the World Health Organization" (Joint Committee, 2021).

Goodness (rightness) "Good" and "right" are at the core of every ethical theory. Theorists may disagree on what is good and bad and right and wrong, but they all strive for goodness and rightness.

Governmental health agencies Health agencies that have authority for certain duties or tasks outlined by the governmental bodies that oversee them.

Graduate research assistantship A graduate student assists faculty with research in return for tuition assistance and/or stipends.

Graduate teaching assistantship A graduate student teaches or assists with teaching courses in the department in return for tuition assistance and/or stipends.

H

Hard money Money used to hire health education specialists and fund their programs that is part of the regular budget of the hiring institution.

Health behavior Those behaviors that impact a person's health.

Health Belief Model (HBM) Addresses the individual's perceptions of the threat posed by a health problem (susceptibility, severity), the benefits of avoiding the threat, and factors influencing the decision to act (barriers, cues to action, and self-efficacy).

Health disparity Higher burden of illness, injury, disability, and/or mortality that is experienced by one group relative to another due to current or historic disadvantage, oppression, or racism, which is manifested through inequitable social, economic, and environmental systems.

Health education "Any combination of planned learning experiences using evidence based practices and/or sound theories that provide the opportunity to acquire knowledge, attitudes, and skills needed [to] adopt and maintain healthy behaviors" (Joint Committee, 2021).

Health education research "A systematic investigation involving the analysis of collected information or data that ultimately is used to enhance health education knowledge or practice, and answers one or more questions about a health-related theory, behavior or phenomenon" (Cottrell & McKenzie, 2011, p. 2) (Chapter 6).

Health education specialist An individual who has met, at a minimum, baccalaureate-level required health education academic preparation qualifications, who serves in a variety of settings, and is able to use appropriate educational strategies and methods to facilitate the development of policies, procedures, interventions, and systems conducive to the health of individuals, groups, and communities.

Health field A term the government describes as being far more encompassing than the "healthcare system." This term is much broader and includes all matters that affect health.

Health literacy The capacity of individuals to access, interpret, and understand basic health information and services, and the skills to use the information and services to promote health.

Health A constellation of factors—economic, social, political, ecological, and physical—that add up to health, high-quality lives for individuals and communities.

Health promotion "Any planned combination of educational, political, environmental, regulatory, or organizational mechanisms that support actions and conditions of living conducive to the health of individuals, groups, and communities" (Joint Committee, 2021).

Healthcare organization Consists of the quantity, quality, arrangement, nature, and relationships of people and resources in the provision of health.

Healthcare settings Clinics, hospitals, and managed care organizations.

Health-field concept A framework that would subdivide the concept into principal elements so that the elements could be studied.

Health-related quality of life (HRQOL) An individual's or a group's perceived physical and mental health over time.

Healthy People First governmental publication that recognized the importance of lifestyle in promoting health and well-being.

Healthy People 2030 The fifth iteration of the Healthy People public health objectives released in 2020 and includes objectives for the year 2030.

Hippocrates The famous Greek physician who came from the Asclepian tradition. He lived from about 460 BCE until 377 BCE.

Holistic philosophy The mind and body disappear as recognizable realities and in their stead comes the acknowledgment of a whole being...man is essentially a unified integrated organism.

Human biology Includes all those aspects of health, both physical and mental, which are developed within the human body as a consequence of the basic biology.

Hygeia Character in the *Iliad*. She was given the power to prevent disease.

I

Index References articles from journals, books, and reports pertaining to topics that fall under the subject headings for which the index was created (e.g., health behavior, physical activity, methamphetamine treatment, or corporate health education/promotion programs).

Individual freedom (equality principle or principle of autonomy) This principle means that people, being individuals with individual differences, must have the freedom to choose their own ways and means of being moral within the framework of the first four basic principles.

Informed consent People—whether patients, research participants, or participants in a health education/promotion program—

are given sufficient information from which to make informed choices about whether they want a certain medical procedure, or to participate in a research project or health education/promotion program.

Innovators The first people to adopt an innovation. They are venturesome, independent, risky, and daring. They want to be the first to do something.

Intention An indication of a person's readiness to perform a given behavior; it is considered to be the immediate antecedent of behavior.

International Union for Health Promotion and Education (IUHPE) Builds and operates an independent, global, professional network of people and institutions to encourage the free exchange of ideas, knowledge, know-how, experiences, and the development of relevant collaborative projects, both at global and regional levels.

Intervention mapping Focuses on planning programs that are based on theory and evidence. It also draws on multiple principles used in the PRECEDE-PROCEED and MATCH models.

J

Justice This principle deals with people treating other people fairly and justly in distributing goodness (benefits) and badness (burdens).

L

Laggards The last ones to get involved in an innovation, if they get involved at all.

Late majority People who are skeptical of an innovation but will finally make a change.

Liberal One who generally supports government programs to attack social and economic problems.

Licensure The process by which an agency or government [usually a state] grants permission to individuals to practice a given profession by certifying that those licensed have attained specific standards of competence.

Life expectancy The average number of years of life remaining for persons who have attained a given age.

Lifestyle Combination of decisions for which individuals have control that affect their health.

Likelihood of taking action The possibility of acting in order to get a particular result.

Local health department (LHD) Has the authority to protect, promote, and enhance the health of people living in a specific geographic area.

M

Macrolevel A general or abstract level that is large in scope or scale.

Maintenance stage The stage in which people work to prevent relapse and consolidate the gains attained during action.

Master Certified Health Education Specialist (MCHES) An advanced level of certification available for certified health education specialists (CHES) who have 5 continuous years as a certified health education specialist or for those with a master's degree in health education or a master's degree in another field with at least 25 semester hours of health education classes. The MCHES exam must be taken and passed to receive this credential.

MAPP Mobilizing for Action through Planning and Partnerships. It is a planning model created by the National Association of County and City Health Officials (NACCHO) to assist local health departments (LHDs) at the city or county level with planning.

MATCH Multilevel Approach To Community Health. This planning model was developed in the late 1980s.

MCHES   Master Certified Health Education Specialist.

Medicaid   A system that assists in the payment of medical bills for the poor.

Medicare   A system that assists in the payment of medical bills for the elderly.

Metaphysics   The study of the nature of reality.

Miasmas theory   A theory that using herbs and incense would perfume the air and supposedly fill the nose crowding out foul, disease causing odors or miasmas.

Microlevel   A general or abstract level that is small in scope or scale.

Model   A composite, a mixture of ideas or concepts taken from any number of theories and used together.

Moderate   One who usually acts in a more situationally specific manner with regard to using tax-supported programs to solve societal problems.

Modifiable risk factors   Changeable or controllable; includes such factors as sedentary lifestyle, smoking, and poor dietary habits—things that individuals can change or control.

Moral   Refers to the making choices and of deciding, judging, justifying and defending those actions or behaviors called moral.

Moral philosophy   Dates back 2,000 plus years to the Greek philosopher Socrates (470–399 BCE). He, and other early philosophers, publicly posed questions and challenged people to think about how they lived.

Moral sensitivity   Being aware that an ethical problem exists and having an understanding of what impact different courses of action may have on the people involved.

Multicausation disease model   Diseases that manifest themselves in people over a period of time and are not caused by a single factor but by combined factors.

Multitasking   The skill of coordinating and completing multiple health education/promotion projects at the same time.

N

National Commission for Health Education Credentialing   Responsible for overseeing and administering the health education certification process.

National Task Force on the Preparation and Practice of Health Educators   The group that oversaw development of the roles and responsibilities of health education specialists and ultimately the CHES credentialing system.

National Wellness Institute   The mission is to enrich the lives and careers of wellness professionals.

Needs assessment   A process that helps program planners determine what health problems might exist in any given group of people, what assets are available in the community to address the health problems, and the overall capacity of the community to address the health issues (McKenzie et al., 2017) (Chapter 6).

Networking   Establishing and maintaining a wide range of contacts in the field that may be of help when looking for a job and in carrying out one's job responsibilities once hired.

Noncommunicable diseases   Those illnesses that cannot be transmitted from an infected person to a susceptible, healthy one.

Nonconsequentialism   See Formalism.

Nongovernmental health agencies   Agencies that are free from governmental interference as long as they comply with the Internal Revenue Service's guidelines for their tax status.

Nonmaleficence   Nonmaleficence refers to the non-infliction of harm to others.

Nonmodifiable risk factors   Nonchangeable or noncontrollable; includes factors such as age, sex, and inherited genes—things that individuals cannot change or do not have control over.

Nurturing public health   Strong, well-resourced public health leaders and capabilities at national, state, and local levels who protect Americans from health threats.

Open-access journals   The "open access" designation means that the article is copyrighted but generally can be used more liberally than articles with more traditional copyrights.

Ownership   Responsibility for the program.

P

Panacea   Character in the *Iliad*. She was given the power to treat disease.

Pandemic   An outbreak over a wide geographic area, without specific geographic boundaries.

Participation   The active involvement of those in the priority population in helping identify, plan, and implement programs to address the health problems they face.

Patient Protection and Affordable Care Act   Through a combination of cost controls, subsidies, and mandates, it expanded healthcare coverage to 20 million uninsured Americans.

Peer-reviewed journal   A journal that publishes original manuscripts only after they have been read by a panel of experts in the field (peer-reviewers) and recommended for publication.

Perceived barriers   A person's estimation of the level of challenge of social, personal, environmental, and economic obstacles to a specified behavior or their desired goal status on that behavior.

Perceived behavioral control   The perception of the difficulty of enacting a behavior.

Perceived benefits   Belief about the positive outcomes associated with a behavior in response to a real or perceived threat.

Perceived seriousness/severity   The negative consequences an individual associates with an event or outcome, such as a diagnosis of cancer. These consequences may relate to an anticipated event that may occur in the future, or to a current situations that were difficult or troubling to the individual and were described by respondents in narrative form such as a pre-existing health problem.

Perceived susceptibility   Belief about the chances of getting a disease or condition.

Perceived threat   Situation that is difficult or troubling to an individual.

Philanthropic foundations   Foundations built on altruistic concern for human welfare and advancement, usually manifested by donations of money, property, or work to needy persons, by endowment of institutions of learning and hospitals, and by generosity to other socially useful purposes.

Philosophy of symmetry   The idea that health has physical, emotional, spiritual, and social components, and each is just as important as the others.

Philosophy   A statement summarizing the attitudes, principles, beliefs, values, and concepts held by an individual or a group.

Popular press publications   Range from weekly summary-type magazines (e.g., *Time, Newsweek, and U.S. News & World Report*), regular articles in newspapers (e.g., Dr. Oz's column), and newspaper supplements (e.g., *Parade*) to monthly magazines (e.g., *Shape, Prevention, and Men's Health*) and tabloids (e.g., *The Star, People, and Us* Weekly).

Population-based approaches   Includes policy development, policy advocacy, organizational change, community development, empowerment of individuals, and economic supports.

Population health   "A cohesive, integrated, and comprehensive approach to health care that considers the distribution of health outcomes within a population, the health determinants that influence distribution of care, and the policies and interventions that affect and are affected by the determinants" (Nash, Fabius, Skoufalos, Clarke, & Horowitz, 2016, p. 448).

Portfolio   A collection of evidence that enables students to demonstrate mastery of desired course or program outcomes/competencies.

Postsecondary institution   Community college, college, or university.

PRECEDE-PROCEED   This model has two components. PRECEDE is an acronym that stands for *p*redisposing, *r*einforcing, and *e*nabling *c*onstructs in *e*ducational/*e*cological *d*iagnosis and *e*valuation. PROCEED stands for *p*olicy, *r*egulatory, and *o*rganizational *c*onstructs in *e*ducational and *e*nvironmental *d*evelopment.

Precontemplation stage   The stage at which there is no intention to change behavior in the foreseeable future.

Preparation stage   The stage in which individuals intend to take steps to change, usually within the next month.

Prevention   The planning for and the measures taken to forestall the onset of a disease or other health problem before the occurrence of undesirable health events.

Primary data   Original data gathered by the health education specialist as part of a needs assessment; this includes data gathered from telephone surveys, focus groups, and interviews.

Primary prevention   Comprises those preventive measures that forestall the onset of illness or injury during the prepathogenesis period (before the disease process begins).

Primary sources   Published studies or eyewitness accounts written by the people who actually conducted the experiments or observed the events in question.

Privacy   The claim of individuals, groups, or institutions to determine for themselves when, how, and to what extent information about them is communicated to others.

Procedural justice   Deals with whether fair procedures were in place and whether those procedures were followed.

Professional ethics   Actions that are right and wrong in the workplace and are of a public matter. Professional moral principles are not statements of taste or preference; they tell practitioners what they ought to do and what they ought not to do.

Professional health associations/ organizations   The mission of these organizations is to promote the high standards of professional practice for their respective profession, thereby improving the health of society by improving the people in the profession.

Promoting Health/Preventing Disease: Objectives for the Nation   A document containing 226 health objectives for the United States to be accomplished during the 1980's. The first of the "Objectives for the Nation" documents which have been updated and published every 10 years.

Public health   "The science and art of preventing disease, prolonging life, and promoting health through the organized efforts and informed choices of society, organizations, communities, and individuals" (Joint Committee, 2021).

Public health agencies   Governmental health agencies, which are usually financed through public tax monies.

Q

Quality assurance   The planned and systematic activities necessary to provide adequate confidence that the product or service will meet given requirements.

Quasi-governmental health agencies   So named because they possess characteristics of both governmental health agencies and nongovernmental agencies.

R

Rate   A measure of the frequency with which an event occurs in a defined population over a specified period of time.

Reduction of threat   The difference between the benefits of and the barriers to something specific.

Refereed   See peer-reviewed journal.

Reform phase of public health The period from 1900 to 1920. During this time, urban areas expanded, and many people lived and worked in deplorable conditions. To address these concerns, federal regulations were passed concerning the food industry, states passed workers' compensation laws, the U.S. Bureau of Mines and the U.S. Department of Labor were created, and the first clinic for occupational diseases was established.

Research ethics Comprises principles and standards that, along with underlying values, guide appropriate conduct relevant to research decisions.

Responsibilities The major categories of performance expectations of a proficient health education specialist.

Risk factors Any attribute, characteristic, or exposure of an individual that increases the likelihood of developing a disease or injury.

Role delineation A process to determine the responsibilities, competencies and sub-competencies of a given profession

Rule of Sufficiency Any strategies chosen must be sufficiently robust, or effective enough, to ensure stated objectives for a health education program have a reasonable chance of being met.

S

School Health Education Evaluation Study Another important study. This study concentrated on the Los Angeles, California, area. Its purpose was to evaluate the effectiveness of school health work in selected schools and colleges in that area.

School Health Education Study A major study of significance to school health education.

School health education/promotion instruction Primarily involves instructing school-age children about health and health-related behaviors.

Secondary data Preexisting data used by a health education specialist in a needs assessment.

Secondary prevention Includes the preventive measures that lead to an early diagnosis and prompt treatment of a disease or an injury to limit disability and prevent more serious pathogenesis.

Secondary sources Usually written by someone who was not present at the event or did not participate as part of the study team. Examples of secondary sources are journal review articles, editorials, and non-eyewitness accounts of events occurring in the community, region, or nation.

Self-efficacy Confidence in one's own ability to perform a certain task or function.

Service learning The "learn by doing" approach to training is common in public health education and provides benefits for both the students and the community organizations being served.

Situational analysis The combination of social and epidemiological assessments of conditions, trends, and priorities with a preliminary scan of determinants, relevant policies, resources, organizational support, and regulations that might anticipate or permit action in advance of a more complete assessment of behavioral, environmental, educational, ecological, and administrative factors.

SMART Social marketing planning framework. It provides a composite of other social marketing models and it has been used from start to finish on multiple occasions in several social marketing interventions.

Smith Papyri The oldest written documents related to health care.

Social capital The relationships and structures within a community, such as civic participation, networks, norms of reciprocity, and trust that promote cooperation of mutual benefit.

Social change philosophy Emphasizes the role of health education specialists in creating social, economic, and political change that benefits the health of individuals and groups.

Social determinants of health Conditions with which people are born, live, learn, work, and play, all of which typically would impact their health outcomes. These conditions and outcomes are shaped by the distribution of money, power, and resources at global, national, and local levels.

Social marketing The application of commercial marketing technologies to the analysis, planning, execution, and evaluation of programs designed to influence the voluntary behavior of target audiences in order to improve their personal welfare and that of their society.

Social media Media that uses the Internet and other technologies to allow for social interaction.

Social network Person-centered web of social relationships.

Society for Public Health Education (SOPHE) Provides global leadership to the profession of health education and health promotion and to promote the health of society.

Society of Health and Physical Educators (SHAPE) The nation's largest membership organization of health and physical education professionals—from pre-K–12 educators to university professors. Their mission is to "advance professional practice and promote research related to health and physical education, physical activity, dance, and sport.

Society of State Leaders of Health and Physical Education A professional association whose members supervise and coordinate programs in health, physical education, and related fields of coordinated school health programs within state departments of education. The mission of The Society is to use advocacy, partnerships, professional development, and resources to build capacity of school health leaders to implement effective health education and physical education policies and practices that support success in school, work and life.

Socio-ecological approach A multilevel, interactive approach that examines how physical, social, political, economic, and cultural dimensions influence behaviors and conditions.

Soft money Money from contracts, grants or foundations used to hire health education specialists and fund their programs. This money is typically limited and time specific. When the funding cycle is ended, the position will be terminated unless additional funding can be obtained.

Specific rate A rate for a particular population subgroup such as for a particular disease (i.e., disease-specific) or for a particular age of people (i.e., age-specific).

Stage theory An ordered set of categories into which people can be classified. It identifies factors that could induce movement from one category to the next.

Sub-Competencies A cluster of simpler but essential related skills or abilities within a competency.

Subjective norm The belief that an important person or group of people will approve and support a particular behavior.

T

Technology Applying scientific knowledge for practical purposes, especially in industry.

Teleological theories This category of ethical theories states that the end *does* justify the means.

Termination The time when individuals who made a change now have zero temptation to return to their old behavior.

Tertiary prevention It is at this level that health education specialists work to retrain, reeducate, and rehabilitate the individual who has already incurred disability, impairment, or dependency.

Tertiary sources Sources that contain information that has been distilled and collected from primary and secondary sources.

Theory of Planned Behavior (TPB) Individuals' intention to perform a given behavior, which is a function of their attitude toward performing the behavior, their beliefs about what relevant others think they should do, and their perception of the ease or difficulty of performing the behavior.

Theory A set of interrelated concepts, definitions, and propositions that presents a *systematic* view of events or situations by specifying relations among variables in order to *explain* and *predict* the events of the situations.

Traditional family A mother, father, and their children.

Transtheoretical Model of Change (TMC) The theory that intentional behavior change "occurs in stages."

Truth telling Honest communication.

Value of life The philosophy that human beings should revere life and accept death.

Variable A quantitative measurement of a construct.

Voluntary health agencies Nonprofit organizations created by concerned citizens to deal with a health need not met by governmental health agencies.

Wellness Whereby an individual actively seeks a collection of preventive practices and processes in which all dimensions of that person's health are addressed to achieve optimal well-being and minimize conditions of illness.

WSCC Whole School, Whole Community, Whole Child Model.

Years of potential life lost (YPLL) A measure of premature mortality and is calculated by subtracting a person's age at death from 75 years.

Index

Note: Page references indicated by *f* are a figure; *t* are a table; *b* are a box and bold page references indicate defined terms.